Lumbar Interbody Fusions

Lumbar Interbody Fusions

Sunil V. Manjila, MD

Staff Neurosurgeon
McLaren Bay Region Medical Center
Bay City, Michigan, USA

Thomas E. Mroz, MD

Director, Center for Spine Health
Director, Clinical Research
Center for Spine Health
Departments of Orthopaedic and Neurological Surgery
Cleveland Clinic
Cleveland, Ohio, USA

Michael P. Steinmetz, MD

Professor and Chairman
Department of Neurosurgery
Cleveland Clinic Lerner College of Medicine
Cleveland Clinic
Cleveland, Ohio, USA

For additional online content visit ExpertConsult.com

ELSEVIER

Edinburgh London New York Oxford Philadelphia St Louis Sydney 2019

ELSEVIER

Notices

Practitioners and researchers must always rely on their own experience and knowledge in evaluating and using any information, methods, compounds or experiments described herein. Because of rapid advances in the medical sciences, in particular, independent verification of diagnoses and drug dosages should be made. To the fullest extent of the law, no responsibility is assumed by Elsevier, authors, editors or contributors for any injury and/or damage to persons or property as a matter of products liability, negligence or otherwise, or from any use or operation of any methods, products, instructions, or ideas contained in the material herein.

ISBN: 978-0-323-47663-8

E-ISBN: 978-0-323-49741-1

Content Strategist: Belinda Kuhn
Content Development Specialist: Sharon Nash
Project Manager: Beula Christopher
Design: Ryan Cook
Illustration Manager: Karen Giacomucci

Printed in China

Last digit is the print number: 9 8 7 6 5 4 3 2 1

Video Contents

Contents

Preface

"No matter what measures are taken, doctors will sometimes falter, and it isn't reasonable to ask that we achieve perfection. What is reasonable is to ask that we never cease to aim for it."

— **Atul Gawande, *Complications: A Surgeon's Notes on an Imperfect Science***

It is a distinct honor and privilege to present the inaugural edition of *Lumbar Interbody Fusions* by Manjila, Mroz, and Steinmetz, showcasing the techniques and nuances in lumbar spine surgery that can improve both safety and efficacy in our operating rooms. This highly technical and contextualized treatise provides a unique and state-of-the-art "single-stop shop" for the reader, whether a novice resident or an expert practitioner, perusing all the major lumbar interbody fusion techniques in its sum and substance. This book will truly serve as a *vade mecum* procedural guide, and a perfect addendum to the conventional pedagogical texts in spine surgery. This book has five intuitive sections and spans 232 pages. Section I provides a primer to the subject with relevant and updated clinical studies, while Section II provides an overview of pertinent surgical anatomy and intraoperative imaging. Section III discusses the surgical options of lumbar interbody fusions with indications, techniques, pearls and pitfalls, with complication avoidance and management. Section IV presents contemporary updates on adjunct instrumentation, implant biomaterials, and biologic options in lumbar fusion, with subsections on integrated implant/screw options and role of spinous process plates, facet screws, and pedicle screws in offering spinal stability. Finally, Section V provides an overview of revision interbody fusions, thoracic and lumbar overlap diseases, and evidence-based reports on lumbar interbody fusions. This practical template gives a 360-degree approach to lumbar spine surgery, providing ample insights and tenets to deal with complex lumbar spine procedures in vexing clinical situations. The authors have infused their vast clinical and surgical experience into what makes for a well-choreographed, rehearsed operation, notably in an era where "10,000 hours of practice to perfection" is cumbersome with current residency training restrictions.

We also thank the publishers at Elsevier for their boundless and unfailing support as well as tireless assistance in bringing out this volume. I would personally like to thank Sharon Nash (Senior Content Development Specialist), Belinda Kuhn (Senior Content Strategist), and Beula Christopher King (Senior Project Manager) for their continued interactions and diligent interventions in bringing out this magnum opus in a timely manner. We welcome your thoughtful comments, suggestions, and criticisms to improve subsequent editions, as we truly believe that surgical training is a mesmerizing art and science, ever-changing and evolving with time and ensuing needs of both patients and the providers.

Sunil V. Manjila, MD

List of Contributors

Vincent J. Alentado, MD
Neurosurgery Resident
Department of Neurosurgery
Indiana University School of Medicine
Indianapolis, Indiana, USA

Neel Anand, MD
Professor of Orthopaedics
Department of Orthopaedics
Cedars-Sinai Spine Center
Los Angeles, California, USA

Mauricio J. Avila, MD
Neurosurgery Resident
Department of Neurological Surgery
University of Arizona
Tucson, Arizona, USA

Ali A. Baaj, MD
Associate Professor
Department of Neurological Surgery
Weill Cornell Medicine
New York, New York, USA

Charles L. Branch Jr., MD
Professor and Chairman
Department of Neurological Surgery
Wake Forest Baptist Medical Center
Winston-Salem, North Carolina, USA

Julie L. Chan, MD PhD
Resident
Department of Neurosurgery
Cedars-Sinai Medical Center
Los Angeles, California, USA

Hsuan-Kan Chang, MD
Clinical Research Fellow
Department of Neurosurgery
University of Miami Miller School of Medicine
Miami, Florida, USA

Peng-Yuan Chang, MD
Clinical Research Fellow
Department of Neurosurgery
University of Miami Miller School of Medicine
Miami, Florida, USA

Jason Cohen, BS
Albert Einstein College of Medicine
Bronx, New York, USA

Ryan Cohen, BS
Boston University School of Medicine
Boston, Massachusetts, USA

Kelly A. Frank, MS
Clinical Research
Spine Institute of Louisiana
Shreveport, Louisiana, USA

Mark B. Frenkel, MD
Neurosurgical Resident
Department of Neurological Surgery
Wake Forest Baptist Medical Center
Winston Salem, North Carolina, USA

Zoher Ghogawala, MD
Professor
Tufts University School of Medicine
Chairman
Department of Neurosurgery
Lahey Hospital and Medical Center
Burlington, Massachusetts, USA

Colin Haines, MD
Clinical Spine Fellow
Cleveland Clinic Center for Spine Health
Cleveland, Ohio, USA

David J. Hart, MD
Associate Professor
Department of Neurological Surgery
Wake Forest Baptist Medical Center
Winston Salem, North Carolina, USA

Roger Härtl, MD
Professor of Neurological Surgery
Director of Spinal Surgery
Department of Neurological Surgery
Weill Cornell Medicine
New York, New York, USA

Hamid Hassanzadeh, MD
Assistant Professor
Department of Orthopaedic Surgery
University of Virginia
Charlottesville, Virginia, USA

Wellington K. Hsu, MD
Clifford C. Raisbeck, MD, Professor of Orthopaedic Surgery
Associate Professor of Orthopaedic Surgery and Neurological Surgery
Northwestern University
Chicago, Illinois, USA

Andre M. Jakoi, MD
Spine Fellow
Department of Orthopaedic Surgery
University of Southern California
Los Angeles, California, USA

Jacob R. Joseph, MD
Resident
Department of Neurosurgery
University of Michigan
Ann Arbor, Michigan, USA

Adam S. Kanter, MD
Chief of Presbyterian Spine Service
Director, Minimally Invasive Spine Program
Department of Neurological Surgery
University of Pittsburgh
Pittsburgh, Pennsylvania, USA

Adam Khalil, MD
Resident
Department of Neurosurgery
Cleveland Clinic
Cleveland, Ohio, USA

John Paul G. Kolcun, BS
Clinical Research Associate
Department of Neurosurgery
University of Miami Miller School of Medicine
Miami, Florida, USA

Ajit A. Krishnaney, MD
Staff Surgeon
Department of Neurosurgery
Cleveland Clinic
Cleveland, Ohio, USA

Abhishek Kumar, MD FRCSC
Assistant Professor
Department of Orthopedic Surgery
Louisiana State University
New Orleans, Louisiana, USA

Shankar A. Kutty, MCh
Consultant Neurosurgeon
NMC Specialty Hospital
Abu Dhabi, United Arab Emirates

Allan D. Levi, MD PhD
Professor and Chair
Department of Neurological Surgery
University of Miami Miller School of Medicine
Jackson Memorial Hospital
Miami, Florida, USA

Sunil V. Manjila, MD
Staff Neurosurgeon
McLaren Bay Region Medical Center
Bay City, Michigan, USA

Glen Manzano, MD
Assistant Professor
Department of Neurological Surgery
University of Miami Miller School of Medicine
Jackson Memorial Hospital
Miami, Florida, USA

Marco C. Mendoza, MD
Resident
Orthopaedic Surgery
Northwestern University
Chicago, Illinois, USA

Thomas E. Mroz, MD
Director, Center for Spine Health
Director, Clinical Research
Center for Spine Health
Departments of Orthopaedic and Neurological Surgery
Cleveland Clinic
Cleveland, Ohio, USA

Rodrigo Navarro-Ramirez, MD
Neurological Surgery Fellow
Department of Neurological Surgery, Weill Cornell Medicine
New York, New York, USA

Pierce D. Nunley, MD
Director, Spine Institute of Louisiana
Spine Institute of Louisiana;
Associate Professor
Louisiana State University Health Science Center Orthopaedics
Shreveport, Louisiana, USA

R. Douglas Orr, MD
Staff
Center for Spine Health
Neurologic Institute
Cleveland Clinic
Cleveland, Ohio, USA

Samuel C. Overley, MD
Orthopedic Surgery Resident
Department of Orthopedic Surgery
Mount Sinai Medical Center
New York, New York, USA

Paul Park, MD
Associate Professor
Department of Neurosurgery
University of Michigan
Ann Arbor, Michigan, USA

Neil N. Patel, MD
Spine Fellow
Department of Orthopaedic Surgery
University of Southern California
Los Angeles, California, USA

Martin H. Pham, MD
Spine Fellow
Department of Neurological Surgery
University of Southern California
Los Angeles, California, USA

Varun Puvanesarajah, MD
Resident
Department of Orthopedic Surgery
John's Hopkins Medical Institute
Baltimore, Maryland, USA

Rabia Qureshi, BS
Clinical Research Fellow
Department of Orthopedic Surgery, Spine Division
University of Virginia School of Medicine
Charlottesville, Virginia, USA

Sheeraz Qureshi, MD
Associate Professor
Department of Orthopedic Surgery
Mount Sinai Medical Center
New York, New York, USA

Jaclyn J. Renfrow, MD
Resident
Department of Neurological Surgery
Wake Forest Baptist Medical Center
Winston-Salem, North Carolina, USA

Angela M. Richardon, MD PhD
Resident
Department of Neurological Surgery
University of Miami Miller School of Medicine
Jackson Memorial Hospital
Miami, Florida, USA

Timothy T. Roberts, MD
Spine Surgeon
Coastal Spine Center
Coastal Orthopedics Sports and Pain Management
Bradenton, Florida, USA

Brett D. Rosenthal, MD
Resident Physician
Orthopaedic Surgery
Northwestern University
Chicago, Illinois, USA

David J. Salvetti, MD
Spine Fellow
Department of Neurological Surgery
University of Pittsburgh
Pittsburgh, Pennsylvania, USA

Jason W. Savage, MD
Staff Spine Surgeon
Cleveland Clinic Center for Spine Health
Cleveland, Ohio, USA

Michael P. Steinmetz, MD
Professor and Chairman
Department of Neurosurgery
Cleveland Clinic Lerner College of Medicine
Cleveland Clinic
Cleveland, Ohio, USA

Zachary J. Tempel, MD
Neurosurgeon
Mayfield Brain and Spine
Mayfield Clinic
Cincinnati, Ohio, USA

Jeffrey C. Wang, MD
Chief, Orthopaedic Spine Service
Co-Director, USC Spine Center
Professor of Orthopaedic and Neurosurgery
University of Southern California
Los Angeles, California, USA

Michael Y. Wang, MD FACS
Professor
Departments of Neurosurgery and Rehabilitation Medicine
University of Miami Miller School of Medicine
Miami, Florida, USA

Robert G. Whitmore, MD, FAANS
Assistant Professor
Tufts University School of Medicine
Department of Neurosurgery
Lahey Hospital and Medical System
Burlington, Massachusetts, USA

Alex M. Witek, MD
Resident
Department of Neurosurgery
Cleveland Clinic
Cleveland, Ohio, USA

Acknowledgments

I would like to acknowledge all the outstanding contributing authors who volunteered their time, effort, and energy in making this work an astounding success. I appreciate all the ideas, suggestions, and guidance from the editorial/publishing team and content developers of Elsevier, and I dedicate this volume to the esteemed readers who will make best use of its contents for the welfare and well-being of our patients all across the world.

Sunil V. Manjila, MD

I would like to acknowledge all of my mentors. Their training and guidance have made this project possible. I would like to further acknowledge present and past partners, collaborators, fellows, residents, and medical students.

Michael P. Steinmetz, MD

I would like to dedicate this book to my mentors, teachers, benefactors, friends, and family, especially my loving sons—Nihal Manjila and Rehan Manjila.

Sunil V. Manjila, MD

I would like to dedicate this book to my wife, Bettina, and my two children, Cameron and Marcus. Editing a book is a challenging endeavor and consumes considerable time. Much of this time is taken away from family. This is not lost on us as editors, and this finished product is a testament to a supportive and loving family.

Michael P. Steinmetz, MD

1 General Indications and Contraindications

SHANKAR A. KUTTY AND SUNIL V. MANJILA

Introduction

This chapter provides an overview of the contemporary literature on lumbar interbody fusion (LIF) instrumentation based on the Spine Patient Outcome Research Trial, Swedish Spinal Stenosis Study, and a recent *New England Journal of Medicine* article on clinical outcomes. Preoperative factors influencing the surgical outcome are discussed, along with five basic tenets of LIF based on: (1) presence and extent of concurrent listhesis at the level of fusion, (2) need for unilateral versus bilateral foraminal decompression, (3) presence of central canal stenosis, (4) loss of coronal and sagittal balance, and (5) the history of prior surgery at the same level or adjacent levels with or without instrumentations. We also discuss the complications of some original LIF approaches with relevant illustrations depicting the successful use of alternate LIF approaches to correct them. The chapter also portrays the synergistic role of novel techniques and technologies that can make modern LIF procedures safer, more feasible, and more efficacious. These LIF techniques require a lot of expertise and can often be hard to do well, especially in reoperations. These operations are very equipment dependent, and it is important to be familiar with all the common LIF techniques in clinical practice and their individual benefits and complications. Clear understanding about the various LIF approaches can equip the spine surgeon especially when dealing with a complication needing implant retrieval from a distinct approach that was performed by another surgeon.

Background

The first recorded surgical attempt at fusion of the spinal column was in 1891, when Hadra attempted cervical interspinous wiring to treat subluxation caused by Potts spine.[1] However, it took another two decades before the first reports of surgery in the lumbosacral spine emerged in 1911, when Russell Hibbs and Fred Albee[2,3] reported on their techniques of spinal fusion to treat tuberculosis. Hibbs used "feathered" (morselized) laminae and spinal processes, which were placed into decorticated facet joints to create the world's first dynamic stabilization. Albee, on the other hand, used tibial grafts between the spinous processes to stimulate fusion. The rationale behind the "posterior fusion" surgery was to prevent deformity, improve stability, and reduce pain. The next major step in development of spinal surgery occurred when Watkins reported the posterolateral intertransverse fusion in 1953.[4]

In 1962 Harrington reported on his series of scoliosis surgery using sublaminar hooks and rods, and the era of spinal instrumentation began.[5] Advances in metallurgy and surgical techniques led to the development of transpedicular, translaminar, corticopedicular, and facet screw systems as well as myriad types of interbody cages made of titanium, polyetheretherketone, and so forth, with variations such as trabecular mesh. Spinal technology grew closely following the prosthetic joint technology; for example, the lessons of enhanced biomechanical pull-out strength and migration resistance offered by porous coating of hip implant (first application of Plasmapore coating of titanium hip prosthesis) in 1986 slowly made its way to the lumbar spine market in 2012 (as the first Plasmapore-coated polyetheretherketone lumbar implant). Continuous improvisation of novel technologies, designs, navigation, and robotics make LIF an ever-evolving area of spine surgery.

Other revolutionizing factors included various osteoinductive and osteoconductive materials being used in bone fusion. A significant step forward was made with the development of recombinant human bone morphogenetic protein (rhBMP). BMPs comprise a group of osteoinductive cytokines that belong to the transforming growth factor beta (TGF-β) superfamily. BMP-2 had been approved by the US Food and Drug Administration (FDA) in 2002 for anterior lumbar interbody fusion (ALIF) based on a pivotal study by Burkus et al.[6] Since its introduction into clinical use, BMP had an immense surge in popularity as spinal surgeons started using osteobiologicals in large numbers to avoid the graft site complications associated with iliac crest grafts. This, in turn, led to reports of many serious complications following off-label use in posterior surgeries, as well as in ALIF. Carragee et al.[7] reported a higher reoperation rate in patients treated with rhBMP-2, mainly to correct graft subsidence. They, among other researchers, found that as many as 20% to 70% of patients had suffered some complications that could be attributed to BMP, including endplate resorption, retrograde ejaculation, seroma formation, bone overgrowth, osteolysis, and an increased risk of cancer.[8,9] The Yale University Open Data Access study[10] was conducted against this background to assess the safety and utility of BMP-2 and found that the incidence of retrograde ejaculation and neurologic complications were equal in both autograft and BMP-augmented ALIF surgeries. It also demonstrated a small increased relative risk of malignancy with the use of rhBMP-2 in posterolateral lumbar surgeries. However, the absolute risk was very low and therefore clinically insignificant. No difference was found between rhBMP-2 and iliac crest graft, but there was a higher rate of ectopic bone formation in these procedures. Based on these findings, judicious use of BMP is now advocated in posterior lumbar surgeries. In transforaminal lumbar interbody fusion (TLIF), a high risk of postoperative radiculitis has been reported; hence, the use of BMP in these cases is not encouraged.[11a] The use of bone marrow aspiration from the exposed lumbar vertebral bodies during the surgery, and then using this aspirate as graft material has been recently reported.[11b] This overcomes the graft site complications as well as the problems associated with the use of BMP-2. Further research is ongoing about the use of growth differentiation factor 5, also known as BMP-14, as an osteogenetic material.

Interbody Fusion: A Primer and Recent Literature

Over the years a number of approaches have been developed for LIF, namely posterior, anterior, axial, transforaminal, lateral, extreme lateral, and oblique lateral. In keeping with the trend toward minimally invasive surgeries, reports of percutaneous attempts at surgical stabilization of the lumbar spine first appeared more than two decades ago.[12,13] Although posterior lumbar fusion via minimally invasive techniques has become commonplace, endoscopic surgeries for TLIF require special training. Even though the exact procedure that is chosen for a particular patient may depend on a number of factors, such as the exact pathology and surgical anatomy of a particular patient and the surgeon's preference, the pathologies that need surgical fusion of the lumbar spine remain broadly the same. These include degenerative diseases, spinal trauma, deformity correction, infections, and tumors.

Interbody fusion is indicated in a subgroup of patients in whom the surgical approach to treat a pathology results in spinal instability or if preexisting instability is present. Spondylolisthesis, the most common indication for interbody fusion, is defined as the horizontal translation of a vertebral body over an adjacent one and was divided into five groups by Newman and Stone,[15] namely, congenital, degenerative, spondylolytic, traumatic, and pathologic. Spondylolisthesis is graded depending on the length of the vertebral body that is not in contact with the adjacent vertebra (extent of slippage). In grade I spondylolisthesis, the area of noncontact is less than 25% of the anteroposterior diameter of the vertebral body on a lateral x-ray study, whereas in grade II, the slip is between 26% and 50%. When the area of noncontact is between 51% and 75%, it is called grade III; in grade IV, the slip is between 76% and 100%. A greater than 100% slip, where the adjacent vertebral bodies are lying totally separated from each other, is designated grade V, or spondyloptosis. Grades I and II are considered low grade, whereas the rest are designated as high-grade spondylolisthesis. The degenerative variant is usually seen in women over the age of 50 years. Low-grade lesions are commonly treated conservatively, and surgery is reserved for those patients who fail to respond or for those who have neurologic deterioration.

The benefit of surgery has been demonstrated repeatedly in various trials, with the Spine Patient Outcomes Research Trial being the most significant study to support surgery for these patients.[16–18] The best surgery indicated in each case of degenerative spondylolisthesis and whether these patients need spinal fusion are still open to debate. Presence of spondylolisthesis in patients with lumbar canal stenosis was considered an indication for fusion surgery, even in stable cases where the slip is less than 3 mm. Recent studies have shown that in the United States approximately half the patients with lumbar spinal stenosis and 96% of those with degenerative spondylolisthesis undergo spinal fusion.[19–21] This view has been challenged by recent studies from Sweden and the United States, which found that the benefit of fusion in patients with stable spondylolisthesis and lumbar spinal stenosis was marginal at best. The Swedish Spinal Stenosis Study was a randomized controlled trial of 247 patients who were divided into fusion and nonfusion groups, with each group containing at least 40 patients with and without degenerative spondylolisthesis (at least 3 mm). At 2- and 5-year follow-ups, no significant difference in outcomes were found in the two groups. The rates of reoperation were also remarkably similar, raising a question about the need for fusion in degenerative spondylolisthesis. In this study, the preoperative evaluation did not include flexion-extension x-ray studies; if this had been done and patients with demonstrable instability were assigned to the fusion group, the results in the nonfusion group vis à vis repeated surgery may have been even better.[22]

However, another study, albeit smaller, published in the same issue of *New England Journal Medicine* mentioned above, found a minimally improved physical outcome in patients who had undergone fusion surgery at 2, 3, and 4 years. This was not considered sufficiently significant to support the higher cost in terms of financial burden, blood loss, operative time, and hospital stay in these patients. Counter-intuitively the reoperation rate was higher in patients who did not undergo fusion even though this study had excluded patients with instability as demonstrated by flexion-extension x-ray study.[23] This apparent confounding factor may be related to the physician approach in the two countries where the studies were done, with physicians in the United States tending to offer revision-with-fusion to those patients who had pain after decompression alone, whereas the threshold for offering revision surgery to a patient with pain, who had already undergone spinal stabilization, may be much higher. The current evidence seems to point to the need for fusion only in those with unstable degenerative spondylolisthesis as shown on flexion-extension x-ray films, patients with destruction of vertebral bodies owing to trauma, infection or tumors, and spinal deformities such as other variants of spondylolisthesis or scoliosis. The need for fusion in neural-foraminal stenosis owing to postsurgical disk prolapse is another contentious area, with no evidence to support improved outcome with fusion.[24]

In isthmic spondylolisthesis, there is a fracture of the pars interarticularis or isthmus, which is the area of the vertebra where the lamina and inferior articular process join the pedicle and the superior articular process. These cases often occur in a patient population that is younger than the typical patient with degenerative spondylolisthesis, which is common in the third to fifth decades. The management strategy is similar, with a 3-month trial of conservative therapy before opting for surgical management, even though some studies have shown a better outcome for surgery in these patients.[25,26] Even in this case, multiple surgical techniques are described to treat isthmic spondylolisthesis, depending on many factors such as lateral foraminal compression, fusion of facets, grade of listhesis, and expertise of surgeon.

Preoperative Factors Influencing Outcome of Spinal Fusion

Although appropriate patient selection and an impeccable technique go far in ensuring the success of spinal stabilization surgeries, a number of comorbid conditions or extraneous factors, such as diabetes mellitus, osteoporosis, and smoking, may affect a good outcome. Patients with diabetes mellitus have a much higher rate of complications following any spinal surgery, with surgical site infections accounting for a majority of problems.[27] A study in 2003 by Glassman et al.[28] showed that the overall complication rates in diabetic patients were over 50%, whereas it was only 21% in controls. Nonunion rates in the diabetic patients ranged between 22% and 26%, whereas it was 5% in controls.[28] A more recent study by Guzman et al.[29] showed that for diabetic patients the mean length of stay increased (~2.5 d), costs were greater (1.3-fold), and there was a greater risk of inpatient mortality (odds ratio = 2.6, $P < .0009$). The ability of cigarette smoke to inhibit fusion was demonstrated in animal studies and fusion rates following surgery have also been found to be lower in patients who smoked. Cessation of smoking at least 6 months prior to a planned surgery may overcome this risk.[30,31] Concomitant rheumatoid arthritis can also increase the risk of complications, such as surgical site infections and implant failure, but fusion rates in patients with rheumatoid arthritis have been reported to be comparable to that of controls.[32] Osteoporosis is known to increase the risk of implant failure and fractures and should be medically managed prior to, or concurrent with, surgery. Bone density index (bone densitometry) prior to an elective surgery in a patient at high risk can assess the chance of graft failure and vertebral body osteoporotic collapse. High risk patients undergoing elective surgery can be assessed by an endocrinologist, as the management strategies of these patients are complex and include not only the use of calcium and vitamin D replacement, but also administration of alendronate, parathyroid hormone, calcitonin and raloxifene,[33,34] with use of a post-operative external bone stimulator.

Tenets of Interbody Fusion

The five basic tenets that govern the type of interbody fusion are (1) the presence and extent of spondylolisthesis; (2) the need for unilateral or bilateral neural foraminal decompression; (3) the presence of coexistent central canal stenosis requiring decompression; (4) the loss of coronal and sagittal balance in relation to the level of disease; and (5) the presence of prior surgery at the same level or adjacent levels with or without instrumentation and/or interbody grafts.

Symptomatic low-grade spondylolisthesis is by far the most common indication for interbody fusion in the lumbar spine. Careful selection of approaches must be directed by goal, lateralization of clinical signs, loss of curvature, and prior surgery, and these must be in relation to the age, gender, and medical condition of the patient. With significant spondylolisthesis and both neural foramina at lower lumbar levels needing to be decompressed, an ALIF can be used, especially if there is no canal stenosis. ALIF is useful for correcting listhesis, especially if the slippage is the cause of central, lateral recess, or foraminal stenosis, as against significant ligamentum flavum hypertrophy with associated large hypertrophic facets. If the patient has circumferential soft tissue canal stenosis resulting in neurogenic claudication rather than radiculopathic symptoms, a TLIF would be a better option.

AxiaLIF can be used if central canal stenosis is not significant, and the foraminal compression does not cause symptomatic radiculopathy. With a predominantly unilateral radiculopathy, a TLIF with wide facetectomy at the side of radiculopathy can be used, with facetal decompression along the symptomatic side. If the surgeon feels that an indirect foraminal decompression is sufficient to treat radiculopathy, a direct lateral (DLIF/lateral lumbar interbody fusion [XLIF]) can be used. There is always a concern about using stand-alone techniques with ALIF, AxiaLIF, and direct lateral approaches, which then would require adjunct instrumentation posteriorly with pedicle screws, facet screws, or cortical/corticopedicular screw placement at those levels.

In reoperations, the following factors must be considered while planning the surgery. Avoid dissecting through the old surgical scar if possible; for example, if there is recurrence after multiple posterior approaches, an ALIF or DLIF can be used, unless the old hardware needs to be revised owing to fracture. A fractured/displaced L4-5 DLIF graft can removed by repeat DLIF or ALIF as the cage is large, whereas a combined TLIF or posterior lumbar interbody fusion (PLIF) might be needed to get the fragmented cage if it has slipped below the level of disk space or is compressing the axilla of nerve root.[2] Always anticipate cerebrospinal fluid leak from a dural tear owing to severe epidural fibrosis from prior surgery, in which case an open approach is preferred over minimally invasive transtubular retractors. It is easier to follow the normal dura mater with an open or mini-open approach compared to transtubular vision.[3] Patients with failed back syndrome are advised to have an electromyography (EMG) to evaluate residual deficits from prior surgery to prognosticate on expected neurologic recovery.[4] Always review the existing hardware using a computed tomography scan, rather than a magnetic resonance image of the lumbosacral spine to rule for fractured implants or haloing around screws (nonunion) or graft dislodgement.[5] Always verify the sagittal/coronal balance (using a full scoliosis film, if needed) and the levels adjacent to the symptomatic one (dynamic x-ray study of flexion and extension).

Continuous EMG and somatosensory evoked potential (SSEP) monitoring during the surgery may be useful in reducing the risk of complications caused by overzealous manipulation.[35–37a] The latest published guidelines on the use of intra-operative monitoring has focused attention on the absence of level I evidence regarding the ability of intraoperative monitoring to prevent (as opposed to diagnosing) injury to the spinal cord during surgery.[37b] We would however, advise a set of electrophysiologic monitoring before and after the patient is positioned prone or lateral, especially the latter after breaking/bending the operating table which causes stretching of the psoas muscle. It may be necessary to monitor the upper lumbar plexus in selected cases.

Each case should be individually assessed for safety and feasibility of each approach; for example, if ALIF in a young male patient runs the risk of retrograde ejaculation, XLIF graft, which migrated into the central canal, can be retrieved only by an XLIF approach because of the larger footprint of the cage. In osteopenic cases with fractured pedicles, an adjunct posterior support can be provided by facet screws, laminar clamps, or even interspinous clamps, depending on the presence of canal stenosis and features of spinal anatomy on imaging. It is important for surgeons to be familiar with these multiple interbody fusion techniques and specific implant retrieval methods in graft failures, as one could potentially encounter a complication from any of these approaches (e.g., graft migration, nonunion, osteomyelitic collapse) in the years to come (Figs. 1.1–1.3).

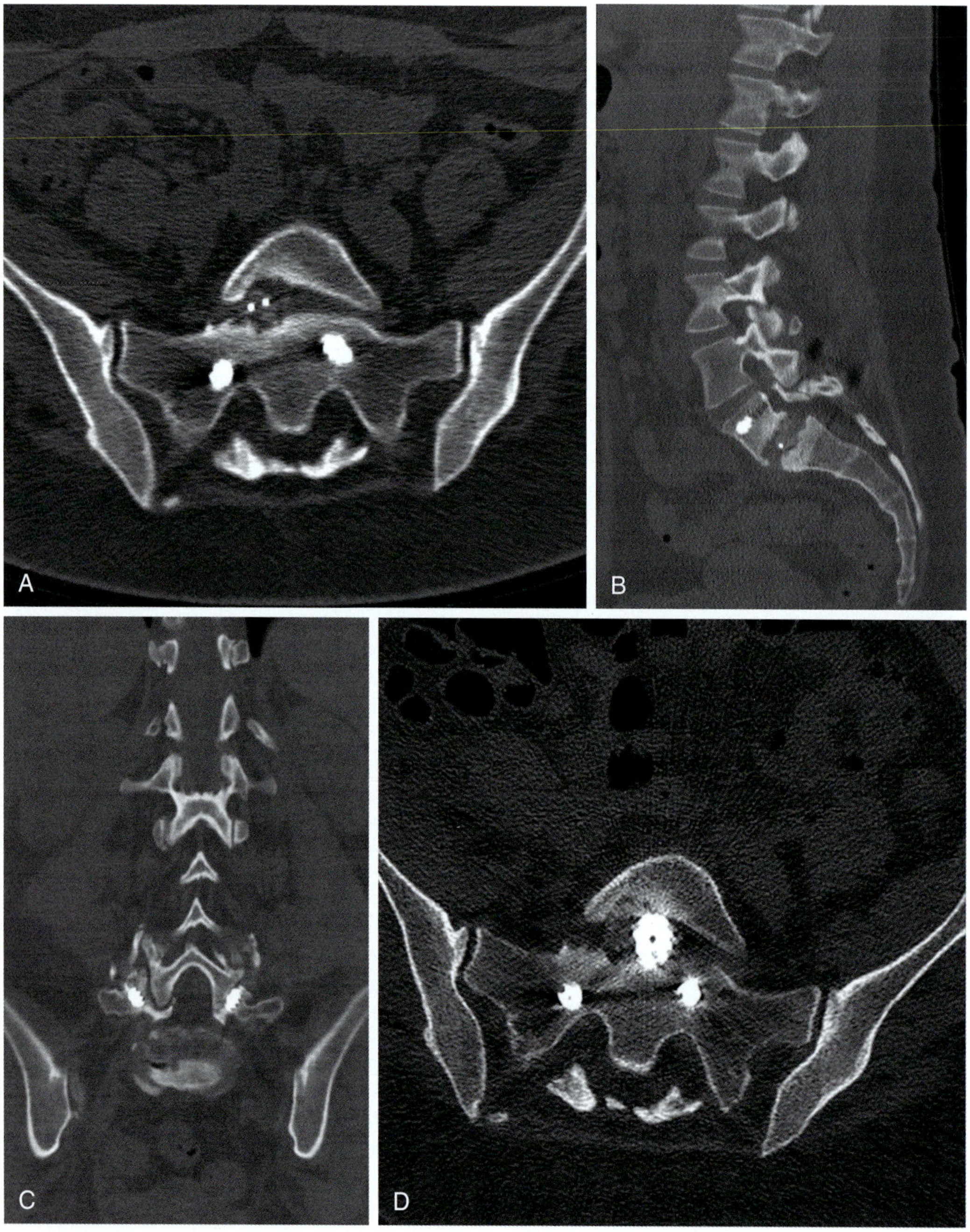

• **Fig. 1.1** **A–C**. Patient with recurrent severe backache and right radiculopathy; computed tomography (CT) scan images of failed fusion L5-S1, graft subsidence, and nonunion. **D–F**. Postoperative CT scan showing removal of old cage, new AxiaLIF rod at L5-S1 with pedicle screw fixation. (Courtesy Jonathan Pace, MD, Department of Neurosurgery, Case Western Reserve University, Cleveland, Ohio and David J. Hart, MD, Department of Neurosurgery, Wake Forest University Baptist Medical Center, Winston-Salem, North Carolina.)

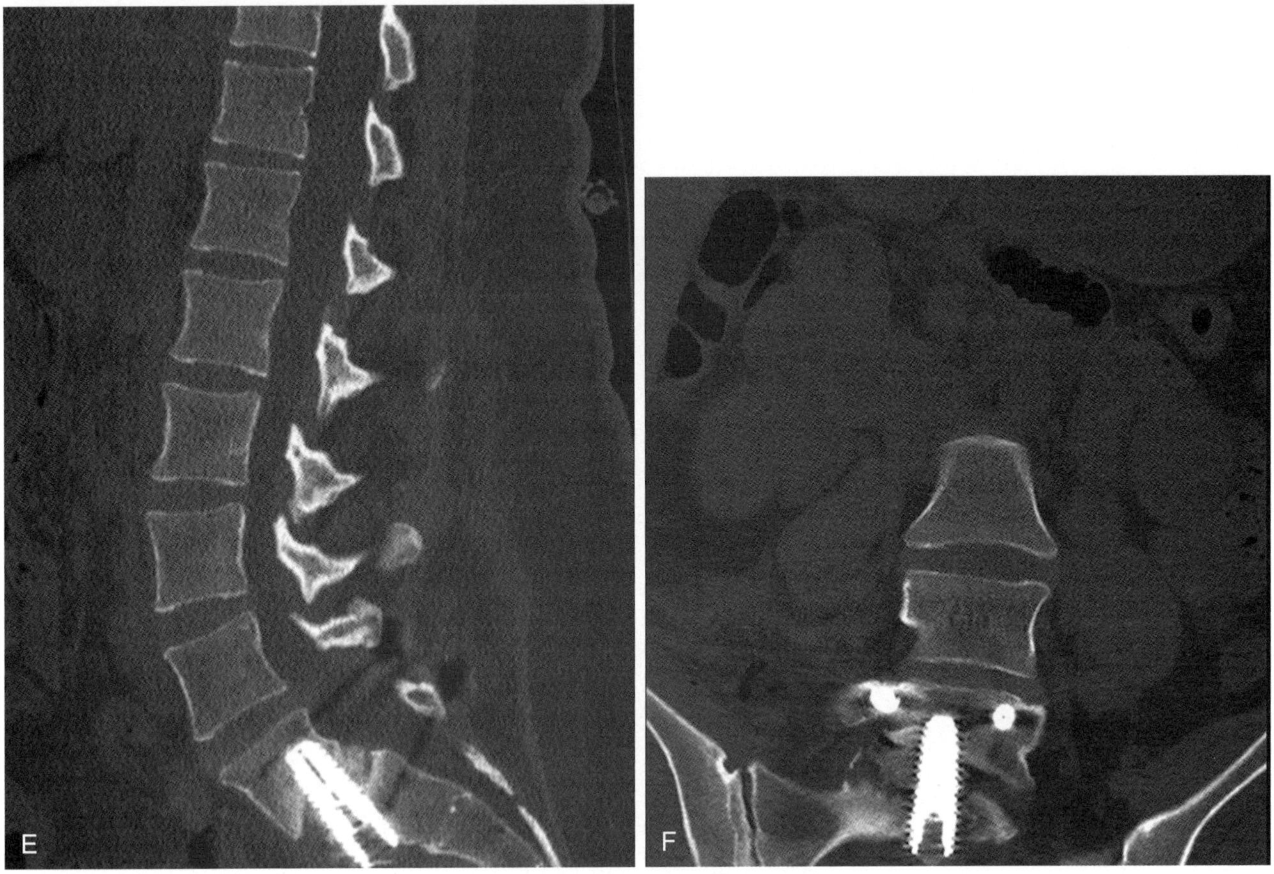

• **Fig. 1.1, cont'd**

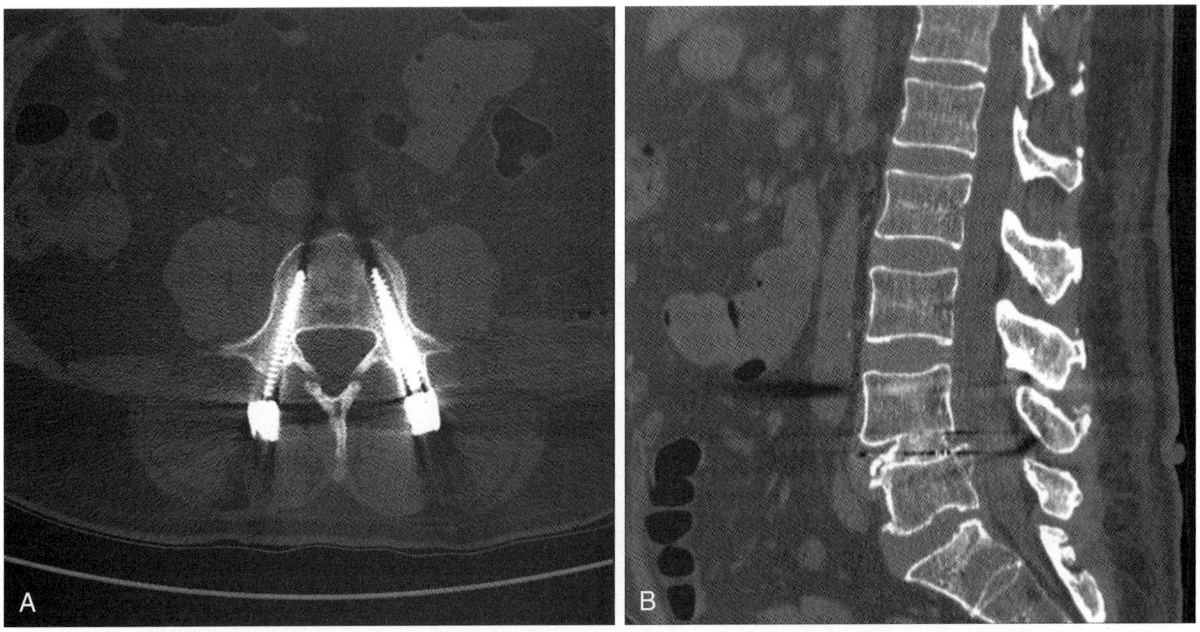

• **Fig. 1.2** **A–C**. Patient with refractory postoperative back pain, computed tomography (CT) scan of spine showing haloing around screws at L4-5 level bilaterally, more on the left with a displaced interbody cage. **D–F**. Postoperative CT scan showing repositioned L4-5 graft, with bigger graft size and a larger diameter pedicle screws. (Courtesy Jonathan Pace, MD, Department of Neurosurgery, Case Western Reserve University, Cleveland, Ohio and David J. Hart, MD, Department of Neurosurgery, Wake Forest University Baptist Medical Center, Winston-Salem, North Carolina.)

Continued

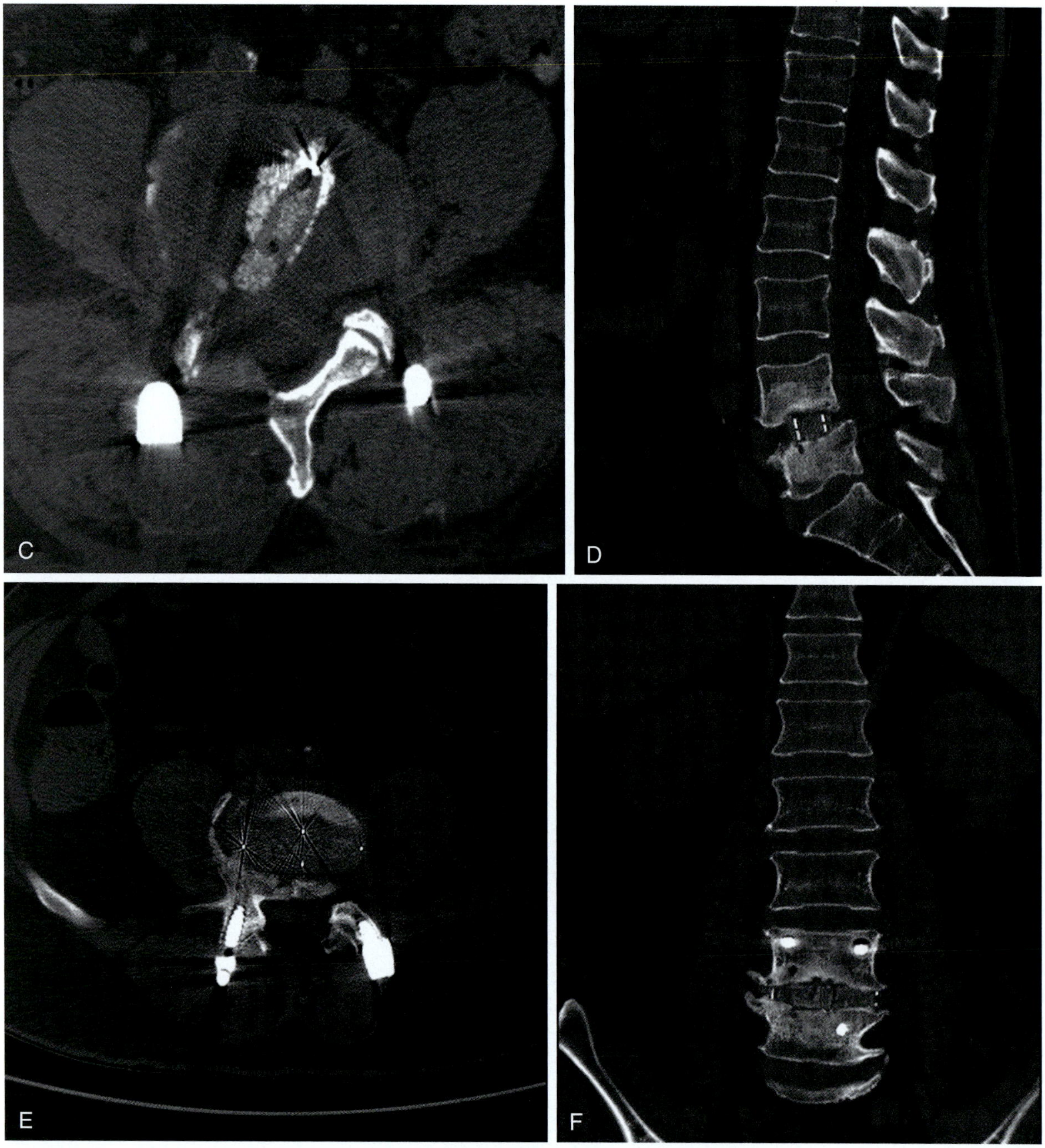

• Fig. 1.2, cont'd

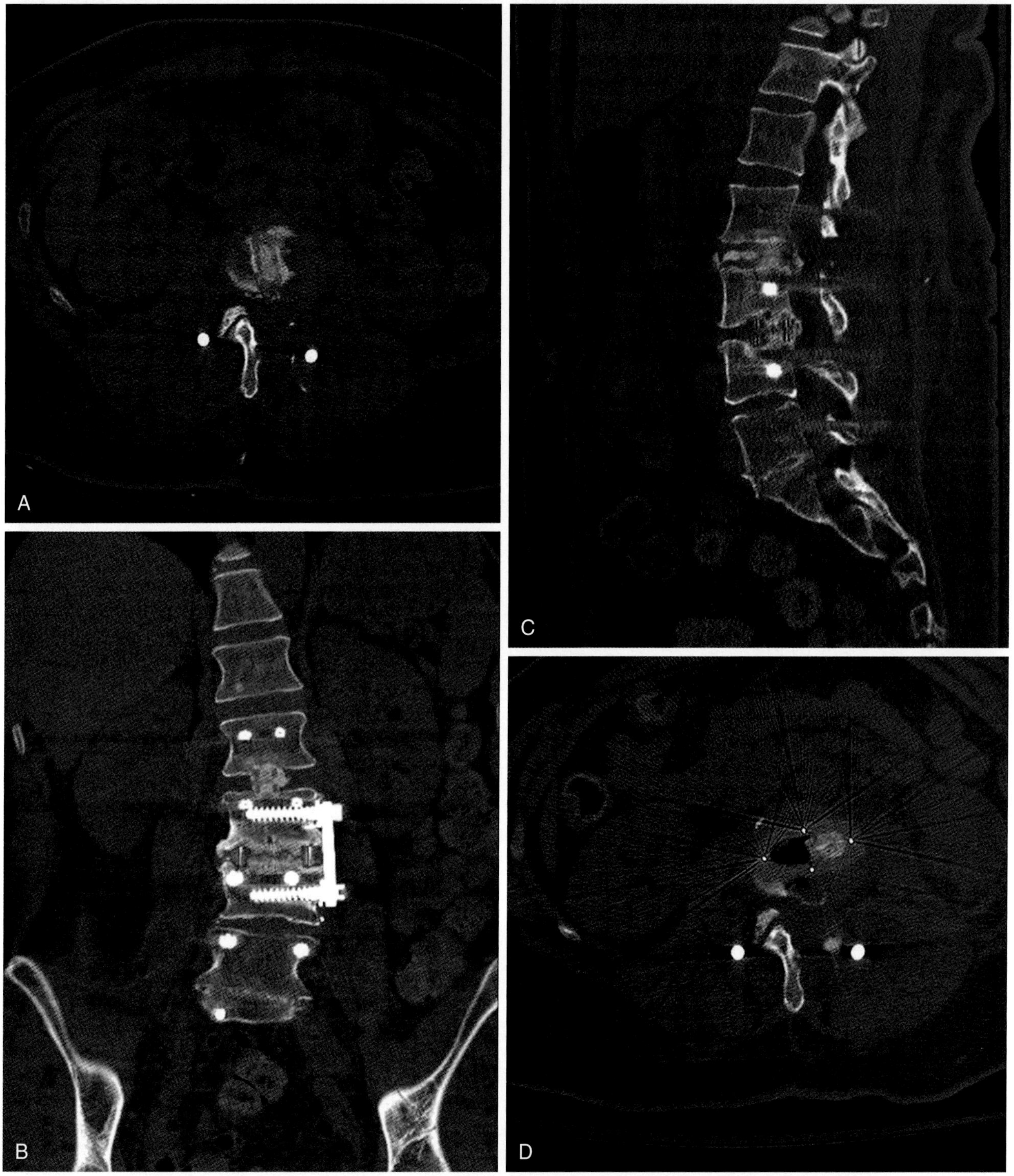

• **Fig. 1.3** **A–C**. Adjacent level disease: Patient with midlumbar backache (prior L3-4 direct lateral fusion with plate, backed with pedicle screws) and new preoperative computed tomography (CT) scan showing a retropulsed and migrated prior L2-3 interbody cage. **D–F**. Postoperative CT scan showing replacement of a larger graft at L2-3 level via direct lateral approach, with pedicle screws with dramatic relief of symptoms. (Courtesy Jonathan Pace, MD, Department of Neurosurgery, Case Western Reserve University, Cleveland, Ohio, and David J. Hart, MD, Department of Neurosurgery, Wake Forest University Baptist Medical Center, Winston-Salem, North Carolina.)

Continued

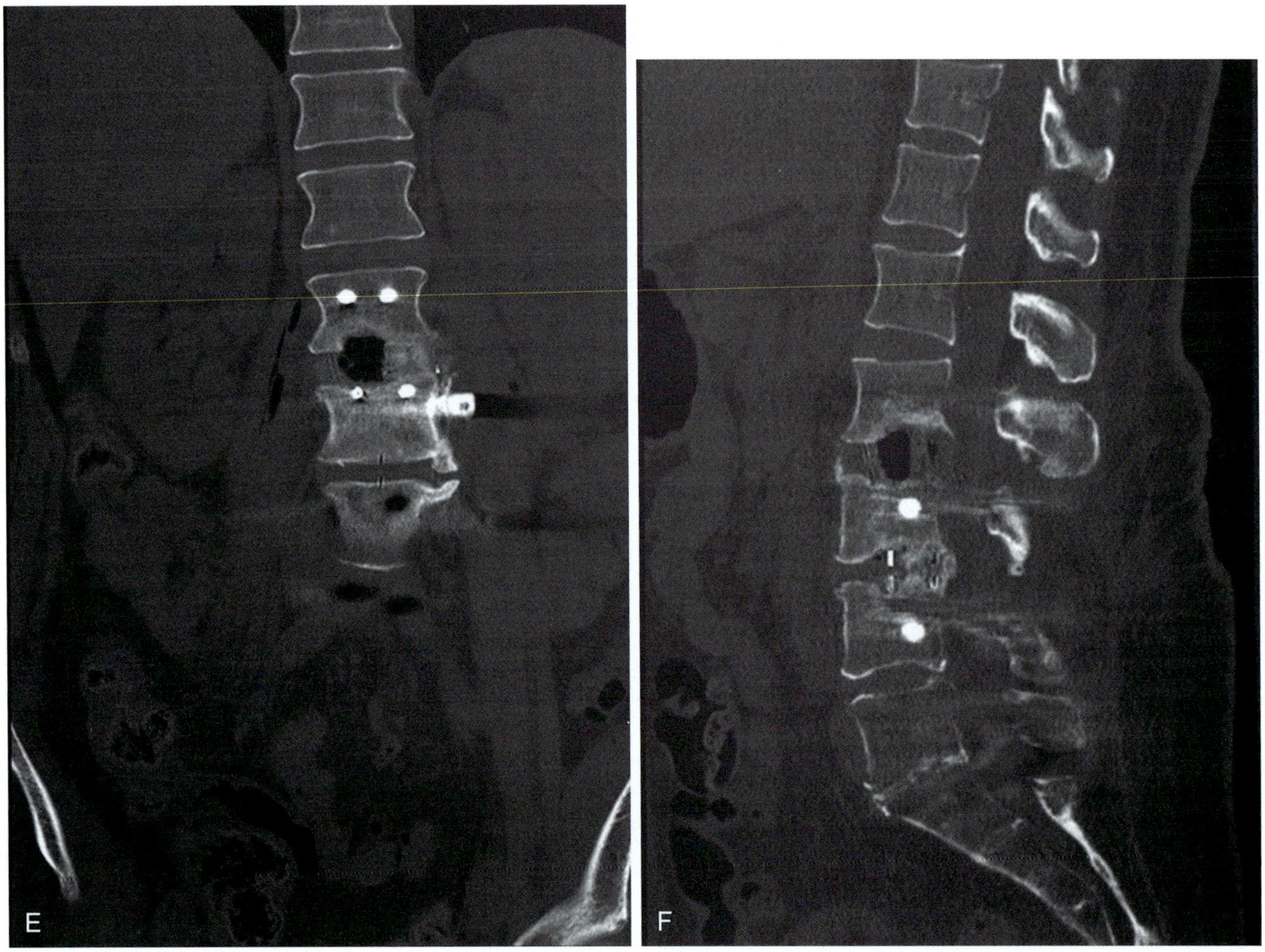

• **Fig. 1.3, cont'd**

Complications Following Lumbar Interbody Fusion Surgery

Acute and delayed complications of any spinal surgery may be associated with LIFs as well. The most devastating complication, of course, is death, and mortality rates following spine surgery have been reported to be between 0.15% and 0.29%.[38,39] Surgical site infections may be superficial or deep, and may necessitate prolonged antibiotic therapy or even the removal of implants.[40] Discitis following surgery is a debilitating, but fortunately rare, complication.[41] Incidental dural tears during surgery may result in postoperative cerebrospinal fluid leak and meningitis and may result in symptomatic adhesive arachnoiditis. A rare, but often irreversible complication is loss of vision owing to compression of the orbits while the patient is positioned prone for lumbar spine surgery.[42]

Neurologic injury may range from injury to the nerve roots to a complete cauda equina syndrome (0.38%).[43] This syndrome could result owing to an injury from a misplaced screw (out of the pedicle), neuropraxia from excessive manipulation during reduction of the spondylolisthesis, or even from direct injury to the neural structures. Postoperative epidural hematoma compressing on the cauda equina or conus medullaris also needs to be ruled out, especially when the neurologic deficit is rapidly worsening in the acute postoperative period. In most cases, a finding of postoperative deficits would mandate an emergent computed tomography scan to rule out hardware failure, malposition, fracture, or migration—treatable causes.[44] Computed tomography or magnetic resonance imaging could be used to assess surgical site hematoma, cerebrospinal fluid leak, and pressure on neural structures. The complications specific to each LIF technique are extensively described in Chapter 2.

Deep vein thrombosis has been reported to occur in as many as 15% to 17% of patients undergoing spine surgery, although the incidence of symptomatic deep venous thromboembolism is much lower. The use of chemoprophylaxis is still controversial owing to the incidence of postoperative epidural hematoma which may cause neurologic deficits. Judicious use of mechanical prophylaxis and early mobilization of patients at high risk may help to mitigate the incidence of symptomatic deep venous thromboembolism. Low-molecular-weight heparin has also been used for the first week in some studies.[45,46]

Ekman et al.[47] followed 111 patients who were randomized to exercise, surgery without fusion, or surgery with spinal instrumentation for a mean of 12.6 years.[47] They found that adjacent segment disk disease was higher in patients with spinal instrumentation, and that it was highest in patients who had laminectomy and spinal stabilization. Semirigid or dynamic stabilization has been attempted to reduce the incidence of this complication, but the results are not yet convincing.[48]

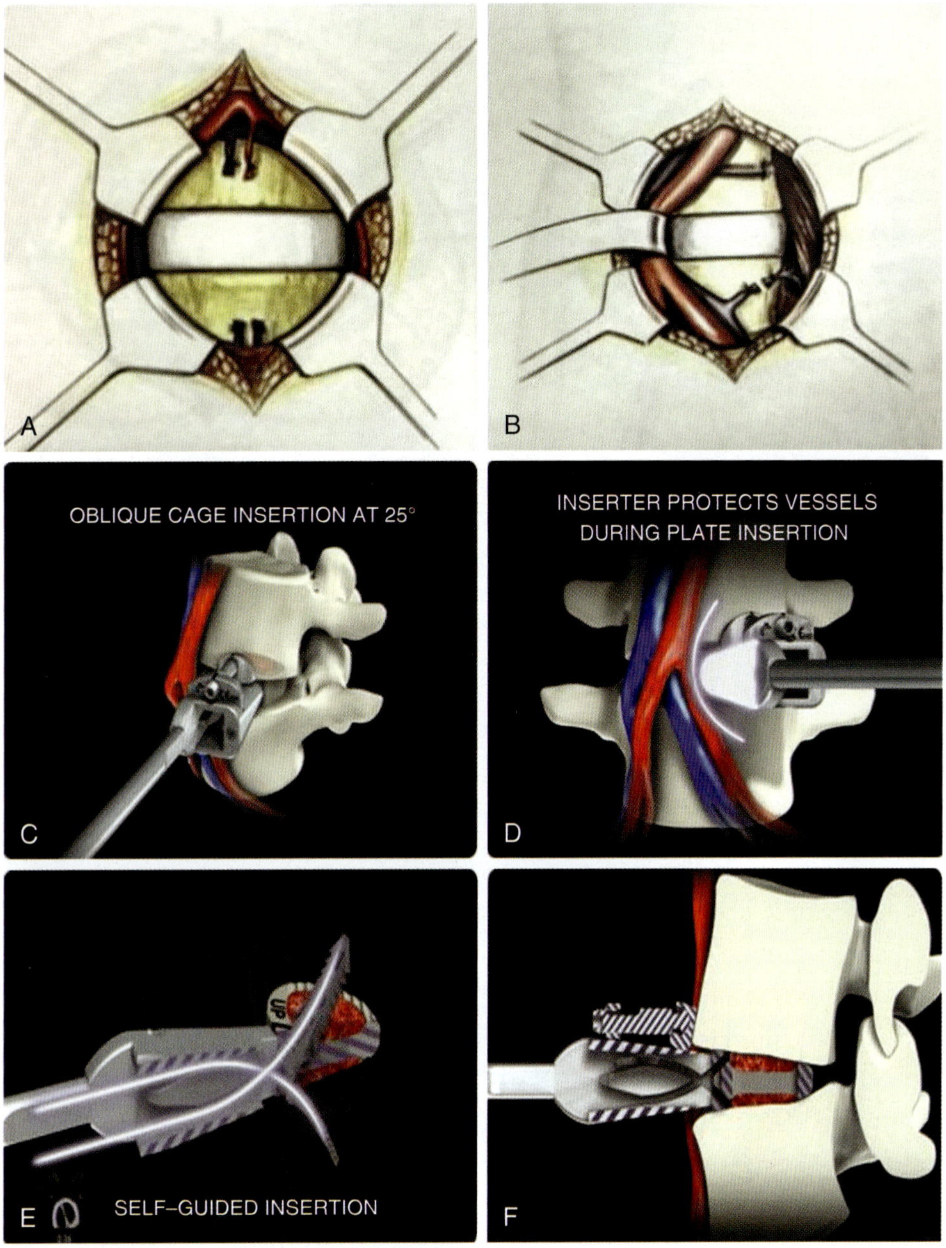

• **Fig. 1.4** A and B. Vessel retraction during anterior retroperitoneal exposure at L5-S1 and L4-5 levels, respectively. **C**. An oblique cage insertion at 25 degrees obviating vessel retraction and ligation-sectioning of its branches. **D**. Use of inserter protecting the large vessels. **E and F**. Anchoring blades with directional serrations to prevent graft back-outs, compared to conventional straight screws. (Figures C–F Courtesy Zimmer Biomet, Warsaw, Indiana, USA.)

Techniques and Technologies in Lumbar Interbody Fusion Surgery

This textbook provides an overview of the novel technologies and techniques involved in modern LIF surgeries. Fig. 1.4 clearly represents the vessel-mobilization strategies at various disk levels during an anterior lumbar interbody exposure and the new oblique-modification technique synergized with appropriate nuances in technology. This is a perfect example of synergistic improvisation in both anatomy-based technique and technology, which also accommodates the straight transpedicular screws easily. Likewise, Fig. 1.5 describes the mini-open modification of TLIF using a "pedicle-based" lateral retractor system, providing an extended lateral view of the disk space, causing lesser muscular and vascular interruption, and also preventing muscle creep from intraoperative shifting of retractor assembly. This technique provides a better visualization of Kambin's triangle during TLIF, providing wider lateral working space and hence safe and easy placement of interbody graft.

Neuronavigation and robotics have emerged as the latest additions to the armamentarium. Fig. 1.6 illustrates intraoperative navigation using interbody graft registration with intraoperative images using O-arm images transferred to a Stealth system. Both two-dimensional and three-dimensional image acquisitions are

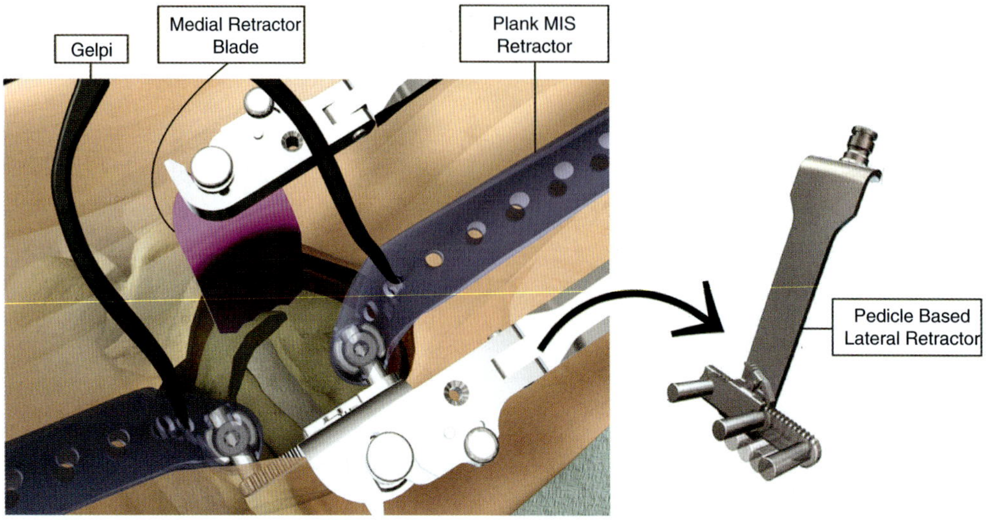

• **Fig. 1.5** Lateral retractor-distractor blade based on pedicle to expose the Kambin's triangle. This lateral retractor, along with a Gelpi self-retaining ratcheted finger-ring retractor, can facilitate extreme lateral dissection by providing a fixed "extreme lateral" point preventing vascular disruption and muscle shifting caused by migration of the retractor assembly. (Courtesy K2M, Inc., Leesburg, Virginia.)

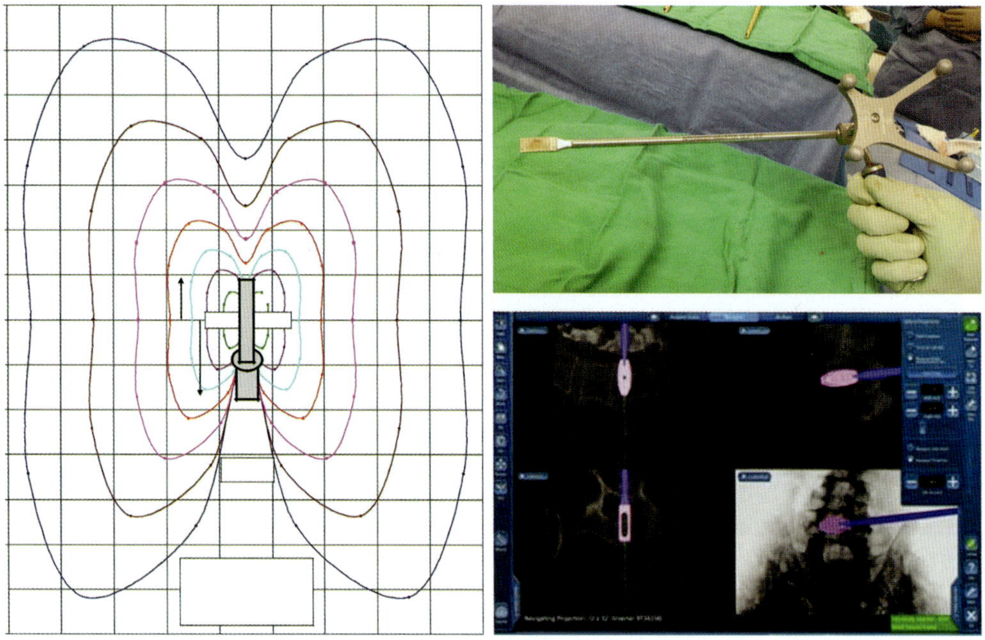

• **Fig. 1.6** O-arm technology for intraoperative spinal navigation and use in lumbar interbody fusion surgery. Note the radiation dose curves around the surgical table. (Images Provided by Medtronic Inc. Incorporates technology developed by Gary K. Michelson, MD.)

possible with surgical personnel situated at least 15 feet away from the patient during image acquisition, minimizing the radiation load for the surgeon and the operating room team. Similarly, there have been many recent FDA–approved devices in spinal robotics marketed for transpedicular access, including MedTech's ROSA and Mazor X, a third-generation robotic system following the original Spine Assist in 2004 and Renaissance system in 2011. However, there is paucity of literature elucidating the efficacy and superiority of using robotic technology in lumbar interbody graft insertion.

Conclusions

Although a century has passed since the first attempt at fusion of the lumbar spine, the relative and absolute indications and contraindications are still a matter of debate. Whereas there is a broad consensus that patients with unstable spondylolisthesis and symptomatic disease need surgical fixation, other scenarios are not so clear-cut as in the presence of associated synovial cysts at that level suggesting mobility. Most surgeons would agree that the following patients would merit surgery for spinal stabilization:

spondylolisthesis with failed medical management, traumatic and neoplastic conditions, postlaminectomy instability, and chronic pain owing to discitis or osteomyelitis. The role of surgical fusion in patients with idiopathic chronic back pain remains controversial, and more studies are required to elucidate the best treatment options for these patients. Technologic improvements will lead the way into the future, with better implants, safer osteogenetic materials, and a concerted move toward minimally invasive surgery with fewer morbidities and reduced hospital stay.

References

1. Hadra BE. The classic: wiring of the vertebrae as a means of immobilization in fracture and Potts disease. Berthold E Hadra. *Clin Orthop.* 1975;112:4–8.
2. Hibbs RA. An operation for progressive spinal deformities. *N Y Med.* 1911;121:1013.
3. Albee FH. Transplantation of a portion of the tibia into the spine for Pott's disease. *JAMA.* 1911;57:855.
4. Watkins MB. Posterolateral fusion of the lumbar and lumbosacral spine. *J Bone Joint Surg Am.* 1953;35:1014–1018.
5. Harrington PR. Treatment of scoliosis. Correction and internal fixation by spine instrumentation. *J Bone Joint Surg Am.* 1962;44:591–610.
6. Burkus JK, Gornet MF, Dickman CA, Zdeblick TA. Anterior lumbar interbody fusion using rhBMP-2 with tapered interbody cages. *J Spinal Disord Tech.* 2002;15(5):337–349.
7. Carragee EJ, Hurwitz EL, Weiner BK. A critical review of recombinant human bone morphogenetic protein-2 trials in spinal surgery: emerging safety concerns and lessons learned. *Spine J.* 2011;11(6):471–491.
8. Hansen SM, Sasso RC. Resorptive response of rhBMP2 simulating infection in an anterior lumbar interbody fusion with a femoral ring. *J Spinal Disord Tech.* 2006;19(2):130–134.
9. Vaidya R, Weir R, Sethi A, et al. Interbody fusion with allograft and rhBMP-2 leads to consistent fusion but early subsidence. *J Bone Joint Surg Br.* 2007;89(3):342–345.
10. Hustedt JW, Blizzard DJ. The controversy surrounding bone morphogenetic proteins in the spine: a review of current research. *Yale J Biol Med.* 2014;87(4):549–561.

11a. Rihn JA, Patel R, Makda J, et al. Complications associated with single-level transforaminal lumbar interbody fusion. *Spine J.* 2009;9(8):623–629.

11b. Mclain RF, Fleming JE, Boehm CA, et al. Aspiration of osteoprogenitor cells for augmenting spinal fusion: comparison of progenitor cell concentrations from the vertebral body and iliac crest. *J Bone Joint Surg Am.* 2005;87(12):2655–2661. https://Doi:10.2106/jbjs.e.00230.

12. Leu HF, Hauser RK. Percutaneous endoscopic lumbar spine fusion. *Neurosurg Clin North Am.* 1996;7:107–117.
13. Kambin P. Diagnostic and therapeutic spinal arthroscopy. *Neurosurg Clin North Am.* 1996;7:65–76.
14. Jacquot F, Gastambide D. Percutaneous endoscopic transforaminal lumbar interbody fusion: is it worth it? *Int Orthop.* 2013;37(8):1507–1510.
15. Newman PH, Stone KH. The etiology of spondylolisthesis. *J Bone Joint Surg Br.* 1963;45:39–59.
16. Weinstein JN, Lurie JD, Tosteson TD, et al. Surgical compared with nonoperative treatment for lumbar degenerative spondylolisthesis. Four-year results in the Spine Patient Outcomes Research Trial (SPORT) randomized and observational cohorts. *J Bone Joint Surg Am.* 2009;91(6):1295–1304.
17. Watters WC, Bono CM, Gilbert TJ, et al. An evidence-based clinical guideline for the diagnosis and treatment of degenerative lumbar spondylolisthesis. *Spine J.* 2009;9:609–614.
18. Herkowitz HN. Degenerative lumbar spondylolisthesis: evolution of surgical management. *Spine J.* 2009;9:605–606.
19. Kepler CK, Vaccaro AR, Hilibrand AS, et al. National trends in the use of fusion techniques to treat degenerative spondylolisthesis. *Spine (Phila Pa 1976).* 2014;39:1584–1589.
20. Bridwell KH, Sedgewick TA, O'Brien MF, et al. The role of fusion and instrumentation in the treatment of degenerative spondylolisthesis with spinal stenosis. *J Spinal Disord.* 1993;6:461–472.
21. Bae HW, Rajaee SS, Kanim LE. Nationwide trends in the surgical management of lumbar spinal stenosis. *Spine.* 2013;38:916–926.
22. Försth P, Ólafsson G, Carlsson T, et al. A randomized, controlled trial of fusion surgery for lumbar spinal stenosis. *N Engl J Med.* 2016; 374:1413–1423.
23. Ghogawala Z, Dziura J, Butler WE, et al. Laminectomy plus fusion versus laminectomy alone for lumbar spondylolisthesis. *N Engl J Med.* 2016;374:1424–1434.
24. Peul WC, Moojen WA. Fusion for lumbar spinal stenosis—safeguard or superfluous surgical implant? Editorial. *N Engl J Med.* 2016;374:1478–1479.
25. Jones TR, Rao RD. Adult isthmic spondylolisthesis. *J Am Acad Orthop Surg.* 2009;17:609–617.
26. Moller H, Hedlund R. Surgery versus conservative management in adult isthmic spondylolisthesis. *Spine.* 2000;25:1711–1715.
27. Bendo JA, Spivak J, Moskovich R, et al. Instrumented posterior arthrodesis of the lumbar spine in patients with diabetes mellitus. *Am J Orthop.* 2000;29:617–620.
28. Glassman SD, Alegre G, Carreon L, et al. Perioperative complications of lumbar instrumentation and fusion in patients with diabetes mellitus. *Spine J.* 2003;3(6):496–501.
29. Guzman JZ, Iatridis JC, Skovrlj B, et al. Outcomes and complications of diabetes mellitus on patients undergoing degenerative lumbar spine surgery. *Spine.* 2014;39(19):1596–1604. https://doi.org/10.1097/BRS.0000000000000482.
30. Lee TC, Ueng SW, Chen HH, et al. The effect of acute smoking on spinal fusion: an experimental study among rabbits. *J Trauma.* 2005;59:402–408.
31. Andersen T, Christensen FB, Laursen M, et al. Smoking as a predictor of negative outcome in lumbar spinal fusion. *Spine.* 2001;26:2623–2628.
32. Crawford CH, Carreon LY, Djurasovic M, et al. Lumbar fusion outcomes in patients with rheumatoid arthritis. *Eur Spine J.* 2008;17:822–825.
33. Kanis JA, Burlet N, Cooper C, et al. European guidance for the diagnosis and management of osteoporosis in postmenopausal women. *Osteoporos Int.* 2008;19:399–428.
34. Xue Q, Li H, Zou X, et al. The influence of alendronate treatment and bone graft volume on posterior-lateral spine fusion in a porcine model. *Spine.* 2005;30:1116–1121.
35. Eccher MA, Ghogawala Z, Steinmetz MP. The possibility of clinical trials in neurophysiologic intraoperative monitoring: a review. *J Clin Neurophysiol.* 2014;31:106–111.
36. Ney JP, van der Goes DN, Watanabe JH. Cost-benefit analysis: intraoperative neurophysiological monitoring in spinal surgeries. *J Clin Neurophysiol.* 2013;30:280–286.

37a. Fehlings MG, Brodke DS, Norvell DC, et al. The evidence for intraoperative neurophysiological monitoring in spine surgery: does it make a difference? *Spine (Phila Pa 1976).* 2010;35:S37–S46.

37b. Hadley MN, Shank CD, Rozzelle CJ, Walters BC. Guidelines for the use of electrophysiological monitoring for surgery of the human spinal column and spinal cord. *Neurosurgery.* 2017;81(5):713–732. https://doi.org/10.1093/neuros/nyx466.

38. Kalanithi PS, Patil CG, Boakye M. National complication rates and disposition after posterior lumbar fusion for acquired spondylolisthesis. *Spine.* 2009;34:1963–1969.
39. Juratli SM, Franklin GM, Mirza SK, et al. Lumbar fusion outcomes in Washington State workers' compensation. *Spine.* 2006;31:2715–2723.

40. Olsen MA, Mayfield J, Lauryssen C, et al. Risk factors for surgical site infection in spinal surgery. *J Neurosurg Spine*. 2003;2:149–155.
41. Chaudhary SB, Vives MJ, Basra SK, et al. Postoperative spinal wound infections and postprocedural diskitis. *J Spinal Cord Med*. 2007;30(5):441–451.
42. Nickels TJ, Manlapaz MR, Farag E. Perioperative visual loss after spine surgery. *World J Orthop*. 2014;5(2):100–106.
43. Cook C, Santos GC, Lima R, et al. Geographic variation in lumbar fusion for degenerative disorders: 1990 to 2000. *Spine J*. 2007;7:552–557.
44. Ogilvie JW. Complications in spondylolisthesis surgery. *Spine*. 2005;30:S97–S101.
45. Glotzbecker MP, Bono CM, Wood KB, et al. Thromboembolic disease in spinal surgery: a systematic review. *Spine (Phila Pa 1976)*. 2009;34(3):291–303.
46. Yang SD, et al. Prevalence and risk factors of deep vein thrombosis in patients after spine surgery: a retrospective case-cohort study. *Sci Rep*. 2015;5:11834.
47. Ekman P, Moller H, Shalabi A, et al. A prospective randomized study on the long-term effect of lumbar fusion on adjacent disc degeneration. *Eur Spine J*. 2009;18:1175–1186.
48. Cakir B, Carazzo C, Schmidt R, et al. Adjacent segment mobility after rigid and Semirigid instrumentation of the lumbar spine. *Spine*. 2009;34:1287–1291.

2

Complications and Avoidance in Lumbar Interbody Fusions

VINCENT J. ALENTADO AND MICHAEL P. STEINMETZ

Introduction

As with any surgical procedure, interbody fusions are associated with unique complications. Given the wide variety of approaches utilized when performing an interbody fusion, it is important to recognize common complications associated with each specific technique. Recognition of these complications allows the surgeon to utilize a more protective surgical approach to limit perioperative complications. Furthermore, recognition of common complications better enables the surgeon to inform patients of the risks of potential surgical treatment.

All pressure points should be padded to avoid peroneal neuropathy with pressure on the lateral leg at the proximal fibula. Care must also be made when positioning the patient in the lateral position. The authors do not advocate aggressive "breaking" of the table when lateral interbody fusion is performed. This aggressive "breaking" or bending the bed with the bed and foot of the bed lowered while the fulcrum at the lumbar spine is raised directly or indirectly has resulted in opening of the space between the iliac crest and rib cage. This was performed at the expense of potential stretching of the lumbar plexus and resultant neuropathy (i.e., ipsilateral thigh pain and/or weakness).

At times intraoperative neuromonitoring is utilized in an attempt to minimize neurological complications following interbody fusion. No high level evidence suggests the usage of these techniques results in improved outcome or decreased complications. Triggered electromyography (EMG) is commonly used during transpsoas direct lateral interbody fusion. Identification of motor nerves may decrease the incidence of weakness following surgery; however, it should be noted that this technique cannot accurately identify sensory nerves.

Posterior Lumbar Interbody Fusion

Posterior lumbar interbody fusion (PLIF) is a technically challenging procedure and therefore is associated with increased complication rates compared with other lumbar fusion techniques. Two of the primary complications of PLIF are nerve root injury and incidental durotomy. The reason for higher rates of these specific complications is owing to the significant traction that must be placed on the thecal sac and nerve roots in order to gain access to the intervertebral space.[1] Furthermore, PLIF requires violation of both facet joints to enable adequate exposure for graft placement.

Nerve Root Injury

Arguably the worst complication that commonly occurs with the PLIF procedure is nerve root injury. The current literature is widely variable in reported rates of nerve root injury with incidences ranging from 0.6% to 24%.[2–5] Davne and Myers[5] reported the lowest rate of nerve root injury at only a 0.6% in their series of 384 PLIF procedures.

Given the high rates and significant morbidity associated with nerve root injury during PLIF, many authors have investigated techniques to lower the rates of this complication. Barnes and colleagues[2] reported a 14% incidence of permanent nerve root injury when using threaded fusion cages compared to a 0% incidence using smaller allograft wedges in their retrospective review of 49 patients. The authors noted their preference for allograft wedges given these findings and their discovery that clinical outcomes were better in the allograft wedge group. Krishna and colleagues[6] noted a 9.7% rate of postoperative neuralgia in patients treated with subtotal facetectomy compared with a 4.9% rate in 226 patients treated with total facetectomy. Although this was not statistically significant, the authors noted their preferred practice of total facetectomy to help prevent nerve root injury. In a separate study, Okuda et al.[7] found a 6.8% rate of postoperative neuralgia with total facetectomy during PLIF.

The aforementioned studies demonstrate the importance of a wide exposure with adequate facetectomy, careful dissection techniques without unnecessary traction of nerve root (especially with canal stenosis at the levels above), and avoidance of oversized grafts in order to minimize the risk of nerve root injury during PLIF. Angled nerve root retractors and direct visualization of the nerve roots at all times can also help prevent neurologic injury during the procedure. A more aggressive total facetectomy can provide an excellent window for graft placement while minimizing the amount of retraction on the nerve root. Triggered EMG, if utilized, may enable assessment of undue retraction during this step of the operation; however, data do not support an improved outcome.

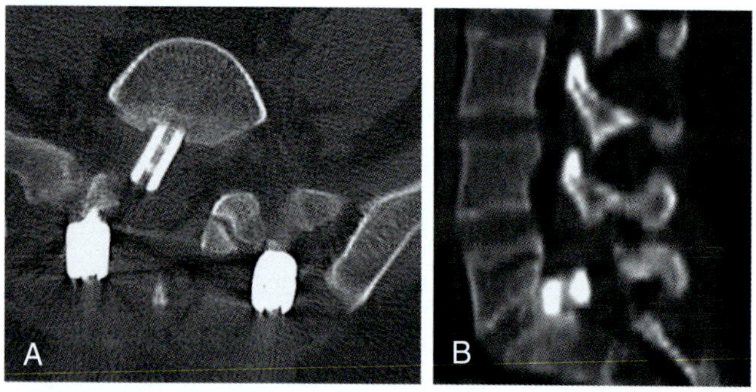

• **Fig. 2.1** Migration of the interbody cage. Axial (A) and sagittal (B) computed tomography (CT) scan of the lumbar spine showing posterior migration of an interbody cage (the first approach), which has resulted in neural compression. (From Benzel E. *Spine Surgery: Techniques, Complication Avoidance, & Management*. 3rd ed Philadelphia: Elsevier Saunders; 2012:539.)

Durotomy

Incidental durotomies are another common complication that occurs at higher rates during PLIF procedures owing to the direct retraction of the thecal sac intraoperatively. Studies have reported rates of durotomies at 9% to 19%, with higher rates occurring during reoperation surgeries owing to dural adhesions.[3,7,8] If a durotomy does occur, it can usually be repaired primarily. However, repair may be more difficult when using a minimally invasive technique.

Graft- and Cage-Related Complications

Graft dislodgement and loosening are other complications associated with PLIF, especially during early use of the technique (Fig. 2.1). The cumulative incidence of graft-related complications is less than 5%.[9] However, the rate of this complication is even lower when posterior pedicle screw stabilization is used with the PLIF procedure. Conversely, total facetectomy is associated with a higher incidence of graft extrusion owing to the decreased stability associated with this technique, but is lessened with the use of screw fixation. When graft-related complications are symptomatic, they require revision surgery, which is technically challenging.

Interbody cage type and positioning have been shown to effect rates of migration, with newer technologies being utilized to decrease the incidence of graft dislodgement (Fig. 2.2).[10] Furthermore, subsidence of the implants may also occur after PLIF, which may result in postoperative neuralgia (Fig. 2.3).[6]

Nonunion

Fusion rates after PLIF are generally high, with studies reporting incidences of 95% to 98%.[7,8,11] However, there is some reported variability with Rivet et al.[12] achieving a fusion rate of only 74% in 42 patients receiving PLIF.

Other Complications

Other complications, including epidural hematoma (1%),[3] wound infections, and other nonimplant-related complications, seem to occur with a similar frequency in PLIF as in other reconstructive spinal operations. Although adjacent segment disease (ASD) is more of an adverse outcome than complication, some studies have demonstrated earlier rates of ASD and revision surgery compared with other cohorts. However, new surgical techniques have been

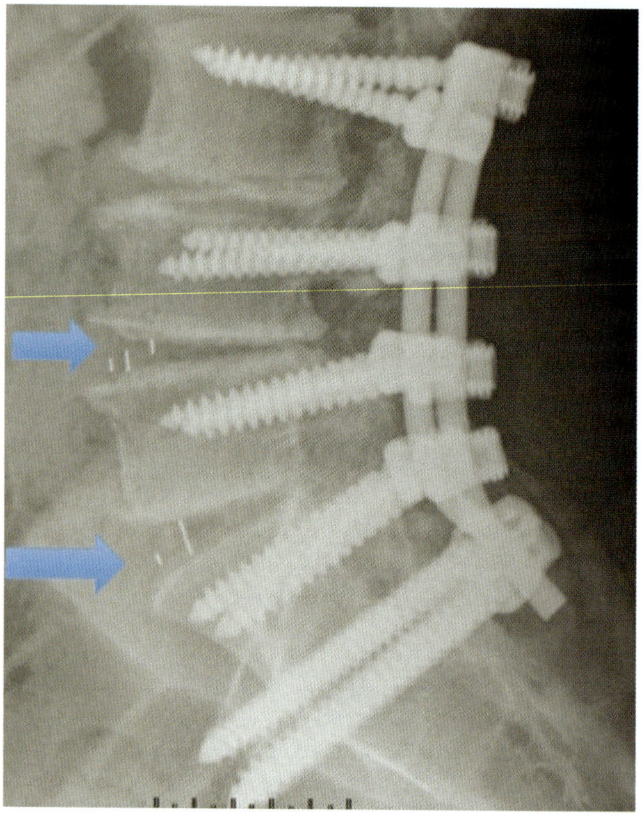

• **Fig. 2.2** Steerable cage placed along the anterior annulus. Newer cage design allows cage placement as anterior as possible. Cages can now be steered and placed along the anterior annulus.

utilized to prevent this development. Lastly, there is a risk of loss of lumbar lordosis. This was much more relevant with the use of older cages; however, careful attention to detail should minimize this complication.

Anterior Lumbar Interbody Fusion

In contrast to PLIF, the anterior lumbar interbody fusion (ALIF) technique can provide the same interbody support without manipulation of the dural or posterior neural structures. However, the ventral approach required during the ALIF procedure often necessitates significant retraction of the iliac vessels, hypogastric nerves, and peritoneum, which may result in direct injury to these structures. Other complications associated with ALIF include an increased risk of deep vein thrombosis (DVT), abdominal wall hernias, and retrograde ejaculation in men.[13]

Vascular Injury

Major blood vessel injuries are rare during ALIF. However, vascular injury to the common iliac vessels occurs at a rate of 1% to 7%, with higher rates occurring during exposure of the L5-S1 level.[14–16] The common iliac vein is very compressible; it lies posterior to the artery such that it can easily be mistaken for soft tissues during exposure. The iliolumbar vein is at higher risk during exposure of the L4-5 level. Some surgeons advocate for controlled ligation of this vessel in all exposures to minimize the risk of inadvertent tearing with retraction.[15,17] To avoid injury of these vessels, self-retaining retractors should not be used on these vessels during exposure.

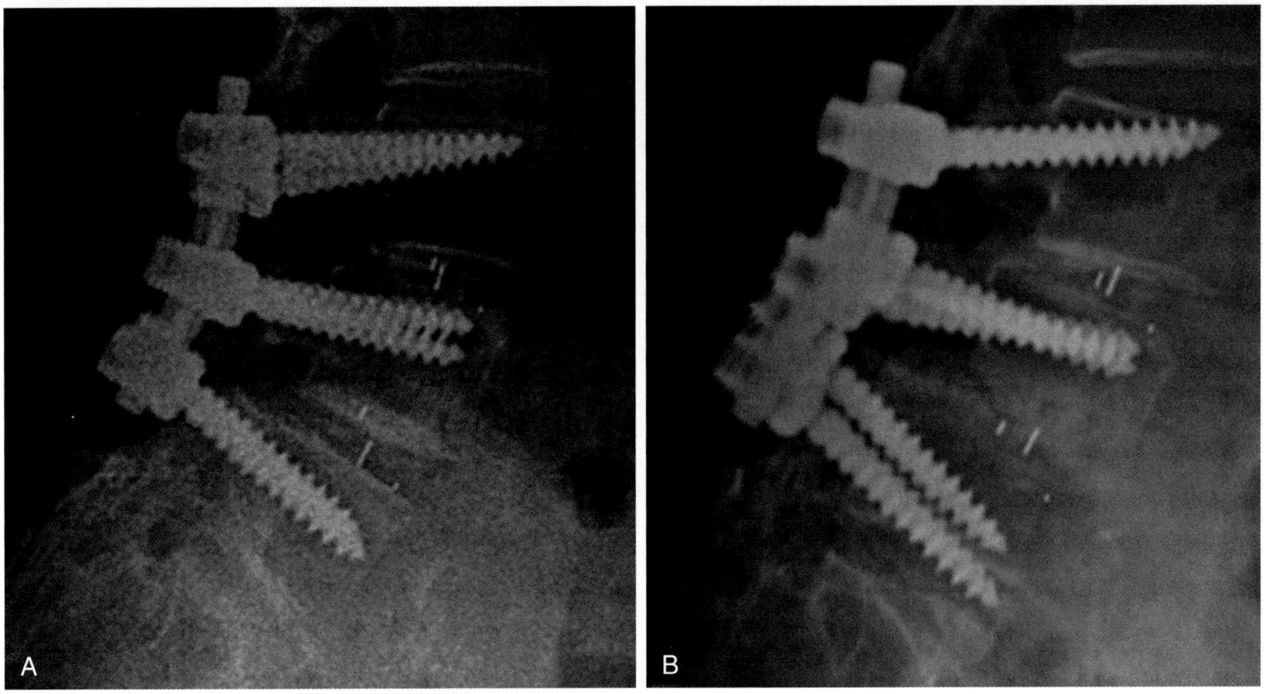

• **Fig. 2.3** Subsidence of the interbody cage. **A**. This patient underwent a two-level interbody fusion, L3-4 and L4-5. **B**. One month after index surgery, the patient developed severe back and leg pain. Lateral radiograph demonstrates subsidence of the L4-5 interbody graft and instability.

Arterial thrombosis secondary to aggressive retraction or arterial injury during ALIF has also been reported.[15,16,18] These occur at a rate of 1%.[15] In contrast, DVT occurs in 1% to 11% of patients receiving ALIF, which is higher than in other fusion procedures.[14,16,19,20] Resultant nonfatal pulmonary embolism (PE) was seen at an incidence of 3% in one study.[20] To avoid thrombosis, retraction should not be prolonged and self-retaining retractors should not be used on vessels. It is important to check the lower extremity pulses bilaterally after the procedure. If thrombosis is suspected, an immediate angiogram or venogram should be obtained.

Intraabdominal Complications

Ventral exposure during ALIF is often performed by vascular or general surgeons to decrease the rate of vascular and intraabominal complications. However, gastrointestinal (GI) tract injuries still occur in 2% of all patients receiving ALIF.[14] GI tract injury rates can be lowered by placing packing behind self-retaining retractors. Furthermore, some surgeons advocate for preoperative bowel preparation, including enema, to help decompress the bowel, theoretically decreasing the rate of bowel injury. A nasogastric tube can also be placed preoperatively to facilitate bowel decompression.

Violation of the peritoneum during the retroperitoneal approach or violation of the transversalis fascia during iliac bone graft harvest can lead to the development of postoperative hernias. Although hernias occur in less than 1% of cases, they can lead to bowel obstruction and/or infaction.[16]

Ileus after ALIF is common with reported incidences of 1% to 8%. However, this complication usually resolves within 1 week of the operation.[14,16,19,21] Prolonged ileus should raise suspicion of a postoperative hernia with bowel obstruction.

Retrograde Ejaculation

Retrograde ejaculation as a result of hypogastric plexus injury has been reported in 0.1% to 8% of ALIF procedures performed on male patients.[14,16,19,21–23] This complication usually occurs after exposure of the L5-S1 level. The mechanism for this complication is secondary to relaxation of the internal sphincter of the bladder with subsequent retrograde flow of ejaculate into the bladder. Avoidance of this complication is possible with good operative technique and anatomical understanding. Inoue et al.[19] noted a decrease in both ileus and retrograde ejaculation with improved surgical technique over the last 13 years in their 27 year study of 350 ALIF patients. Over the last 13 years, no patients had ileus or retrograde ejaculation.

The prevertebral sympathetic plexus runs along the anterolateral edge of the vertebral bodies before traversing over the aortic bifurcation and common iliac vessels and forming the hypogastric plexus. Blunt dissection must be utilized to mobilize the more cephalad prevertebral plexus before the hypogastric plexus can be adequately exposed.[24] Furthermore, aggressive electrocautery should be minimized during the approach of the caudal lumbar spine.

If retrograde ejaculation does occur, patients may be counseled that 25% to 88% of patients suffering from this complication have spontaneous resolution by the end of the second year.[19]

Neurologic Complications

Major neurologic complications during ALIF are rare because the epidural space is not entered and no attempt is made to decompress the neural elements during the procedure. However, injuries to the genitofemoral or ilioinguinal nerves may occur after ALIF, with some authors reporting rates as high as 15%.[21,25] Injuries to these nerves are characterized by postoperative numbness in the groin and/or medial thigh. This complication is most common in patients who undergo ALIF procedures at the upper lumbar levels. Usually, these nerve palsies resolve spontaneously.

A sympathomimetic dysfunction occurs in 7% to 14% of patients undergoing ALIF procedures.[14,21] Patients with this complication note that the lower extremity of the side of operation is warmer and possibly more swollen than the contralateral lower extremity. This complication also resolves over time.

Graft- and Cage-Related Complications

Graft collapse after ALIF occurs in 1% to 2% of patients.[25] This complication usually results from excessive removal of subchondral bone from the adjacent vertebral body endplates. This collapse may result in a kyphotic spinal deformity. Graft absorption may also occur, especially in smokers, although this complication is rare.[25]

Graft dislodgement occurs in 1% of patients receiving ALIF.[25] Such graft displacements can be minimized by using a ventral plate or posterior pedicle fixation to enhance stability.

The aforementioned complication may be minimized by the addition of anterior or posterior instrumentation. Biologics may also have both a positive and negative effect. Bone morphogenetic protein-2 (BMP-2) has been demonstrated to result in early osteolysis, which may result in subsidence or graft collapse if performed in a stand-alone ALIF. This may be minimized with the use of posterior instrumentation.

Nonunion

Pseudoarthrosis after ALIF is reported at highly variable rates, ranging from 3% to 58%[25] (Fig. 2.4). Higher rates of nonunion are seen in patients who smoke more than one pack of cigarettes daily.[25] Nonunion may also be minimized with the use of biologics, such as BMP-2, and the addition of spinal instrumentation.

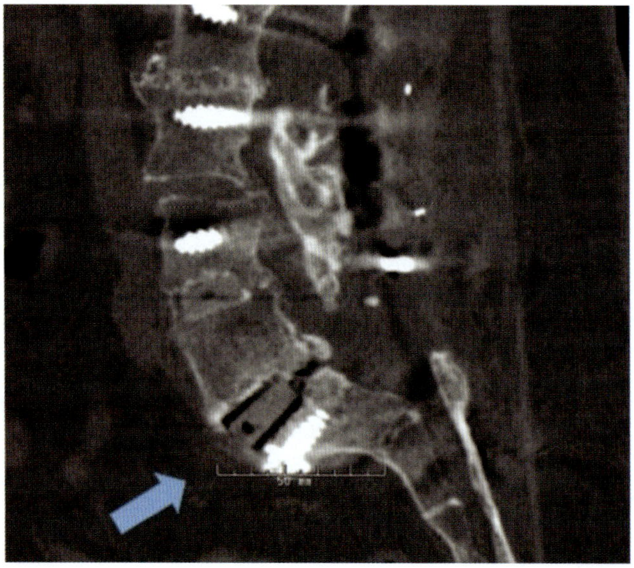

• **Fig. 2.4** Nonunion of the interbody graft. Two years following multilevel fusion for scoliosis, this patient presented with increasing back pain. The patient demonstrates a clear nonunion at the L5-S1 interbody graft. Lucency is clear around the graft *(arrow)*.

Other Complications

Urinary retention after ALIF has been reported in 5% to 28% of cases, but is usually temporary and may be related to narcotic use.[21]

Postoperative infections of the iliac crest donor site occur in 1% to 9% of all ALIF procedures.[20,21] These are best prevented by avoiding the use of foreign materials in the wound and using perioperative antibiotics, copious irrigation, and maintaining intraoperative hemostasis.

Flynn et al.[23] noted impotence in 2% of patients receiving ALIF, but this was deemed nonorganic and patients were treated with psychotherapy.

Translumbar Interbody Fusion

To avoid the complications associated with ALIF and PLIF procedures, Harms and Rolinger[26] described the posterior transforaminal lumbar interbody fusion (TLIF) technique. As TLIF does not require anterior abdominal wall exposure, it avoids all of the vascular, abdominal wall, and autonomic complications of ALIF. Furthermore, exposure and retraction of the thecal sac are minimal compared with the PLIF procedure. Therefore, TLIF can be performed more safely in the upper lumbar spine owing to the lower risk of conus medullaris retraction and injury. The lessened retraction of the thecal sac also makes TLIF better suited for revision cases where there may be significant epidural adhesions and scarring. Furthermore, if a unilateral approach is used, the contralateral lamina, facet joint, and pars can be spared, which provides increased surface area for fusion.[26]

Neurologic Deficit

Neurologic deficits are among the most common complications resulting from TLIF. Neurologic deficits lasting longer than 3 months after surgery occur in 4% of patients undergoing minimally invasive TLIF.[27] Case of contralateral radiculopathy after unilateral TLIF have been reported.[28,29] This complication is hypothesized to occur secondary to asymptomatic contralateral stenosis that is exacerbated by the increased segmental lordosis resulting from the TLIF procedure.

Graft Dislodgement

Graft dislodgement is an infrequent complication following TLIF (see Fig. 2.1). Anecdotal reports suggest cage migration after TLIF may not cause neural compression, or necessitate revision surgery, as often as after PLIF.[30]

NonUnion

Achievement of fusion at 1 year after TLIF ranges from 80% to 98%, with lower fusion rates seen in multilevel fusions.[31,32]

EXtreme Lateral Interbody Fusion (XLIF: Direct Lateral Approach)

The extreme lateral interbody fusion (XLIF) procedure was first described by Ozgur et al.[33] in 2006. The XLIF procedure allows anterior access to the disk space without the complication of an anterior abdominal procedure. As this is a newer procedure, the literature examining complications is sparse. The most common complications seen with the XLIF technique are transient groin and thigh paresthesias secondary to injury of the genitofemoral nerve.

Neurologic Complications

The reported incidence of paresthesias after XLIF is extremely variable with incidences ranging from 0.7% to 62.7%.[34–37] These paresthesias are usually located in the groin and thigh owing to injury of the genitofemoral nerve. In most cases, the paresthesias improve within 4 to 12 weeks postoperatively, with more than 90% recovering by 1 year.[34–37] In addition to paresthesias, transient psoas or quadriceps weakness occurs at a rate of 1% to 24% after XLIF.[35,37,38]

Cummock et al.[35] noted a higher rate of thigh pain, numbness, and weakness after L4-5 surgery in their review of 59 patients receiving XLIF. However, this was not a statistically significant difference, possibly owing to low sample size. Because of the potential for higher neurologic complication rates at this level, Rodgers and colleagues[38] opted to give patients 10 mg of IV dexamethasone intraoperatively during L4-5 XLIF procedures. The authors noted a significantly lower rate of paresthesias in patients given dexamethasone compared with patients who did not receive it during XLIF of the L4-5 level.

The natural history of these injuries is favorable. Most cases of weakness, numbness, or paresthesias are usually resolved by six months postoperatively.

To avoid neurologic injury after XLIF, it is imperative to perform careful dissection, avoid tension on the muscle, and perform gentle dilation to the disk space. Furthermore, dilation should not be greater than the minimum required for diskectomy. Neurologic monitoring may also decrease the risk of nerve injury. Lastly, less "breaking of the table" has been theorized to decrease the incidence of ipsilateral lumbar plexus injury. Originally, ipsilateral hip flexor/knee extensor weakness, numbness, and/or pain was thought to be caused by dissection through the psoas muscle; however, it is currently thought more likely to be caused by stretching the lumbar plexus during positioning.

Graft Dislodgement

As with ALIF, direct lateral approaches utilize large interbody grafts. These grafts may be secured in the interbody space via a lateral plate, screw rod construct, or integrated screw plate design. Alternatively, they may be secured via posterior pedicle, facet screws, or spinous process plate. Dislocations of these large XLIF grafts are more likely to cause severe deficits if posterior migration occurs. If this does occur, the graft must be removed via open or direct lateral approach.

Other Complications

Postoperative ileus occurs at a rate of 1% after XLIF.[38] As with the ALIF procedure, most cases of ileus resolve within a week after surgery. Rodgers and colleagues[38] also described one incidence of gastric volvulus in their series of 600 patients.

Postoperative hernias may occur after XLIF if the peritoneum is violated during the procedure. The incidence of this complication is 0.3%.[38] Postoperative retroperitoneal hematomas occur at a rate of 0.3% to 5% after XLIF, most commonly occurring within the psoas muscle.[34–36,38]

For all interbody fusions, care must be taken in patients with advanced osteoporosis. In fact, interbody fusion with a structural graft should be avoided in such circumstances in the authors' opinion. The rate of subsidence, construct failure, and nonunion are greater than the benefits of this surgical technique (authors' opinion). Surgery may be indicated for discitis, which fails to be effectively treated with antibiotics. In this situation, diskectomy may be required to effectively debride the disk space. A structural interbody graft should be not placed in this situation, especially polyetheretherketone (PEEK), but rather autograft packed in the disk space.

Conclusion

Interbody fusion is effective for successful treatment of a number of lumbar pathologies. It has been shown to result in improved fusion rates and segmental alignment. A number of complications may be seen following each specific interbody technique. These complications may be mitigated by careful patient selection and careful attention to detail.

References

1. Cole CD, McCall TD, Schmidt MH, et al. Comparison of low back fusion techniques: transforaminal lumbar interbody fusion (TLIF) or posterior lumbar interbody fusion (PLIF) approaches. *Curr Rev Musculoskelet Med.* 2009;2(2):118–126. https://doi.org/10.1007/s12178-009-9053-8.
2. Barnes B, Rodts GE, Haid RW, et al. Allograft implants for posterior lumbar interbody fusion: results comparing cylindrical dowels and impacted wedges. *Neurosurgery.* 2002;51(5):1191–1198. discussion 1198.
3. Hosono N, Namekata M, Makino T, et al. Perioperative complications of primary posterior lumbar interbody fusion for nonisthmic spondylolisthesis: analysis of risk factors. *J Neurosurg Spine.* 2008;9(5):403–407. https://doi.org/10.3171/SPI.2008.9.11.403.
4. Elias WJ, Simmons NE, Kaptain GJ, et al. Complications of posterior lumbar interbody fusion when using a titanium threaded cage device. *J Neurosurg.* 2000;93(suppl 1):45–52.
5. Davne SH, Myers DL. Complications of lumbar spinal fusion with transpedicular instrumentation. *Spine.* 1992;17(suppl 6):S184–S189.
6. Krishna M, Pollock RD, Bhatia C. Incidence, etiology, classification, and management of neuralgia after posterior lumbar interbody fusion surgery in 226 patients. *Spine J Off J North Am Spine Soc.* 2008;8(2):374–379. https://doi.org/10.1016/j.spinee.2006.09.004.
7. Okuda S, Miyauchi A, Oda T, et al. Surgical complications of posterior lumbar interbody fusion with total facetectomy in 251 patients. *J Neurosurg Spine.* 2006;4(4):304–309. https://doi.org/10.3171/spi.2006.4.4.304.
8. Brantigan JW, Steffee AD, Lewis ML, et al. Lumbar interbody fusion using the Brantigan I/F cage for posterior lumbar interbody fusion and the variable pedicle screw placement system: two-year results from a Food and Drug Administration investigational device exemption clinical trial. *Spine.* 2000;25(11):1437–1446.
9. Zhang Q, Yuan Z, Zhou M, et al. A comparison of posterior lumbar interbody fusion and transforaminal lumbar interbody fusion: a literature review and meta-analysis. *BMC Musculoskelet Disord.* 2014;15(1):367. https://doi.org/10.1186/1471-2474-15-367.
10. Imagama S, Kawakami N, Matsubara Y, et al. Preventive effect of artificial ligamentous stabilization on the upper adjacent segment impairment following posterior lumbar interbody fusion. *Spine.* 2009;34(25):2775–2781. https://doi.org/10.1097/BRS.0b013e3181b4b1c2.
11. Kim K-T, Lee S-H, Lee Y-H, et al. Clinical outcomes of 3 fusion methods through the posterior approach in the lumbar spine. *Spine.* 2006;31(12):1351–1357. discussion 1358. https://doi.org/10.1097/01.brs.0000218635.14571.55.

12. Rivet DJ, Jeck D, Brennan J, et al. Clinical outcomes and complications associated with pedicle screw fixation-augmented lumbar interbody fusion. *J Neurosurg Spine*. 2004;1(3):261–266. https://doi.org/10.3171/spi.2004.1.3.0261.
13. Mummaneni PV, Haid RW, Rodts GE. Lumbar interbody fusion: state-of-the-art technical advances. Invited submission from the Joint Section Meeting on Disorders of the Spine and Peripheral Nerves, March 2004. *J Neurosurg Spine*. 2004;1(1):24–30. https://doi.org/10.3171/spi.2004.1.1.0024.
14. Rajaraman V, Vingan R, Roth P, Heary RF, Conklin L, Jacobs GB. Visceral and vascular complications resulting from anterior lumbar interbody fusion. *J Neurosurg*. 1999;91(suppl 1):60–64.
15. Brau S. Vascular injury during anterior lumbar surgery*1. *Spine J*. 2004;4(4):409–412. https://doi.org/10.1016/j.spinee.2003.12.003.
16. Brau SA. Mini-open approach to the spine for anterior lumbar interbody fusion: description of the procedure, results and complications. *Spine J Off J North Am Spine Soc*. 2002;2(3):216–223.
17. Kozak JA, Heilman AE, O'Brien JP. Anterior lumbar fusion options. Technique and graft materials. *Clin Orthop*. 1994;(300):45–51.
18. Hackenberg L, Liljenqvist U, Halm H, et al. Occlusion of the left common iliac artery and consecutive thromboembolism of the left popliteal artery following anterior lumbar interbody fusion. *J Spinal Disord*. 2001;14(4):365–368.
19. Inoue S, Watanabe T, Hirose A, et al. Anterior discectomy and interbody fusion for lumbar disc herniation. A review of 350 cases. *Clin Orthop*. 1984;(183):22–31.
20. Kozak JA, O'Brien JP. Simultaneous combined anterior and posterior fusion. An independent analysis of a treatment for the disabled low-back pain patient. *Spine*. 1990;15(4):322–328.
21. Chow SP, Leong JC, Ma A, et al. Anterior spinal fusion or deranged lumbar intervertebral disc. *Spine*. 1980;5(5):452–458.
22. Christensen FB, Bünger CE. Retrograde ejaculation after retroperitoneal lower lumbar interbody fusion. *Int Orthop*. 1997;21(3):176–180.
23. Flynn JC, Price CT. Sexual complications of anterior fusion of the lumbar spine. *Spine*. 1984;9(5):489–492.
24. Johnson RM, McGuire EJ. Urogenital complications of anterior approaches to the lumbar spine. *Clin Orthop*. 1981;(154):114–118.
25. Loguidice VA, Johnson RG, Guyer RD, et al. Anterior lumbar interbody fusion. *Spine*. 1988;13(3):366–369.
26. Harms J, Rolinger H. A one-stager procedure in operative treatment of spondylolistheses: dorsal traction-reposition and anterior fusion (author's transl). *Z Für Orthop Ihre Grenzgeb*. 1982;120(3):343–347. https://doi.org/10.1055/s-2008-1051624.
27. Villavicencio AT, Burneikiene S, Bulsara KR, et al. Perioperative complications in transforaminal lumbar interbody fusion versus anterior-posterior reconstruction for lumbar disc degeneration and instability. *J Spinal Disord Tech*. 2006;19(2):92–97. https://doi.org/10.1097/01.bsd.0000185277.14484.4e.
28. Hunt T, Shen FH, Shaffrey CI, et al. Contralateral radiculopathy after transforaminal lumbar interbody fusion. *Eur Spine J Off Publ Eur Spine Soc Eur Spinal Deform Soc Eur Sect Cerv Spine Res Soc*. 2007;16(suppl 3):311–314. https://doi.org/10.1007/s00586-007-0387-x.
29. Jang K-M, Park S-W, Kim Y-B, et al. Acute contralateral radiculopathy after unilateral transforaminal lumbar interbody fusion. *J Korean Neurosurg Soc*. 2015;58(4):350–356. https://doi.org/10.3340/jkns.2015.58.4.350.
30. Aoki Y, Yamagata M, Nakajima F, et al. Posterior migration of fusion cages in degenerative lumbar disease treated with transforaminal lumbar interbody fusion: a report of three patients. *Spine*. 2009;34(1):E54–E58. https://doi.org/10.1097/BRS.0b013e3181918aae.
31. Peng CWB, Yue WM, Poh SY, et al. Clinical and radiological outcomes of minimally invasive versus open transforaminal lumbar interbody fusion. *Spine*. 2009;34(13):1385–1389. https://doi.org/10.1097/BRS.0b013e3181a4e3be.
32. Dhall SS, Wang MY, Mummaneni PV. Clinical and radiographic comparison of mini-open transforaminal lumbar interbody fusion with open transforaminal lumbar interbody fusion in 42 patients with long-term follow-up. *J Neurosurg Spine*. 2008;9(6):560–565. https://doi.org/10.3171/SPI.2008.9.08142.
33. Ozgur BM, Aryan HE, Pimenta L, et al. Extreme Lateral Interbody Fusion (XLIF): a novel surgical technique for anterior lumbar interbody fusion. *Spine J Off J North Am Spine Soc*. 2006;6(4):435–443. https://doi.org/10.1016/j.spinee.2005.08.012.
34. Bergey DL, Villavicencio AT, Goldstein T, et al. Endoscopic lateral transpsoas approach to the lumbar spine. *Spine*. 2004;29(15):1681–1688.
35. Cummock MD, Vanni S, Levi AD, et al. An analysis of postoperative thigh symptoms after minimally invasive transpsoas lumbar interbody fusion. *J Neurosurg Spine*. 2011;15(1):11–18. https://doi.org/10.3171/2011.2.SPINE10374.
36. Moller DJ, Slimack NP, Acosta FL, et al. Minimally invasive lateral lumbar interbody fusion and transpsoas approach-related morbidity. *Neurosurg Focus*. 2011;31(4):E4. https://doi.org/10.3171/2011.7.FOCUS11137.
37. Khajavi K, Shen A, Hutchison A. Substantial clinical benefit of minimally invasive lateral interbody fusion for degenerative spondylolisthesis. *Eur Spine J Off Publ Eur Spine Soc Eur Spinal Deform Soc Eur Sect Cerv Spine Res Soc*. 2015;24(suppl 3):314–321. https://doi.org/10.1007/s00586-015-3841-1.
38. Rodgers WB, Gerber EJ, Patterson J. Intraoperative and early postoperative complications in extreme lateral interbody fusion: an analysis of 600 cases. *Spine*. 2011;36(1):26–32. https://doi.org/10.1097/BRS.0b013e3181e1040a.

3

Relevant Surgical Anatomy of the Dorsal Lumbar Spine

ALEX M. WITEK, ADAM KHALIL, AND AJIT A. KRISHNANEY

Introduction

The typical lumbar spine consists of five vertebrae that are connected in series and permit motion between each segment. Each lumbar vertebra is an anatomically complex structure that consists of multiple distinct subunits. Adjacent vertebrae are connected through the disk space anteriorly and the paired zygapophyseal (facet) joints posteriorly. Further stability is provided by a variety of supporting ligaments. The lumbar spinal canal houses the conus medullaris rostrally, along with the emerging cauda equina, with each lumbar nerve root extending caudally and exiting the canal through its neural foramen directly below the same-numbered pedicle. Understanding the anatomic relationships between these neural structures and the neighboring vertebral bone, disk, and ligament is key to performing effective and safe posterior interbody fusion.

Illustrated views of a lumbar vertebra are provided in Figs. 3.1 and 3.2. The most ventral part of each vertebra is the vertebral body, a cylindrically shaped unit that serves to support axial loads. The vertebral bodies become progressively larger in a cranial –o-caudal direction. In the lumbar spine, where the bodies are largest, the average vertebral body height is 27 mm and is similar among all lumbar levels. In the axial plane, the anterior-posterior length is greater than the transverse width, and the bodies are longer and wider at either endplate than at their cranial-caudal midpoint. The transverse width and mid-sagittal length of the vertebral bodies increase progressively from L1 (29 mm wide and 40 mm long at the cranial-caudal midpoint) to L5 (32 mm wide and 46 mm long).[1] The endplate is composed of cortical bone and is slightly concave. Its central portion is thinnest and porous, whereas the outer portion (the apophyseal ring) is thicker and stronger.[2]

The pedicles are oriented primarily in an anterior-to-posterior direction and connect the vertebral body to the dorsal elements. Each pedicle is angled medially in the axial plane from posterior to anterior, and this angle increases progressively from L1 (average medial angulation of 11 degrees) to L5 (30 degrees). The transverse pedicle width also increases progressively from L1 (8.7 mm average width) to L5 (18 mm). The sagittal pedicle height displays an opposite relationship, decreasing slightly from L1 (15.4 mm) to L5 (14 mm).[3] With the exception of L5, which has especially wide pedicles, the lumbar pedicles are taller than they are wide, and it is therefore the transverse width of the pedicle that limits its instrumentation.

The pedicle is connected to the dorsal vertebral elements at the junction of the superior articulating process (SAP) and the pars interarticularis ("pars"). The pars connects the SAP and pedicle to the lamina and the inferior articulating process (IAP). The lamina is a sheet-like subunit that forms the dorsal roof of the spinal canal. In the sagittal plane, it slopes posteriorly from superior to inferior; in the axial plane, it is angled posteriorly from lateral to medial, with an apex at the midline. When viewed in the coronal plane, the lamina is tall and narrow at the superior lumbar levels and becomes shorter and wider as it goes down to the lower lumbar levels. Between the SAP and IAP, the lamina is contiguous with the pars interarticularis, which forms the narrowest point along the lateral edge of the dorsal vertebra. The spinous process is oriented in the midline sagittal plane and projects dorsally from the lamina with downward angulation, lying slightly below its corresponding vertebral body and overlying the subjacent interlaminar space. The spinous process is the most dorsal part of the vertebra and the first bone encountered during posterior midline surgical exposure. The paired transverse processes originate from the junction of the pedicle with the SAP and project laterally.

The zygapophyseal (facet) joints are paired synovial joints that allow for articulation of the posterior portion of the vertebrae. Each facet joint consists of the IAP from the rostral vertebra (e.g., L4) and the SAP of the caudal vertebra (e.g., L5). Each of the apposed articular surfaces consists of smooth cortical bone covered with a layer of hyaline cartilage. The joint space contains synovial fluid and is enclosed posteriorly by a fibrous capsule.[4] The facet joints in the lumbar spine are angled anteriorly (i.e., anterior-superior to posterior-inferior) in the sagittal plane, and medially (i.e., posterior-lateral to anterior-medial) in the axial plane. This orientation allows significant flexion/extension and moderate lateral bending, but minimal axial rotation.[5,6] The facet joint angle in the axial plane (with respect to midline) decreases progressively at each level from rostral to caudal, such

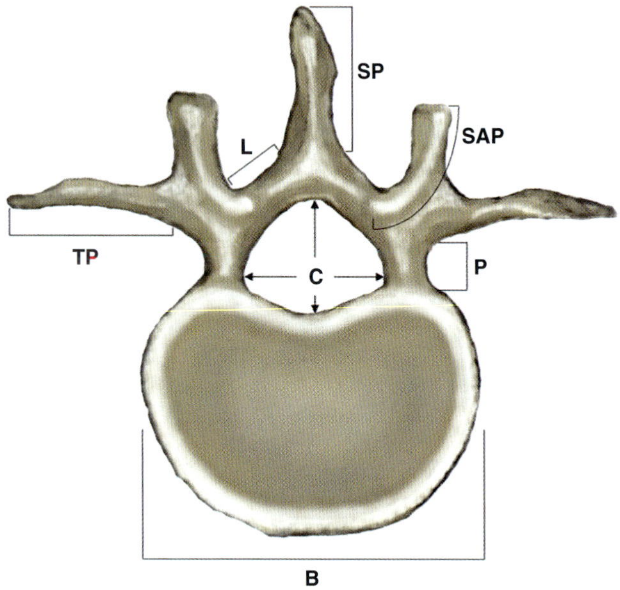

• **Fig. 3.1** Superior view of a lumbar vertebra. *B,* Vertebral body; *C,* spinal canal; *L,* lamina; *P,* pedicle; *SAP,* superior articulating process; *SP,* spinous process.

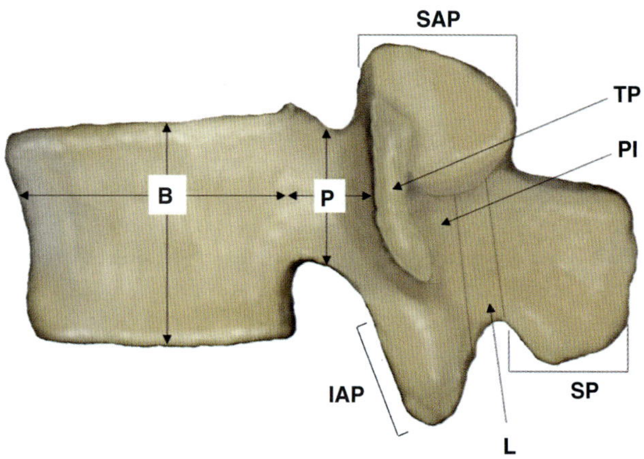

• **Fig. 3.2** Lateral view of a lumbar vertebra. *B,* Vertebral body; *C,* spinal canal; *IAP,* inferior articulating process; *L,* lamina; *P,* pedicle; *PI,* pars interarticularis; *SAP,* superior articulating process; *SP,* spinous process; *TP,* transverse process.

that the upper lumbar facet joints are oriented more in the sagittal plane and the lower facets are more coronally oriented.[4,6–9] The articular surface is curved so that the posterior portion of the joint is more sagittally oriented and the most anterior portion is more coronally oriented, which makes the SAP articular surface concave, and the IAP surface convex. A clear understanding of facetal anatomy is mandatory to optimize bone drilling, especially during open and minimally invasive transforaminal lumbar interbody fusion (TLIF) surgeries.

The lumbar spine contains several ligaments that interconnect and stabilize the vertebrae: anterior and posterior longitudinal ligaments (ALL and PLL), supraspinous and interspinous ligaments, as well as the ligamentum flavum. The ALL runs vertically along the anterior edge of the spinal column and provides resistance to extension. The PLL runs vertically along the posterior aspect of the vertebral bodies (i.e., the ventral border of the spinal canal) and provides resistance to flexion. The PLL is narrowest behind the vertebral bodies and widens as it crosses each disk space. The ligamentum flavum ('yellow ligament,' named so owing to its color) is a discontinuous ligament that bridges the interlaminar space and forms part of the dorsal border of the spinal canal. The ligamentum flavum has its origin on the superior dorsal edge of the caudal lamina and inserts onto the inferior ventral edge of the superior lamina. It provides resistance to flexion at each level. The ligamentum flavum is surgically relevant because it is often hypertrophied in the degenerative spine, in which case it can cause compression of the central canal and lateral recess, and removal of this compressive ligament is key to an effective decompressive surgery. During laminectomy, the ligamentum protects the dura from violation during exposure and bone removal. Because of its discontinuity, the upper half of the lamina has no ligamentum ventrally between the bone and dura, a crucial anatomic landmark in tubular surgical procedures. The surgeon must also be aware that in patients who have undergone previous operations, the ligamentum flavum may be absent at a given level, a point of caution in reexploratory surgeries where inadvertent dural tears may occur. The lumbar interspinous ligament is discontinuous and spans the interval between spinous processes in the sagittal plane, whereas the supraspinous ligament is a continuous structure that runs in the midline along the dorsal edge of the spinous process; both provide resistance to flexion.[10] In lumbar surgical procedures, it is important to preserve the interspinous ligaments wherever possible, to avoid unnecessary iatrogenic instability.

The intervertebral disk allows for transmission of axial loads between vertebral bodies while permitting motion at each segment. The disk consists of three main components: the annulus fibrosis, the outer ring composed of type I collagen, and fibrocartilage arranged in concentric lamellae; the nucleus pulposis, an amorphous inner core composed of water, type II collagen, and proteoglycans; and the cartilaginous endplates, which are composed of hyaline cartilage lining the bony endplates.[11,12] Mean disk height increases progressively from L1-2 (8 mm) to a maximum at L4-5 (11 mm) before decreasing slightly at L5-S1, but there is significant variation among individuals and disk height is a dynamic property that varies with loading conditions.[13] Significant loss of height can be found with degeneration of the disk.[14] The disk is clinically and surgically relevant because degeneration and herniation can narrow the spinal canal, lateral recesses, and foramina and lead to symptomatic compression of neural elements (such as neurogenic claudication, radiculopathy, or cauda equina syndrome). Removal of ectopic disk material is therefore a principal component of many surgical interventions. There are 23 disks in the typical spine, one at each level from C2-3 through L5-S1, and these disk spaces are relevant to interbody fusion, as they serve as the site of arthrodesis. In this setting, it is important to perform a thorough diskectomy including removal of the cartilaginous endplates, to allow for sufficient exposure of the bony endplate and placement of ample bone graft to create optimal conditions for fusion.

The sacrum deserves brief mention because it articulates with the lumbar spine and is often instrumented in the setting of lumbar fusion. The sacrum is composed of five fused vertebrae that are arranged in a kyphotic shape and are tilted anteriorly in the sagittal plane. The rostral laminae are fused, with no interlaminar space, and the median sacral crest represents the fused former spinous processes. The posterior neuroforamina are arranged in paired vertical rows on each side and are the sites of exit of the dorsal rami from the spinal canal. S1 has a superior endplate and SAPs that are similar to those of the lumbar vertebrae, which allow it to articulate with L5 via the intervertebral disk and facet joints. S1 varies from the lumbar vertebrae in that the body and pedicles are flanked on each side by large alae. The S1 pedicle lies between the SAP and the S1 foramen.[15] The S1 pedicles are unique from those of the lumbar vertebrae in that they are taller (21 mm),[16] lack a lateral cortex (given that the pedicle is continuous with the ala), and allow for a shorter cortex-to-cortex screw trajectory. This means that S1 pedicle screws tend to be shorter and have less cortical bone surrounding them, making them more susceptible to pullout or toggling. Strategies for optimizing pullout strength given these limitations include bicortical purchase through the ventral S1 cortex, or tricortical purchase by directing the screw to the apex of the sacral promontory.[17] S1 pedicle screws are at a further disadvantage when at the caudal end of a long construct given the long moment arm applied above the L5-S1 level. Iliac screws or additional points of sacral fixation may be helpful in this scenario.

The lumbar spinal canal has a triangular shape when viewed in the axial plane. It has a flat anterior edge formed by the posterior wall of the vertebral body and the PLL. The posterior edges of the canal meet at an apex in the midline, and are formed by the lamina and facet on each side, and the underlying ligamentum flavum. The canal's transverse width is greater than its anterior-posterior height. The height remains relatively constant among levels in the lumbar spine (17 mm), whereas the width increases progressively from L1 (22 mm) to L5 (26 mm).[1] The epidural space within the canal contains fat and a venous plexus that is most prominent ventrally. The venous plexus must often be coagulated in order to access the disk space and to retract the thecal sac and nerve root medially.

The neural foramen serves as the exit site for the nerve root and is frequently the site of symptomatic compression from degenerative pathology. When viewed in the sagittal plan, the foramen exhibits a keyhole shape, with a wider and circular upper portion and a narrower lower portion (Fig. 3.3). The upper portion is bordered anteriorly by the vertebral body and superiorly by the pedicle of the same numbered vertebra. The inferior portion of the foramen is bordered anteriorly by the disk and inferiorly by the pedicle of the subjacent vertebra. The foramen is bordered dorsally by the ventral aspect of the facet joint (primarily the SAP, which lies anterior to the IAP) and its underlying ligamentum flavum.

The important neural structures of the lumbar spine include the lower spinal cord, conus medullaris, and nerve roots. In normal adults, the conus terminates at the L1 level on average, with a range of T12 to L2/3,[18] but in pathologic conditions it can lie much lower. Below the conus, the nerve roots of the more caudal levels form the cauda equina and travel caudally within the spinal canal. As a root nears its same-numbered vertebral level, it courses laterally into the lateral recess and exits the dura at or just below the superjacent disk space (i.e., the L3 nerve root exits the dura at the level of the L2-3 disk space). The extradural nerve root then travels in an inferolateral direction and exits the spinal canal just below the same-numbered pedicle.

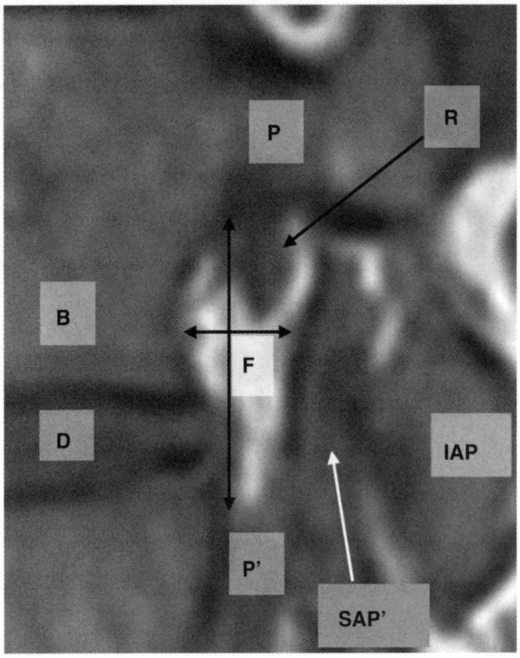

• **Fig. 3.3** T2-weighted sagittal magnetic resonance image (MRI) of the lumbar spine, demonstrating the position of the nerve root *(R)* in the superior aspect of the foramen *(F)*. The foramen is bordered superiorly by the pedicle *(P)*, anteriorly by the posterior vertebral body *(B)* and intervertebral disk *(D)*, inferiorly of the pedicle of the vertebra below *(P')*, and posteriorly by the superior articulating process of the vertebra below *(SAP')*. The inferior articulating process *(IAP)* lies posterior to the SAP, and these two processes articulate to form the facet joint.

A standard open approach posterior lumbar interbody fusion (PLIF) or transforaminal lumbar interbody fusion (TLIF) begins with a midline skin incision and subperiosteal exposure of the dorsal spinal elements (Figs. 3.3 and 3.4). Unlike posterolateral fusion, it is not necessary to expose the lateral aspects of the facet joints and the transverse processes when performing interbody fusion. The location of the deeper structures (such as the pedicle, neural foramen, and intervertebral disk) can be inferred from this superficial anatomy (Fig. 3.5). The dorsal projection of the pedicle is located on the SAP (or inferior half of the facet joint), at the junction of the SAP with the transverse process and pars. The disk space lies deep to the inferior articulating process (or superior half of the facet joint) and the inferior edge of the lamina. The neural foramen lies deep to the pars, and the exiting nerve root passes through the superior portion of the foramen, just below the pedicle, as it travels laterally.

The most important anatomic relationship in the setting of lumbar interbody fusion is that of the lateral edge of the thecal sac, the exiting nerve root, the posterolateral aspect of the intervertebral disk (IVD), and the traversing nerve root that exits at the subjacent level. This relationship is demonstrated in Fig. 3.6. The IVD lies close to the subjacent pedicle (average distance of 3 mm), whereas a significant gap exists between the disk and the superjacent pedicle (average distance of 10 mm).[19] The corridor for diskectomy and placement of graft and implant is a trapezoid-shaped window whose superior margin is formed by the exiting nerve root, medial margin by the lateral edge of the thecal sac and shoulder of the traversing nerve root, and

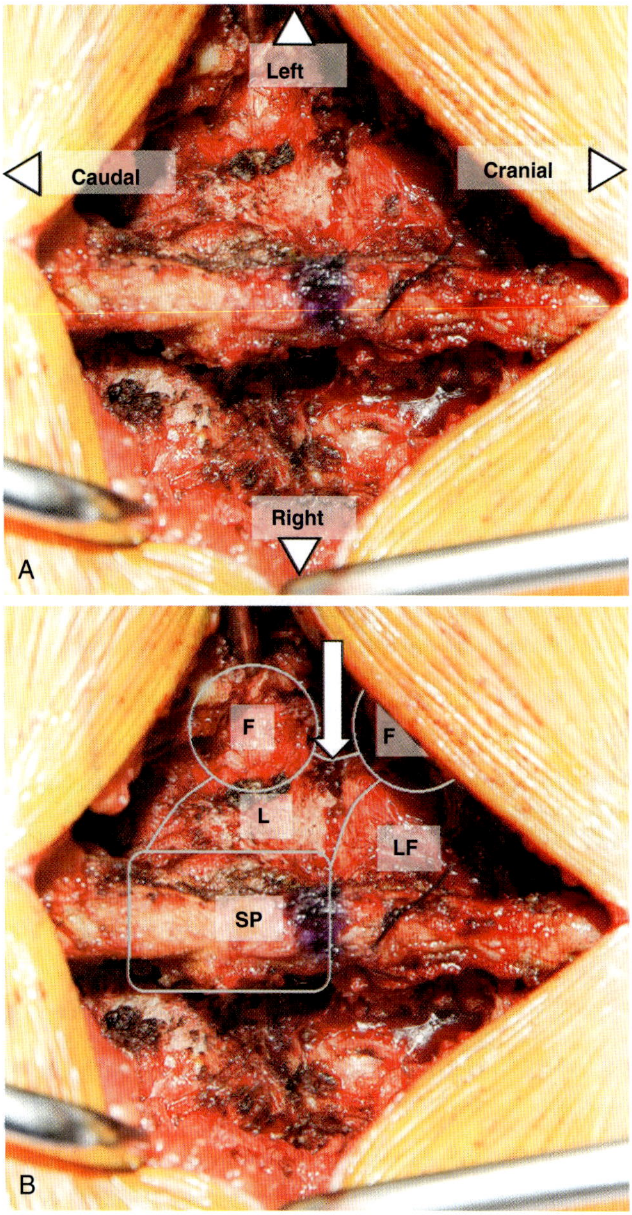

• **Fig. 3.4** **A**. Surgeon's view of the dorsal spinal elements following a midline incision and subperiosteal elevation of the paraspinal muscles. The directions *(left, right, cranial, caudal)* have been labeled for orientation. **B**. The spinal elements of the index level have been outlined and labeled for easier visualization. The spinous process *(SP)* lies in the midline. The lamina *(L)* slopes downward where it meets the pars interarticularis (*arrow*) and the facet joint capsules *(F)*. Ligamentum flavum *(LF)* separates the lamina of this level from that of the vertebra above.

inferior margin by the pedicle of the subjacent level. It is the method for establishing this window that differentiates TLIF from PLIF. PLIF consists of a wide laminectomy and medial facetectomy. The remaining IAP constricts the working corridor along its lateral edge. This may necessitate moderate retraction of the thecal sac medially to create ample working room, and may limit the surgeon's ability to angle medially upon entering the disk space. For this reason, PLIF often involves bilateral disk space access and implant placement. In contrast to this, the TLIF technique involves complete removal of the facet to

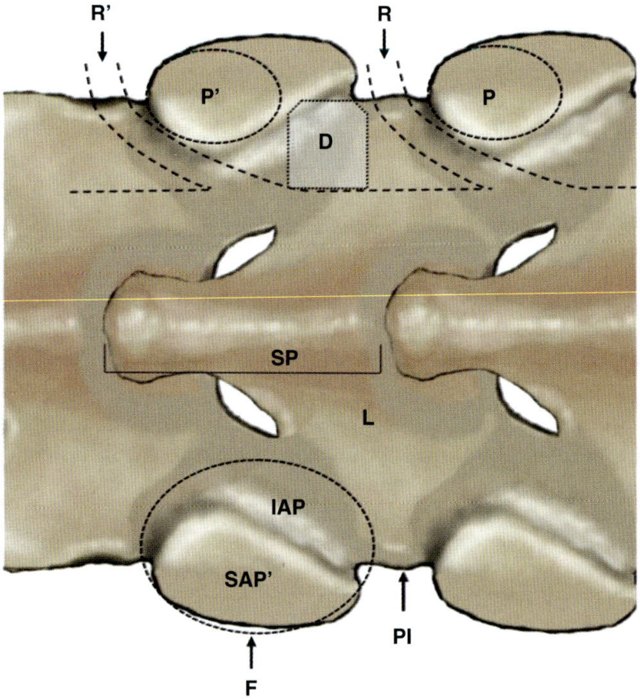

• **Fig. 3.5** Posterior view of the dorsal lumbar spine (*SP*, spinous process; *L*, lamina; *SAP'*, superior articulating process of the subjacent vertebra; *PI*, pars interarticularis; *IAP*, inferior articulating process). The IAP and SAP′ combine to form the facet joint *(F)*. The *dashed lines* toward the left of the spine represent the projections of deeper structures, including the same-numbered pedicle *(P)*, exiting nerve root (R), intervertebral disk *(D)*, subjacent pedicle *(P')*, and traversing nerve root *(R')*.

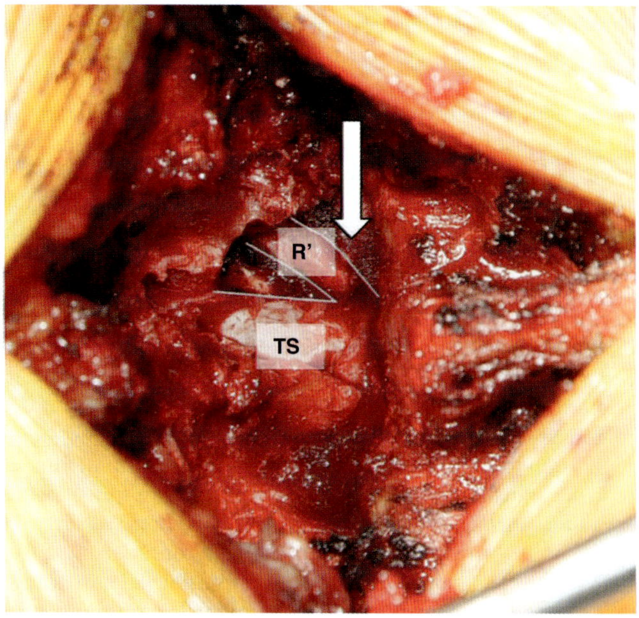

• **Fig. 3.6** Removal of the inferior articulating process and pars significantly improves the degree of lateral exposure compared to laminectomy alone. The traversing nerve root *(R')* is seen as it exits the thecal sac *(TS)* and travels inferolaterally on its way to the foramen of the level below. The posterolateral aspect of the intervertebral disk *(arrow)* is seen ventral to the thecal sac and nerve root.

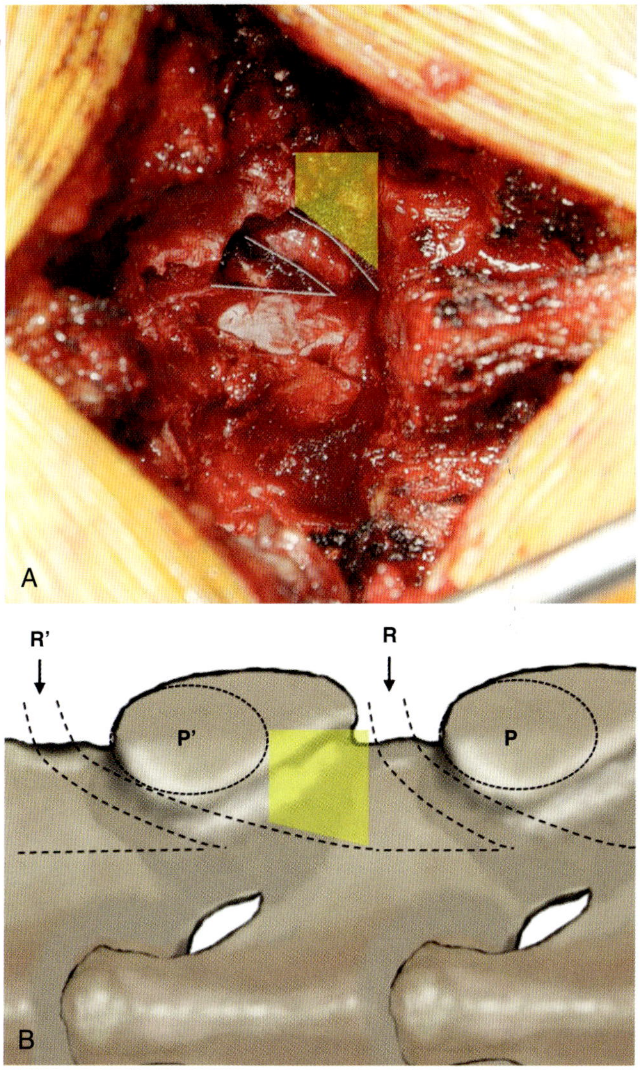

• **Fig. 3.7** A. The transforaminal lumbar interbody fusion (TLIF) exposure creates a trapezoid-shaped window (*highlighted in yellow*) to the posterolateral disk space. This window, which serves as the site of entry into the disk space, is bordered medially by the thecal sac and traversing nerve root, inferiorly by the pedicle of the vertebra below, and superolaterally by the exiting nerve root (not well visualized in this photograph). This window can be widened by gently retracting the shoulder of the traversing nerve root medially. **B**. Illustrated view of the TLIF window (*highlighted in yellow*), demonstrating the relationship of the disk space to the exiting nerve root (*R*), traversing nerve root (*R'*), same-numbered pedicle (*P*), and subjacent pedicle (*P'*), as well as to the overlying bony structures. Note that the window for accessing the disk space lies directly below the inferior articulating process.

create a wider window whose lateral border extends to the exiting nerve root as it slopes gently downward in its lateral course (Fig. 3.7). Access to the disk space can therefore be obtained with minimal or no medial retraction of the thecal sac. The wider exposure allows the surgeon to angle more medially and across the midline within the disk space, perform a thorough diskectomy, and place a biomechanical cage in the midline, all through unilateral disk space access.

Another important anatomic detail relevant to posterior interbody fusion is the structure of the IVD and its relationship to surrounding structures. The biomechanical cage should ideally be placed as anterior as possible within the disk space. This allows for maximal lordosis and places the cage at the ring apophysis, where the endplates are strongest. Meanwhile, the anterior annulus fibrosis should be kept intact because it serves as a barrier to prevent ventral extrusion of the implant and bone graft, and also prevents violation of the structures that lie ventral to the disk space, most importantly the aorta, inferior vena cava, and the iliac arteries and veins. The distance from the posterior site of opening of the annulus fibrosis to the ventral disk margin varies from 36 to 47 mm, with lower levels having slightly longer disk spaces.[19] This serves as a guide for the maximal depth of insertion of instruments within the disk space to avoid violating the anterior annulus; in general, a 3-cm depth should be safe.

The dorsal surgical anatomy of the normal lumbar spine can be altered by a variety of conditions. Facet hypertrophy can obscure the local anatomy and add difficulty to pedicle screw placement. Spondylolisthesis in the setting of a pars defect alters the normal SAP-pars-IAP relationship. In this case, the rostral facet joint lies more anterior and inferiorly than expected, and often the joints appear directly apposed when viewed dorsally (Fig. 3.8). The anteroposterior diameter of the spinal canal and the neural foramina are typically narrowed at the level of spondylolisthesis. Severe loss of disk height can make it difficult to obtain access to the disk space when performing interbody fusion. Scoliosis imparts a coronal curvature to the spine so that the pedicles on the concave side lie closer to one another than on the convex side, as well as a rotational component that alters the normal angle of the pedicles in the axial plane. This alteration of the normal anatomy adds difficulty to pedicle screw placement in patients with scoliosis. Nerve root anomalies, such as conjoined nerve roots, closely adjacent roots, and extradural anastomoses,[20] may increase the risk of nerve root injury if unrecognized by the surgeon. Rib abnormalities at the thoracolumbar junction, such as an absent 12th rib or an extra lumbar rib, occur in approximately 8% of patients,[21] and for this reason the ribs are not a reliable reference for the purpose of surgical localization. The presence of a lumbosacral transitional vertebrae is another factor that can complicate localization of the correct surgical level, and occurs in approximately 16% of the population.[22]

Conclusion

The lumbar spine is an anatomically complex structure. Knowledge of the normal dorsal lumbar anatomy, as well as awareness of common variants, are essential to performing posterior interbody fusion. This knowledge allows for careful preoperative planning, adequate decompression, placement of biomechanically optimal interbody cages and posterior instrumentation, creation of optimal conditions for arthrodesis, and avoidance of complications.

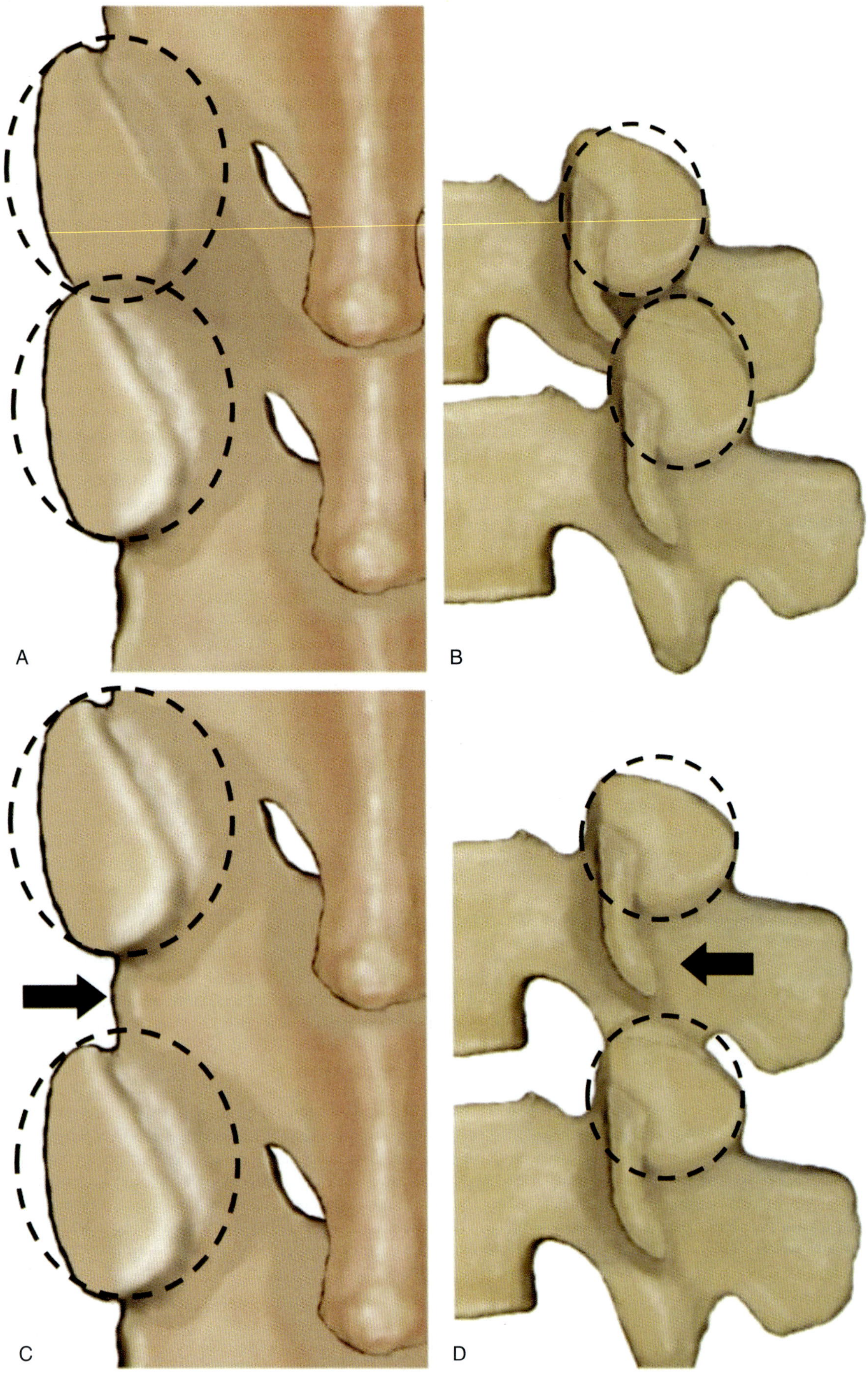

• **Fig. 3.8** Illustration of isthmic spondylolisthesis. Posterior (A) and lateral (B) views demonstrate that the superior facet joint is shifted ventrally and inferiorly with respect to the inferior facet joint, and the defective pars interarticularis is elongated. A normal facet joint is shown for comparison, with (C) posterior and (D) lateral views demonstrating the normal relationship of the facet joints to the pars interarticularis *(arrow)*.

References

1. Berry JL, Moran JM, Berg WS, et al. A morphometric study of human lumbar and selected thoracic vertebrae. *Spine (Phila Pa 1976)*. 1987;12(4):362–367.
2. Grant JP, Oxland TR, Dvorak MF. Mapping the structural properties of the lumbosacral vertebral endplates. *Spine (Phila Pa 1976)*. 2001;26(8):889–896. https://doi.org/10.1097/00007632-200104150-00012.
3. Zindrick MR, Wiltse LL, Doornik A, et al. Analysis of the morphometric characteristics of the thoracic and lumbar pedicles. *Spine (Phila Pa 1976)*. 1987;12(2):160–166.
4. Taylor JR, Twomey LT. Age changes in lumbar zygapophyseal joints. Observations on structure and function. *Spine (Phila Pa 1976)*. 1986;11(7):739–745. https://doi.org/10.1097/00007632-198609000-00014.
5. White AA, Panjabi MM. The basic kinematics of the human spine. A review of past and current knowledge. *Spine (Phila Pa 1976)*. 1978;3(1):12–20. https://doi.org/10.1097/00007632-197803000-00003.
6. Ahmed AM, Duncan NA, Burke DL. The effect of facet geometry on the axial torque-rotation response of lumbar motion segments. *Spine (Phila Pa 1976)*. 1990;15(5):391–401. https://doi.org/10.1097/00007632-199005000-00010.
7. Panjabi MM, White AA. Basic biomechanics of the spine. *Neurosurgery*. 1980;7(1):76–93. https://doi.org/10.1016/0268-0890(89)90038-8.
8. Van Schaik JP, Verbiest H, Van Schaik FD. The orientation of laminae and facet joints in the lower lumbar spine. *Spine (Phila Pa 1976)*. 1985;10(1):59-63.
9. Benzel EC. Biomechanically relevant anatomy and material properties of the spine and associated elements. In: *Biomechanics of Spine Stabilization*. 2nd ed. New York: Thieme; 2001:1–18.
10. Lollis SS. Applied anatomy of the thoracic and lumbar spine. In: Steinmetz MP, Benzel EC, eds. *Benzel's Spine Surgery: Techniques, Complication Avoidance, and Management*. 4th ed. Philadelphia: Elsevier; 2017:95–113. https://doi.org/10.1016/B978-0-323-40030-5.00009-5.
11. Liu JKC. Intervertebral disc: anatomy, physiology, and aging. In: Steinmetz MP, Benzel EC, eds. *Benzel's Spine Surgery: Techniques, Complication Avoidance, and Management*. 4th ed. Philadelphia: Elsevier; 2017:119–123. https://doi.org/10.1016/B978-0-323-40030-5.00011-3.
12. Buckwalter JA. Aging and degeneration of the human intervertebral disc. *Spine (Phila Pa 1976)*. 1995;20(11):1307–1314.
13. Koeller W, Meier W, Hartmann F. Biomechanical properties of human intervertebral discs subjected to axial dynamic compression. A comparison of lumbar and thoracic discs. *Spine (Phila Pa 1976)*. 1984;9(7):725–733.
14. Yu S, Haughton VM, Sether LA, et al. Criteria for classifying normal and degenerated lumbar intervertebral disks. *Radiology*. 1989;170(2):523–526. https://doi.org/10.1148/radiology.170.2.2911680.
15. Finnan R, Archdeacon M. Applied anatomy of the sacral spine. In: Steinmetz MP, Benzel EC, eds. *Benzel's Spine Surgery: Techniques, Complication Avoidance, and Management*. 4th ed. Philadelphia: Elsevier; 2017:114–118. https://doi.org/10.1016/B978-0-323-40030-5.00010-1.
16. Başaloğlu H, Turgut M, Taşer FA, et al. Morphometry of the sacrum for clinical use. *Surg Radiol Anat*. 2005;27(6):467–471. https://doi.org/10.1007/s00276-005-0036-1.
17. Lehman RA, Kuklo TR, Belmont PJ, et al. Advantage of pedicle screw fixation directed into the apex of the sacral promontory over bicortical fixation: a biomechanical analysis. *Spine (Phila Pa 1976)*. 2002;27(8):806–811. https://doi.org/10.1097/00007632-200204150-00006.
18. Wilson DA, Prince JR. John Caffey award. MR imaging determination of the location of the normal conus medullaris throughout childhood. *AJR Am J Roentgenol*. 1989;152(5):1029–1032. https://doi.org/10.2214/ajr.152.5.1029.
19. Arslan M, Cömert A, Açar Hİ, et al. Neurovascular structures adjacent to the lumbar intervertebral discs: an anatomical study of their morphometry and relationships. *J Neurosurg Spine*. 2011;14(5):630–638. https://doi.org/10.3171/2010.11.SPINE09149.
20. Kadish LJ, Simmons EH. Anomalies of the lumbosacral nerve roots. An anatomical investigation and myelographic study. *J Bone Joint Surg Br*. 1984;66(3):411–416.
21. Merks JHM, Smets AM, Van Rijn RR, et al. Prevalence of rib anomalies in normal Caucasian children and childhood cancer patients. *Eur J Med Genet*. 2005;48(2):113–129. https://doi.org/10.1016/j.ejmg.2005.01.029.
22. Tang M, Yang X, Yang S, et al. Lumbosacral transitional vertebra in a population-based study of 5860 individuals: prevalence and relationship to low back pain. *Eur J Radiol*. 2014;83(9):1679–1682. https://doi.org/10.1016/j.ejrad.2014.05.036.

4

Relevant Surgical Anatomy of the Lateral and Anterior Lumbar Spine

ANGELA M. RICHARDON, GLEN MANZANO, AND ALLAN D. LEVI

Introduction

Anterior and lateral approaches to the lumbar spine are performed with increasing frequency and for a wider range of indications. To avoid complications and maximize patient outcomes, a clear understanding of the anatomy encountered during these approaches is necessary. Here we consider the bony, vascular, and neural anatomy most pertinent to the anterior and lateral transpsoas approaches.

Bony and Ligamentous Anatomy

The lumbar spine consists of five kidney-shaped vertebral bodies bordered by the thoracic spine above and the sacrum below (Fig. 4.1). These five vertebral bodies typically have a combined lordosis of 20 to 45 degrees.[1] Each vertebral body consists of a central depression surrounded by an apophyseal ring. The intervertebral disk sits in this depression between adjacent vertebral bodies. The pedicles, lamina, and spinous process form the boundaries of the spinal canal and compose the posterior elements. Facet joints link the superior and inferior articulating processes of adjacent vertebral bodies posteriorly. These posterior elements are not visualized during anterior or lateral approaches to the spine (Fig. 4.2).

Anterior approaches allow direct visualization of the anterior lumbar spine and typically allow intervention at the L4-5 and the L5-S1 disk spaces. The lateral approaches typically utilize dilators and minimal access retractor systems with fluoroscopic visualization of the exact position of the retractor. Direct visualization and neural monitoring form a critical component of safe access to the lumbar spine. Not all levels of the lumbar spine (e.g., L5-S1) can be accessed via a lateral transpsoas approach. Careful preoperative evaluation with a lateral x-ray demonstrating the position of the iliac crests in relation to the vertebral bodies will help determine the lowest accessible disk space. Superior disk space access may be limited by the ribcage or diaphragm, although modifications of the approach may still allow access.

The ligaments most commonly encountered in anterior and lateral approaches to the lumbar spine are the anterior longitudinal ligament and the posterior longitudinal ligament. The anterior longitudinal ligament spans the entire spine and increases in width along the rostral-caudal axis. This multi-layered ligament is encountered early in the anterior approach and must be divided to access the disk space. In lateral approaches it provides a protective layer between the disk space and the large vessels located immediately anteriorly that are not directly visualized. This ligament also provides an anterior tension band preventing hyperextension when left in situ; however, with care, release of this ligament can allow for greater correction of sagittal deformity.[2] Although the posterior longitudinal ligament does not contribute to stability to the extent of the anterior longitudinal ligament, it prevents herniation of nucleus pulposus centrally into the spinal canal. This ligament is not disrupted in either the anterior or lateral approaches but defines a plane posteriorly between the disk space and the spinal canal. The contralateral ligament is routinely released during lateral approaches and care must be taken during left-sided approaches to prevent the interbody graft from injuring vessels on the contralateral side. This risk is increased in patients with deformity, especially with axial rotation, as the vessels may lie outside their usual location.[3]

Musculature of the Lumbar Spine

In anterior approaches the spinal musculature is not violated. Instead, the muscle layers divided are those of the abdominal wall. Closure of these layers and the fascia is important to prevent the development of true abdominal wall hernias. These are to be distinguished from abdominal wall pseudo hernias that are caused by abdominal wall weakness secondary to a neural injury (e.g., subcostal nerve). Lateral approaches also spare the paraspinous muscles but do require passing through the psoas muscle. The psoas muscle originates from the transverse processes and lateral vertebral bodies of L1-5 and along with the iliacus muscle inserts into the femur after passing under the posterior inguinal ligament (Fig. 4.3).

Vascular Anatomy

Large Vessels of the Retroperitoneum

Anterior to the vertebral bodies, in close proximity within the retroperitoneal space, lie the aorta, its terminal branches, and the inferior vena cava (IVC). The close anatomic relationship of these large vessels to the lumbar spine places them at greater risk during lateral and anterior approaches than in posterior approaches. Cadaveric and radiologic studies have sought to describe more thoroughly these anatomic relationships in an attempt to define a safe working corridor as injuries to these vessels can cause serious morbidity and even death.[4]

True anterior retroperitoneal lumbar spine approaches typically involve a paramedian or low abdominal incision to gain access to the retroperitoneum.

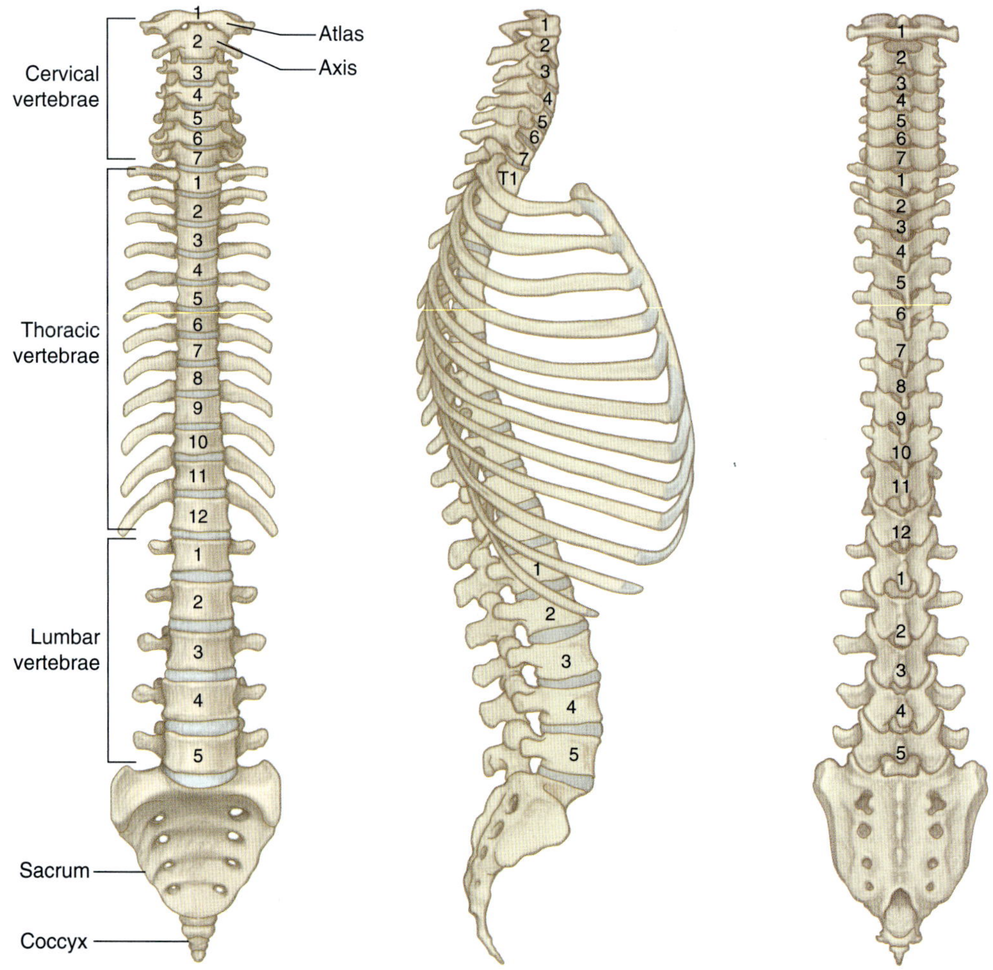

• **Fig. 4.1** Coronal and sagittal views of the bony anatomy of the spine. (From Benzel E. *Spine Surgery: Techniques, Complication Avoidance, & Management*, 3rd ed. Philadelphia: Elsevier Saunders; 2012: Figure 32-1.)

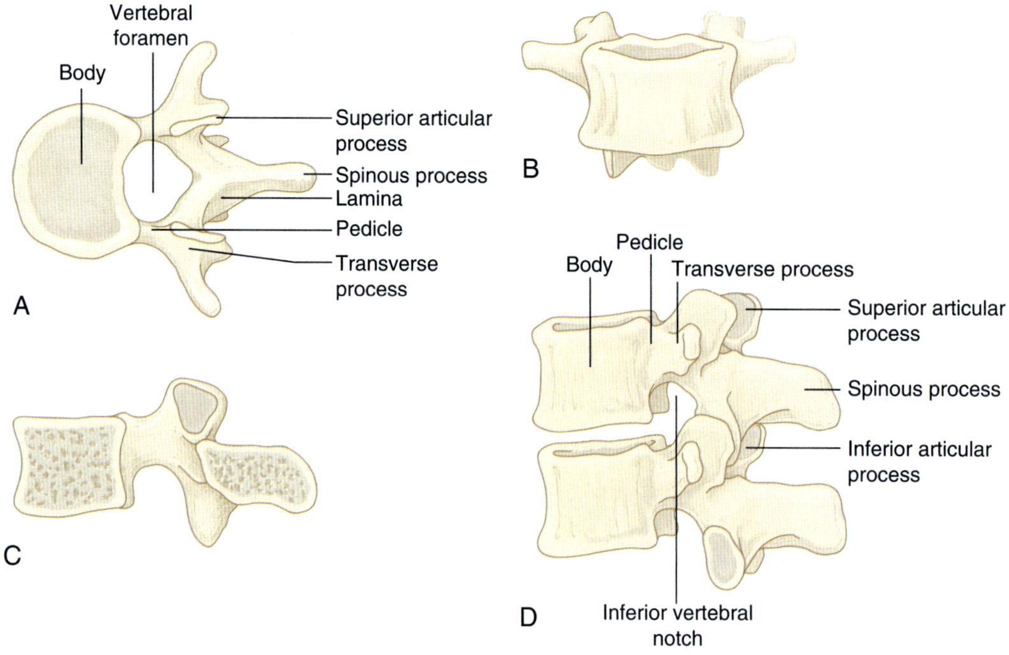

• **Fig. 4.2** Lumbar vertebral bodies from superior (A), anterior (B), midsagittal (C), and lateral (D) views. (From Benzel E. *Spine Surgery: Techniques, Complication Avoidance, & Management*, 3rd ed. Philadelphia: Elsevier Saunders; 2012: Figure 36-2.)

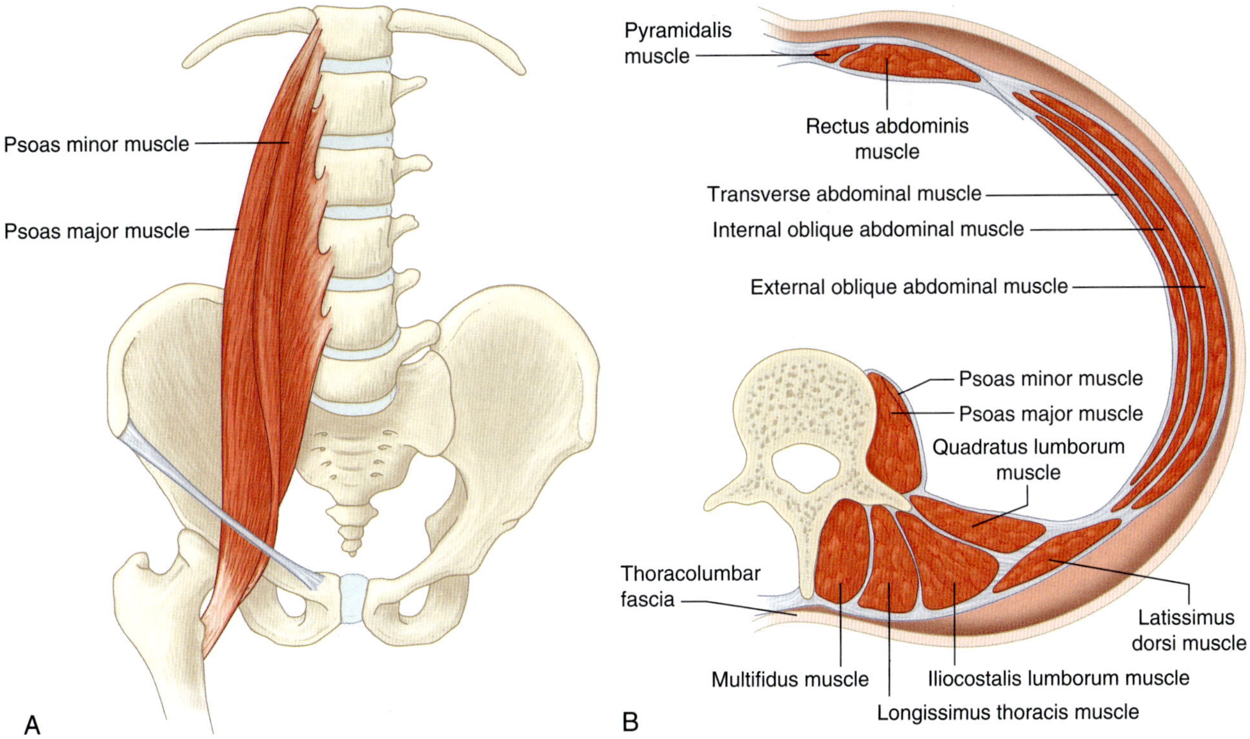

• **Fig. 4.3** Muscular anatomy of relevance for lateral and anterior approaches – (A) the psoas muscles extending from the spine and passing under the inguinal ligament to insert on the femur. (B) Axial section showing mediolateral orientation of erector spinae and psoas muscles. (From Benzel E. Spine Surgery: Techniques, Complication Avoidance, & Management, 3rd ed. Philadelphia: Elsevier Saunders; 2012: Figures 36-6 and 36-7b.)

Access to the L5-S1 disk space is through a working corridor developed between the common iliac arteries and veins after sacrificing the median sacral artery. At L4-5, a left-sided approach is usually preferred, which involves retraction of the aorta to gain access to the mid-line disk space.

The aorta descends along the ventromedial spine only 2.1 cm from the center of the intervertebral disk.[5] This large vessel begins at the fourth thoracic vertebra and continues to the fourth lumbar vertebra where it divides into the two common iliac arteries. The common iliac veins join ventral to the fifth lumbar vertebra forming the IVC. This vessel parallels the path of the aorta traveling along the right anterior aspect of the lumbar vertebrae, with a mean of 1.4 cm between the vessel and the center of the intervertebral disk.[5] The IVC migrates posteriorly and laterally with caudal progression from L1 to L5. The iliolumbar vein crosses from the IVC at the level of the L5 vertebral body crossing the psoas muscle. In approaches that require dissection at L4-5, this vein is usually ligated and divided to the left of the left common iliac vein (Fig. 4.4).

Analysis of the location of the IVC in magnetic resonance images of 48 individuals demonstrated that in 70% the position of this vessel at the L4-5 disk level would place it at risk during a right-sided lateral approach.[6] Additionally, the right common iliac vein can lie draped across the anterolateral corner of the disk space, precluding safe entry at this point.[5] During anterior lumbar interbody fusion, the disk space associated with the highest risk of vascular complication is the L4-5 disk space with reported vascular injury rates of 2% to 15%. At this level the left iliac artery is at risk since it must be mobilized for adequate exposure of the disk space. The iliac veins are also susceptible to injury at this level as they are mobilized.[4] The left iliac vein and iliocaval junction lie in close proximity to the center of the disk space at L5-S1 and are thus at risk for injury in the anterior approach to this level.[7] Anatomic variations in the relative positions of the aorta and the IVC have been described (Fig. 4.5). The aorta typically lies ventral to the IVC and slightly to the left. Owing to this variation in the course of the aorta, IVC, their relative positions, and the location of the bifurcation, many authors advocate preoperative imaging to thoroughly define the vascular anatomy of each patient.

Arterial Supply to the Spine

Lumbar arteries are direct branches of the aorta that run across the vertebral body, approximately 4 mm on average, below the inferior endplate of the superior intervertebral disk space (Fig. 4.6).[5] These vessels originate near the midpoint of the vertebral body and pass under the sympathetic chain and onto the muscles of the abdominal wall forming numerous anastomoses with each other and lower posterior intercostal, subcostal, iliolumbar, deep circumflex iliac, and inferior epigastric arteries. The spinal branches pierce the dura in the vicinity of the dorsal root ganglia and are named according to their termination: radicular if the vessel terminates along the root, radiculopial if it anastomosis with the pial vessels of the spinal cord, radiculomedullary if it anastomoses with the anterior spinal artery. The artery of Adamkiewicz is the largest radiculomedullary artery and may originate between the ninth intercostal (thoracic) artery and the second lumbar artery, most commonly on the left side. Cadaveric studies have shown little variation in the course of the lumbar arteries, although the number present varied (2–4).[8] Injury to even these small vessels can lead to complications. Santillan et al.[9] reported a vascular

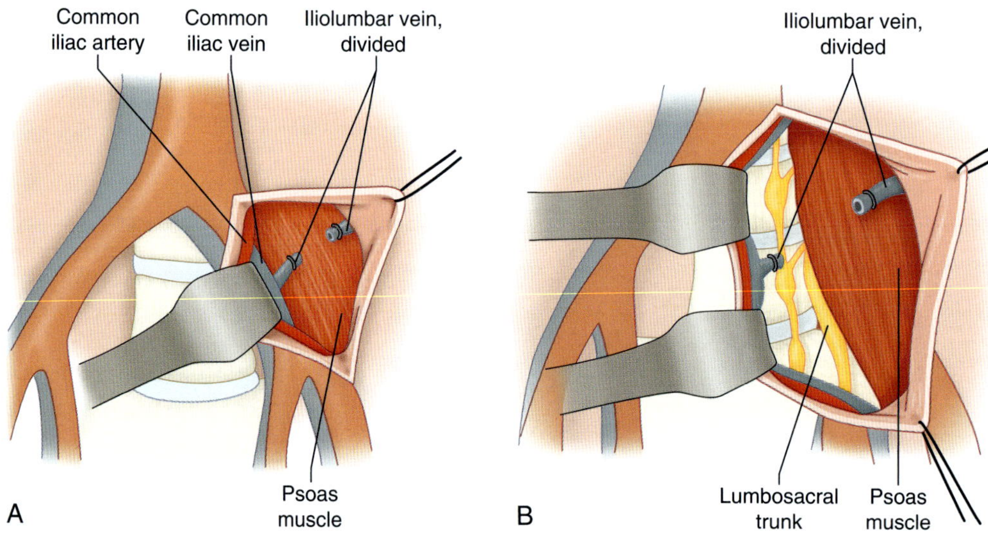

• **Fig. 4.4** A. The iliolumbar vein is seen on the surface of the psoas muscle in the anterior approach to the spine. **B**. After ligating and dividing this vein, access to the disk spaces is enhanced. (From Benzel E. *Spine Surgery: Techniques, Complication Avoidance, & Management*. 3rd ed. Philadelphia: Elsevier Saunders; 2012; Figure 55-3.)

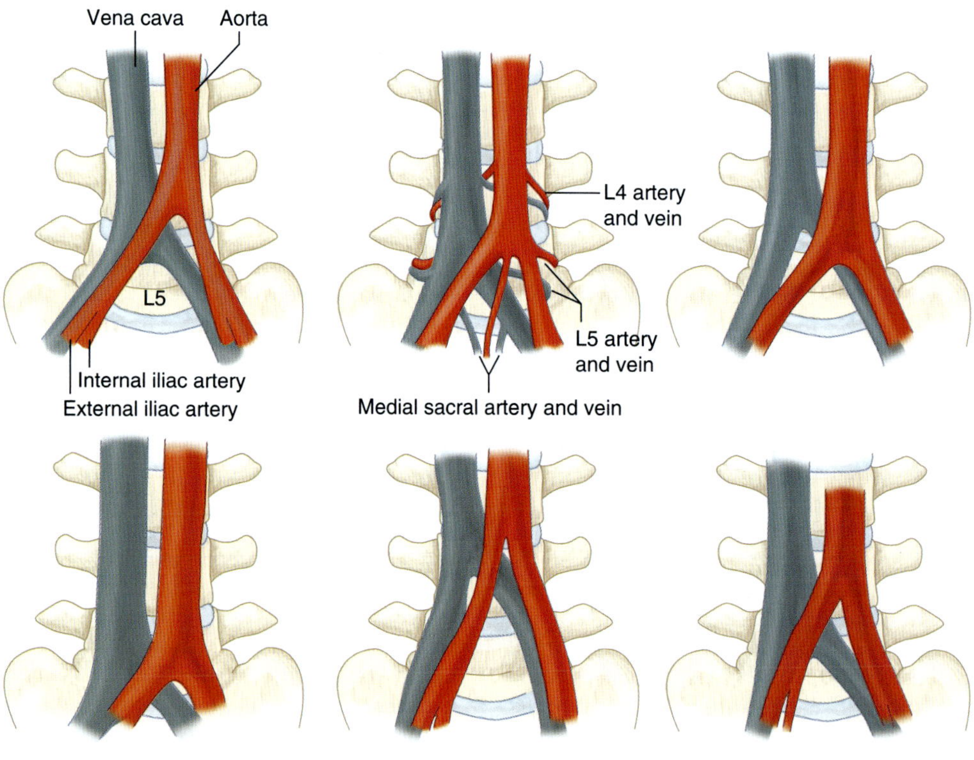

• **Fig. 4.5** Anterior view of the lumbar spine demonstrating anatomical variation in the location of the aorta, inferior vena cava, and their branches. (From Benzel E. *Spine Surgery: Techniques, Complication Avoidance, & Management*, ed 3, Philadelphia: Elsevier Saunders; 2012; Figure 36-12.)

injury of the left L2 segmental artery after an L2-3 eXtreme lateral interbody fusion procedure thought to be caused by the lateral expandable split retractor blade. The injury was discovered 48 hours postoperatively when the patient became hemodynamically unstable and a computed tomography scan showed a large left retroperitoneal hematoma. Immediately, the patient underwent a successful endovascular embolization of a left L-2 segmental artery pseudoaneurysm.[9]

Venous Drainage of the Spine

A large valveless venous plexus is responsible for drainage of the spine (Fig. 4.7). This plexus has external and epidural

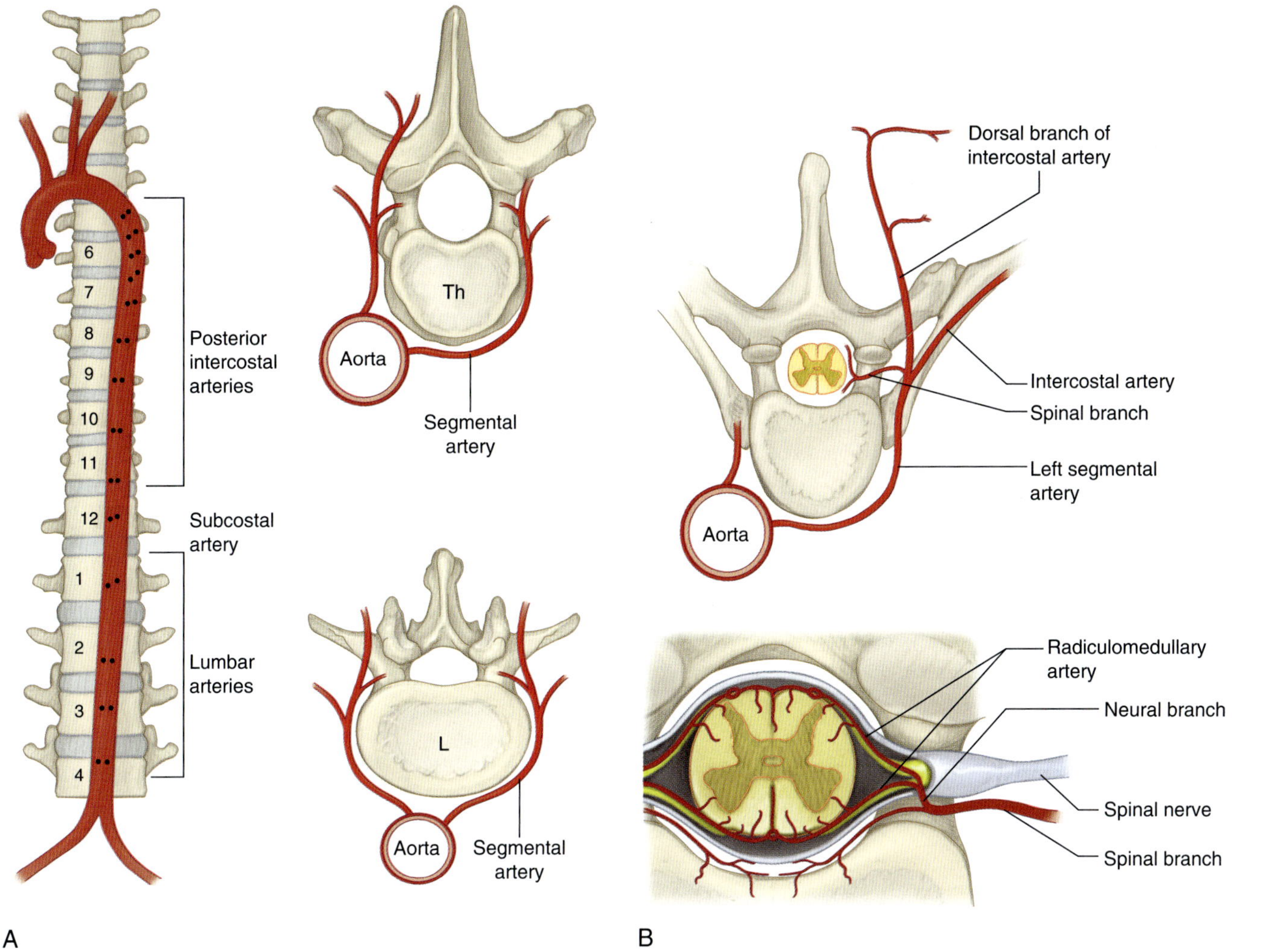

• **Fig. 4.6** A. Arterial supply to the spine. The aorta originating on the anterolateral left side of the thoracic spine and crossing to a more medial location. **B.** The segmental and spinal branches passing around the vertebral body and entering the dura at the site of the nerve root. (From Benzel E. *Spine Surgery: Techniques, Complication Avoidance, & Management*. 3rd ed. Philadelphia: Elsevier Saunders; 2012; Figure 32-24.)

components, and has portions both ventrally and dorsally. Intradural venous drainage is performed by the radiculomedullary veins which feed into the anterior and posterior spinal veins. The venous system closely parallels the arterial system. The lumbar veins travel with the lumbar arteries but with greater variation in course and number. Cadaveric studies frequently identify veins on the left side.[8]

Urinary System

The kidneys and the ureters lie within the retroperitoneal space in proximity to the spine and may also be at risk during the lateral and anterior approaches. The left kidney is more caudal than the right with the upper pole on the left at the level of T11-12 and the lower pole at L2-3. The upper pole of the right kidney is typically at T12-L1, and the lower pole at L3-4.[10] The ureters exit the renal pelvis and travel posterolaterally on the anterior surface of the psoas muscle. The right ureter courses along the right aspect of the IVC and crosses the external iliac artery as it enters the pelvis. The left ureter crosses over the common iliac artery.[11] Vigilance in identifying the ureter may help prevent injury by dissection during the approach or by retraction.

Neural Anatomy

In the average adult the spinal cord terminates at the L1 level, giving rise to the conus medullaris and the nerve roots of the cauda equina. As the dorsal and ventral roots exit the spinal cord, they join to form the spinal nerve in the dural sleeve. This nerve then exits below the pedicle with the same number (Fig. 4.8). These nerves then join to form the lumbar plexus within the psoas major and give rise to the sensory and motor innervation of the abdomen and proximal leg (Fig. 4.9). The ilioinguinal and iliohypogastric nerves originate from L1 and pass laterally and anteriorly into the abdomen. The genitofemoral nerve (from L1 and L2) exits the ventral psoas and later divides into two femoral and genital branches, lateral to the common and iliac arteries. The lateral femoral cutaneous nerve arises from the L1 and L2 roots. The largest branches of the lumbar plexus, which provide motor function to the proximal leg, are the obturator and femoral nerves, which arise from L2, L3, and L4. L4 and L5 combine to form the lumbosacral trunk and join the first sacral nerve. The obturator nerve lies medial to the psoas and is not at risk during lateral transpsoas approaches. The femoral nerve is very much at risk, particularly at the L4-5 level.

Defining a Safe Corridor

With the growing popularity of minimally invasive approaches where visualization of the regional anatomy is limited, many authors have attempted to define safe corridors to allow access to the spine with minimal risk of complications. After the spinal nerves exit the lateral foramen, they traverse the lateral surface of the spine and form the plexus within the psoas muscle. The minimally invasive lateral approach to the lumbar spine requires traversing the ipsilateral psoas muscle with, dilators and retractors; the location of the nerves and plexus places them at risk during this approach. Both cadaveric and radiographic studies have been performed in attempts to define a safe working corridor for this approach. This surgical approach was mimicked in cadavers; in 25% of mimicked cases, nerve damage occurred owing to piercing either a lumbar nerve root or the genitofemoral nerve. Dilation of the retractor resulted in stretch on the lumbar nerve roots in all cases.[12] One simple scheme describing the anatomy divides the psoas muscle into thirds. The sympathetic chain travels in the anterior one-third of the psoas muscle; the genitofemoral nerve is in the middle third. Perforating branches of the lumbar nerve roots can be found in all thirds.

Other studies have divided the vertebral body into six zones: A is the most anterior at the anterior border of the vertebral body, followed by zones 1–4, and then zone P, the most posterior defined as the posterior border of the vertebral body.[13] The more superior disk levels have a larger safe zone than at L4-5 where only the anterior fourth (zone 1) is safe for a right-sided approach, whereas zones 2 and 3 define the safe corridor in a left-sided approach.[6,13]

Radiographic and cadaveric studies have increased our knowledge of the anatomy and normal variants of the lumbar spine and surrounding structures. One cadaveric study measured the ratio of the distance from the posterior endplate of the disk space to the total length of the disk space. This study demonstrated the ventral migration of the lumbosacral plexus from the posterior border of the disk space at L1-2 (ratio = 0) to a more anterior position (ratio = 0.28) at L4-5 moving caudally through the lumbar spine. The safe working zone at L2-3 and L3-4 is in the anterior three-fourth of the disk space but with the ventral migration of the plexus, this decreases to the anterior two-thirds at L4-5. At this level the nerve root is at the greatest risk of injury.[14] Another study focused on the neural structures, identifing zone 3 as a safe area for an approach from L1-2, L2-3, and L3-4. However, at L4-5 the safe area of approach was the border between zone 2 and zone 3, at the midpoint of the vertebral body. Specific analysis of the

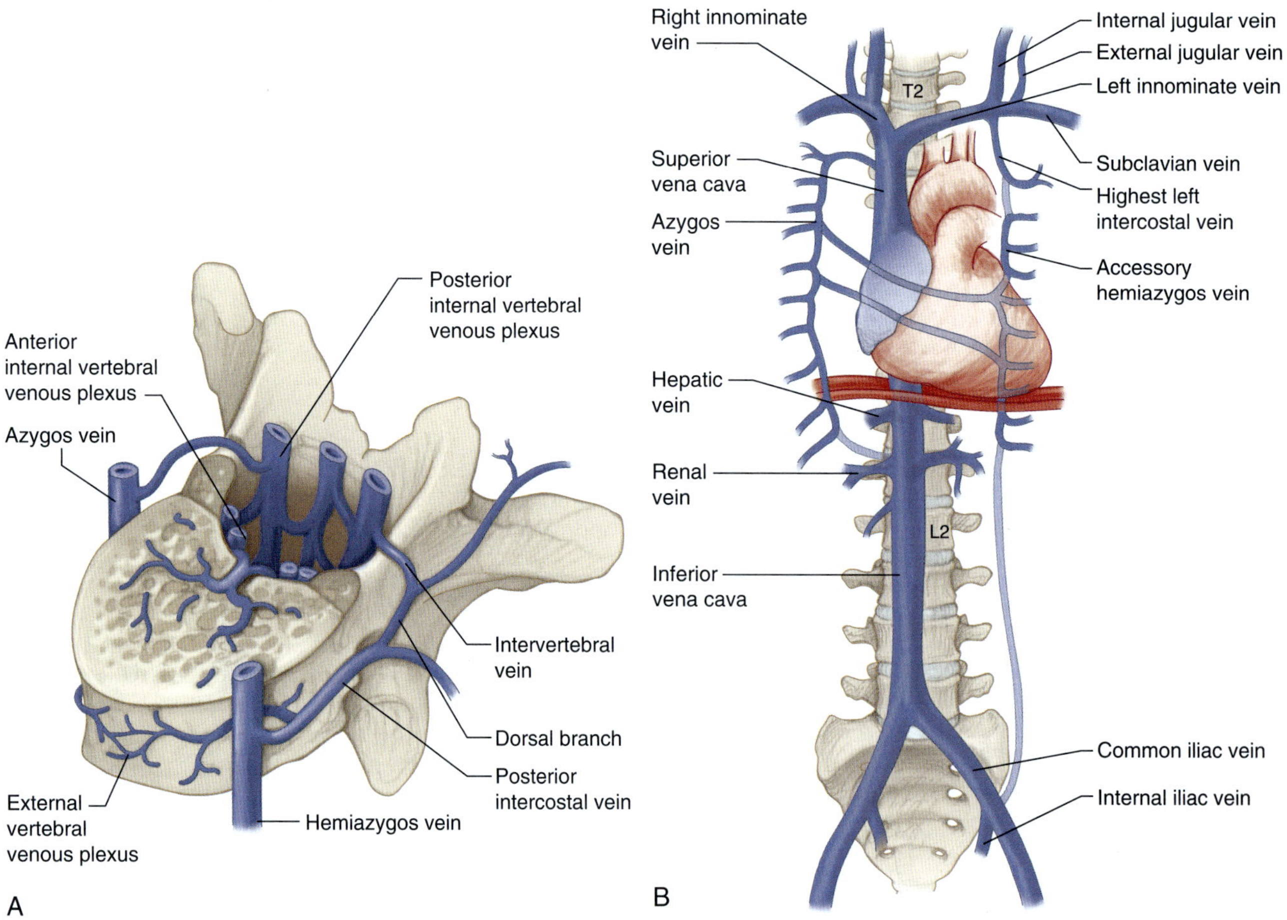

• **Fig. 4.7** Venous drainage of the spine. **A**. The internal and external venous plexuses in relation to the vertebral body. **B**. The inferior vena cava passes on the anterolateral surface of the lumbar spine, to the right of midline. (From Benzel E. *Spine Surgery: Techniques, Complication Avoidance, & Management*, 3rd ed. Philadelphia: Elsevier Saunders; 2012; Figure 32-27.)

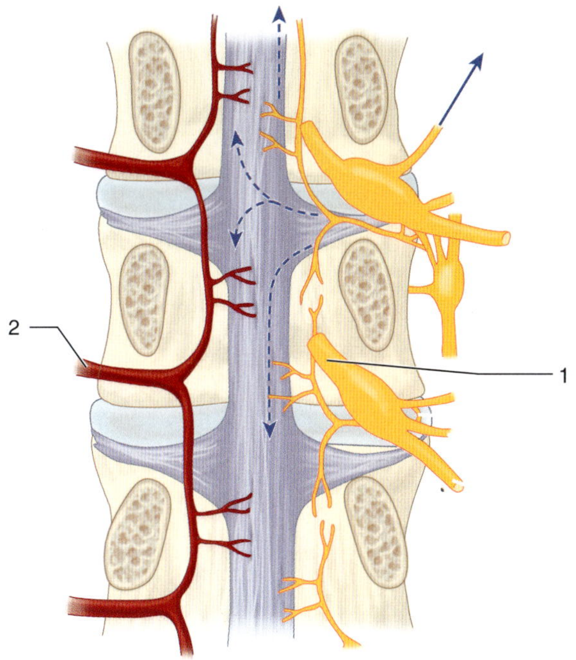

• **Fig. 4.8** Vascular and neural anatomy *(posterior view).* The nerve root (1) exits under the pedicle of the same number. The spinal branch (2) enters under the pedicle, in proximity to the nerve root. (From Benzel E. *Spine Surgery: Techniques, Complication Avoidance, & Management*, 3rd ed. Philadelphia: Elsevier Saunders; 2012; Figure 32-20.)

genitofemoral nerve localized it to zone 2 at L2-3, and zone 1 and L3-4 and L4-5.[15] In another cadaver study the authors used 8 mm as their definition of a safe radius, to allow space for the dilators and distraction instruments. In levels rostral to L4-5, the nerve roots and trunks were greater than 8 mm from the midpoint of the disk space. At L4-5, however, in 25% of dissections the neural structures were present within 8 mm of the center of the disk space.[16] Radiographic studies examining the position of the large vessels anteriorly and the nerves posterolaterally have confirmed these findings. The percentage of the vertebral body believed to be safe from potential injury to neurovascular structures decreases from rostral to caudal with one author reporting 48% at L1-2 to 13% at L4-5.[17] This precipitous decline is owing to the posterior migration of the anteriorly located vascular structures and the anterior migration of the nerves of the plexus relative to the vertebral body.

In addition to cadaveric and radiographic studies, clinical experience also informs us of the risk of these approaches. At L4-5 the risk of femoral nerve injury in one single-center study was 4.8% using a lateral approach; in contrast, the overall risk of femoral nerve injury when considering the lateral approach to any level was 1.7%.[18] This study highlights the increased risk at L4-5 in clinical practice—correlating with what was described. This same study also reports five attempted lateral interbody fusions that were aborted owing to the anterior location of the motor nerve in the psoas, preventing access to the disk space (success rate 98% at L3-4, 92% at L4-5).[18] Analysis of the preoperative imaging in conjunction with expertise in the anatomy of the lumbar spine and knowledge of common variants is key to avoiding neurovascular complications.

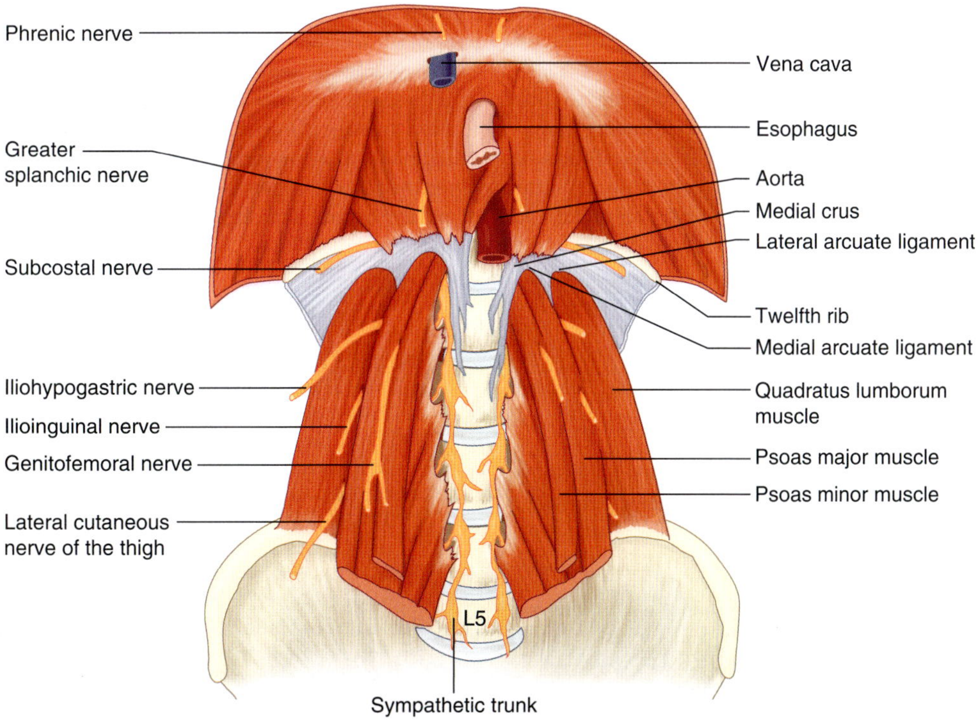

• **Fig. 4.9** The spine as seen *(anterior view)* with the blood vessels removed. The sympathetic chain is on the anterior surface. The nerves of the lumbar plexus are seen exiting from the psoas major. (From Benzel E. *Spine Surgery: Techniques, Complication Avoidance, & Management*, 3rd ed. Philadelphia: Elsevier Saunders; 2012; Figure 36-11.)

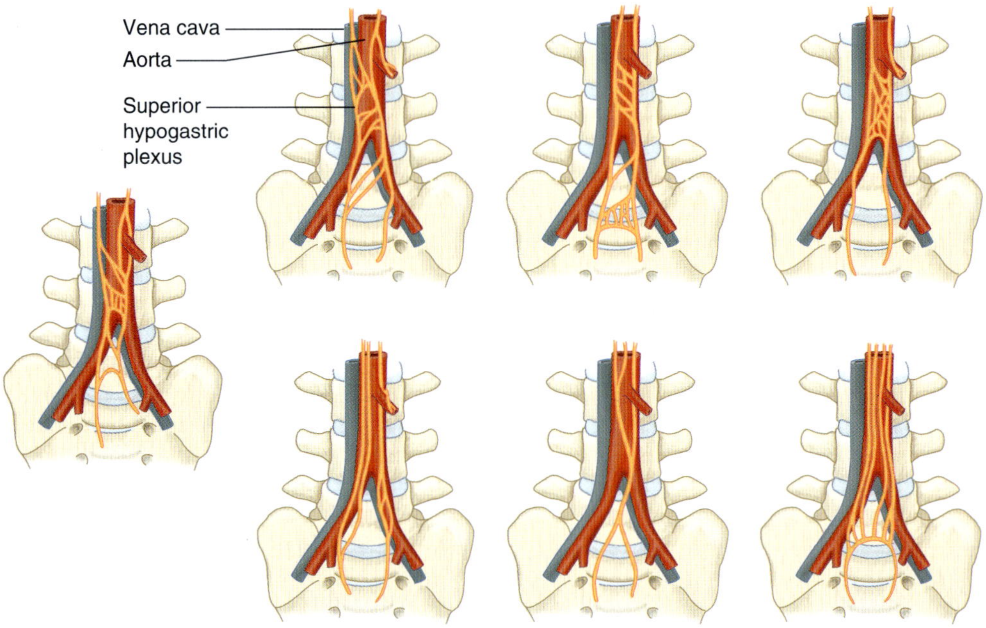

• **Fig. 4.10** The superior hypogastric plexus and variations. (From Benzel E. *Spine Surgery: Techniques, Complication Avoidance, & Management*, 3rd ed., Philadelphia: Elsevier Saunders; 2012; Figure 36-9.)

Hypogastric Plexus

Retrograde ejaculation is an often-discussed complication of anterior lumbar interbody fusions that can occur with damage to the superior hypogastric plexus. This plexus lies on the ventral surface of the aorta and within its bifurcation, extending from the level of L4 to S1, with variation between individuals (Fig. 4.10). This prevertebral plexus receives both sympathetic and parasympathetic contributions from lumbar and sacral autonomic nerves.[19] In males this plexus innervates the bladder, vas deferens, and seminal vesicles, with damage to this structure preventing closure of the bladder neck during ejaculation with resultant retrograde ejaculation. The likelihood of injury can be reduced by avoidance of electrocautery, blunt dissection, and careful retraction of the plexus from left to right.[20]

Conclusion

Modern approaches to the lumbar spine allow the surgeon to approach from nearly any angle, allowing the approach to be tailored to the patient's particular pathology and needs. It is important to account for the unique risk profiles of each approach in planning surgery–preparing for possible complications, and minimizing risk. In the lateral transpsoas approach, cognizance of the width of the approach corridor as it narrows from rostral to caudal will allow for the avoidance of neurologic or vascular complications. This corridor progressively narrows as the neural structures migrate from posterior to anterior along the vertebral bodies and the vascular structures migrate to lie along the anterior surface of the vertebral bodies. The greatest risk for injury is at L4-5; however, this level may be successfully treated with experience and knowledge of the anatomy in many cases.

References

1. Lin RM, Jou IM, Yu CY. Lumbar lordosis: normal adults. *J Formos Med Assoc*. 1992;91(3):329–333.
2. Deukmedjian AR, Dakwar E, Ahmadian A, et al. Early outcomes of minimally invasive anterior longitudinal ligament release for correction of sagittal imbalance in patients with adult spinal deformity. *ScientificWorldJournal*. 2012;2012:789698. https://doi.org/10.1100/2012/789698.
3. Regev GJ, Haloman S, Chen L, et al. Incidence and prevention of intervertebral cage overhang with minimally invasive lateral approach fusions. *Spine (Phila Pa 1976)*. 2010;35(14):1406–1411. https://doi.org/10.1097/BRS.0b013e3181c20fb5.
4. Assina R, Majmundar NJ, Herschman Y, et al. First report of major vascular injury due to lateral transpsoas approach leading to fatality. *J Neurosurg Spine*. 2014;21(5):794–798. https://doi.org/10.3171/2014.7.SPINE131146.
5. Alkadhim M, Zoccali C, Abbasifard S, et al. The surgical vascular anatomy of the minimally invasive lateral lumbar interbody approach: a cadaveric and radiographic analysis. *Eur Spine J*. 2015;24(suppl 7):906–911. https://doi.org/10.1007/s00586-015-4267-5.
6. Hu WK, He SS, Zhang SC, et al. An MRI study of psoas major and abdominal large vessels with respect to the X/DLIF approach. *Eur Spine J*. 2011;20(4):557–562. https://doi.org/10.1007/s00586-010-1609-1.
7. Capellades J, Pellise F, Rovira A, et al. Magnetic resonance anatomic study of iliocava junction and left iliac vein positions related to L5-S1 disc. *Spine (Phila Pa 1976)*. 2000;25(13):1695–1700.
8. Baniel J, Foster RS, Donohue JP. Surgical anatomy of the lumbar vessels: implications for retroperitoneal surgery. *J Urol*. 1995;153(5):1422–1425.
9. Santillan A, Patsalides A, Gobin YP. Endovascular embolization of iatrogenic lumbar artery pseudoaneurysm following extreme lateral interbody fusion (XLIF). *Vasc Endovascular Surg*. 2010;44(7):601–603. https://doi.org/10.1177/1538574410374655.

10. Currarino G, Winchester P. Position of the kidneys relative to the spine, with emphasis on children. *Am J Roentgenol Radium Ther Nucl Med.* 1965;95(2):409–412.
11. Chan JK, Morrow J, Manetta A. Prevention of ureteral injuries in gynecologic surgery. *Am J Obstet Gynecol.* 2003;188(5):1273–1277. PubMed PMID: 12748497.
12. Banagan K, Gelb D, Poelstra K, Ludwig S. Anatomic mapping of lumbar nerve roots during a direct lateral transpsoas approach to the spine: a cadaveric study. *Spine (Phila Pa 1976).* 2011;36(11):E687–E691. https://doi.org/10.1097/BRS.0b013e3181ec5911. PubMed PMID: 21217450.
13. Moro T, Kikuchi S, Konno S, et al. An anatomic study of the lumbar plexus with respect to retroperitoneal endoscopic surgery. *Spine (Phila Pa 1976).* 2003;28(5):423–428; discussion 7–8. https://doi.org/10.1097/01.BRS.0000049226.87064.3B.
14. Benglis DM, Vanni S, Levi AD. An anatomical study of the lumbosacral plexus as related to the minimally invasive transpsoas approach to the lumbar spine. *J Neurosurg Spine.* 2009;10(2):139–144. https://doi.org/10.3171/2008.10.SPI08479.
15. Uribe JS, Arredondo N, Dakwar E, et al. Defining the safe working zones using the minimally invasive lateral retroperitoneal transpsoas approach: an anatomical study. *J Neurosurg Spine.* 2010;13(2):260–266. https://doi.org/10.3171/2010.3.SPINE09766.
16. Park DK, Lee MJ, Lin EL, et al. The relationship of intrapsoas nerves during a transpsoas approach to the lumbar spine: anatomic study. *J Spinal Disord Tech.* 2010;23(4):223–228. https://doi.org/10.1097/BSD.0b013e3181a9d540.
17. Regev GJ, Chen L, Dhawan M, et al. Morphometric analysis of the ventral nerve roots and retroperitoneal vessels with respect to the minimally invasive lateral approach in normal and deformed spines. *Spine (Phila Pa 1976).* 2009;34(12):1330–1335. https://doi.org/10.1097/BRS.0b013e3181a029e1.
18. Cahill KS, Martinez JL, Wang MY, et al. Motor nerve injuries following the minimally invasive lateral transpsoas approach. *J Neurosurg Spine.* 2012;17(3):227–231. https://doi.org/10.3171/2012.5.SPINE1288.
19. Lu S, Xu YQ, Chang S, et al. Clinical anatomy study of autonomic nerve with respective to the anterior approach lumbar surgery. *Surg Radiol Anat.* 2009;31(6):425–430. https://doi.org/10.1007/s00276-009-0461-7.
20. Johnson RM, McGuire EJ. Urogenital complications of anterior approaches to the lumbar spine. *Clin Orthop Relat Res.* 1981; 154:114–118.

5

Intraoperative Image-Guided Navigation for Lumbar Interbody Fusion

VARUN PUVANESARAJAH, RABIA QURESHI, AND HAMID HASSANZADEH

Introduction

Minimally invasive spine surgery has gained much popularity in recent years owing to the reductions in patient morbidity, length of hospital stay, and costs. Although these short-term outcomes have seen marked improvements, there has been little improvement in the long-term outcomes when comparing minimally invasive lumbar interbody fusion (MIS-LIF) to open techniques.[1]

When first developed, MIS-LIF required extensive fluoroscopy to ensure accurate interbody cage placement and extensive imaging for the percutaneous placement of pedicle screws. The consequent accumulation of radiation from many of these minimally invasive procedures may result in dangerous radiation dosages to the surgeons who perform these procedures.[2,3] As such, there has been an increased development and use of navigation-based techniques that rely on the use of intraoperatively acquired images with subsequent image registration allowing for navigation of interbody cage and percutaneous screw placement.[4] This approach exposes surgeons to much less radiation while maintaining comparable accuracy.

In this chapter, we review various advanced imaging modalities related to both accurate interbody cage and associated pedicle screw placement in the lumbar spine.

Fluoroscopy

Prior to the advent of advanced imaging modalities relying on computer-aided image processing and registration, fluoroscopy was utilized to ensure proper cage placement. This method requires successive anterior-posterior and lateral C-arm images to ensure that the cage is inserted orthogonal to the disk space. In patients with deformity or multilevel degenerative disease, ensuring a perfect orthogonal position can require tilting the table to acquire appropriate images; consequently, with the repetitive imaging, there can be significant radiation exposure. Additionally, the accuracy of cage and pedicle screw placement has been a concern, particularly in comparison to more open techniques where visualization is much easier.

Given the increased exposure to large amounts of low-level radiation that can result from high case volumes, several studies have aimed to quantify the average surgeon radiation exposure during MIS-LIF cases. Regarding lateral lumbar interbody fusion (LLIF) cases, Taher et al.[5] found that during eighteen cases fusing a mean 2.4 levels, average total fluoroscopy time was 88.7 seconds, including fluoroscopy at the beginning of the case to ensure accurate positioning. Of note, significant increases in radiation exposure were noted in unprotected areas when compared to the dosimeter located under the lead apron of the primary surgeon.[5] Bindal et al.[3] observed an average fluoroscopy time of 101 seconds during minimally invasive transforaminal interbody fusion (MIS-TLIF), with radiation exposures that were generally improved in a later study by Funao et al., who used a one-shot fluoroscopy technique in an attempt to lessen or reduce surgeon radiation exposure.[2] Other similar low-dose fluoroscopy protocols have been developed to decrease radiation exposure during MIS-TLIF cases.[6]

The significance of such radiation exposures to the surgeon is unclear, although various authors have suggested that exposures may have a more critical impact on younger surgeons who are beginning their practice and have a lifetime of fluoroscopy-dependent spine procedures ahead of them. With this in mind, Taher et al. calculated that 2700 LLIF procedures theoretically could be performed each year without exceeding standards for "safe" occupational radiation exposure.[5] Although this may be true, an interest in reducing surgeon radiation exposure persists.

Stereotactic Navigation

To alleviate the concerns of increases in surgeon radiation exposure and of the placement accuracy of both pedicle screws and interbody cages, there has been a recent push toward the development of technologies that utilize imaging to register an image at the start of the procedure to be used as a reference for navigating instruments. Radiation exposure to surgeons and ancillary personnel is thereby theoretically reduced, as the images taken at the beginning of the procedure for image registration do not require the close proximity of staff. As the procedure progresses and is fully navigated, surgeon visibility improves, ideally also improving the accuracy of placement and addressing both concerns.

Imaging modalities that have been used for the generation of these reference images include intraoperative C-arm fluoroscopy and computed tomography (CT) scans via either an O-arm or another intraoperative CT scanner (Fig. 5.1).[7] In MIS-LIF cases, there is the added benefit of using image registration methods that can be performed after positioning and draping, to decrease navigation error owing to the changes of patient positioning. One general drawback of using navigated instrumentation is increased set-up time, although this may not be a significant issue as time

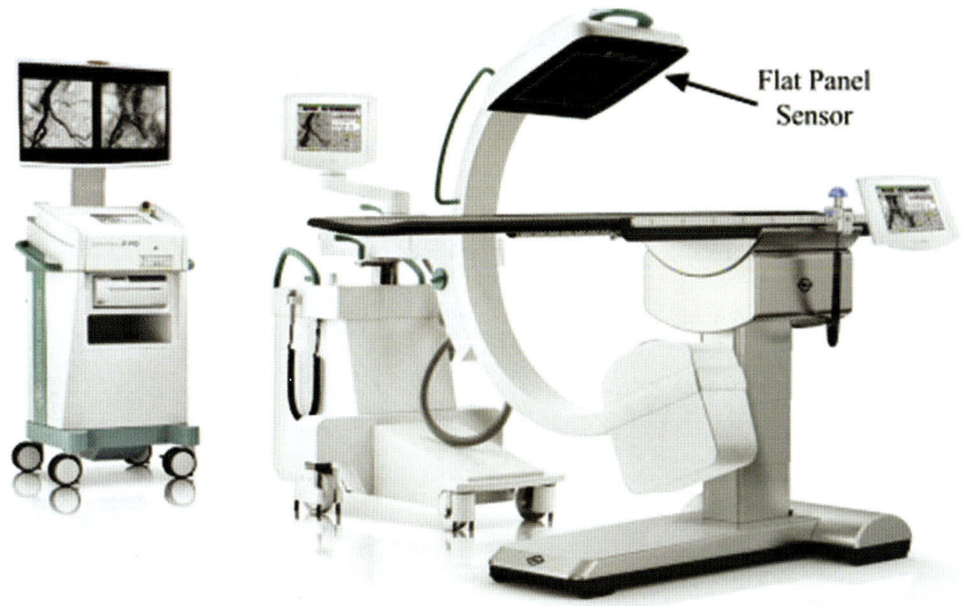

• **Fig. 5.1** Portable fan beam computed tomography scanner. (Courtesy of Ziehm Imaging GmbH, Nuremberg, Germany; with permission.)

expense can be avoided later in the procedure by obviating the need for repeated fluoroscopy.

Modern 3D Image Acquisition Systems

Navigated interbody and pedicle screw placement requires intraoperative image registration using a dynamic reference frame to allow for effective three-dimensional triangulation of instruments. In general, positioning depends on the approach (supine for posterior approach interbody fusion, left lateral with knees and hips flexed for lateral interbody fusion) and sterile draping occurs following induction of anesthesia as during a non-navigated case. Notably, however, draping must include the site of dynamic reference frame placement, and these frame placement sites include adjacent spinous processes, the iliac crest, and skin during the posterior approach cases and the anterior and posterior superior iliac spines during lateral approaches.

Placement of the dynamic reference frame during posterior minimally invasive approaches to interbody fusion has been investigated in detail as many options exist for bony fixation, including the iliac crest[8,9] and cephalad spinous processes,[1,10] during posterior approach cases. Cho et al.[4] investigated the use of cutaneously fixed dynamic reference frames to avoid significant issues that can occur with traditional fixation to bony landmarks. For example, if the reference frame is affixed to the spinous process at the level of the surgical site or on the posterior superior iliac spine, there is a higher possibility of decreasing the already small working field and possibly causing metal artifact. And despite the fact that most reference markers are made from titanium, artifact can commonly occur. However, placing the reference frame at a separate spinous process necessitates a separate incision. Cho et al.[4] found that using a dynamic reference frame affixed to the skin overlying the sacral hiatus allowed acceptable navigation of pedicle screw accuracy during mini-open TLIF. This finding held up despite the potential drawbacks associated with increased dynamic reference frame distance from the pathology and possibly lower stability than fixation to bone.

After sterile placement of the dynamic reference frame, intraoperative three-dimensional imaging is taken, performed via fluoroscopy (i.e., Siemens Iso-C^{3d}, ARCADIS Orbic 3D) or CT scans (i.e., Medtronic O-arm). Images are then registered using the associated navigation system. During this early image registration phase, surgeons and ancillary staff can opt for more stringent radiation protection protocols to minimize radiation exposure. These include moving far from the field and using more extensive lead shielding. Following image registration, the surgical procedure can continue as previously performed, replacing active C-arm action shots with direct navigation of all instruments.

Interbody Cage Placement

Several studies have investigated the use of computer-aided navigation during interbody cage insertion. For example, Drazin et al.[11] describe LLIF via an O-arm linked to the Stealth-Station TREON System (Medtronic Sofamor Danek). Their technique involved the use of a dynamic reference frame attached to a pin that is inserted into the posterior superior iliac spine. Use of the O-arm intraoperatively allows for sterile draping of the patient and full positioning prior to image acquisition and registration, thereby decreasing the chance of error from altering the orientation of the dynamic reference frame to the patient's spine (Fig. 5.2). Park[12] described a similar technique for LLIF that also relied on the use of an O-arm and a similar tracking system, although it included minor changes in retractor positioning and reference frame location. Park advocated the use of the anterior superior iliac spine for placement of the reference frame, although it may slightly increase the risk of injury to the lateral femoral cutaneous nerve. In a series of eight patients, however, Park did not observe any instances of iatrogenic nerve injury. Additionally, on postoperative fluoroscopy, all cages were noted to be placed within the anterior three quarters of the disk space in question, indicating acceptable accuracy as well.[12]

Similar accuracy was demonstrated in a cadaver study comparing conventional fluoroscopy with navigation using registered fluoroscopic images for a direct lateral approach to cage insertion.[13]

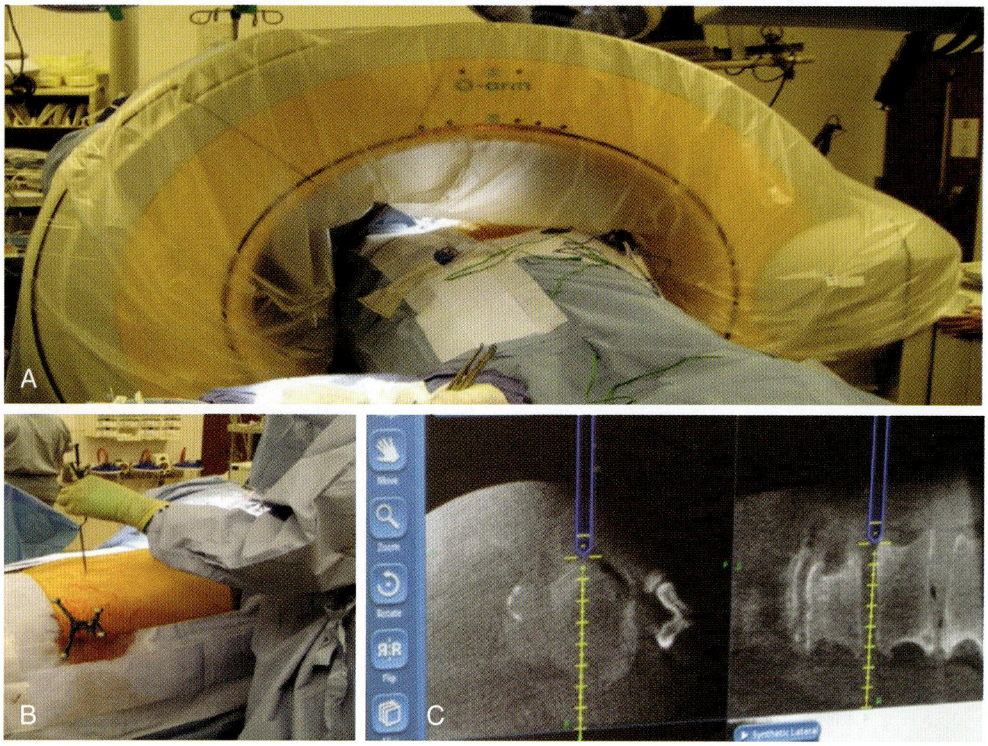

• **Fig. 5.2** Intraoperative use of O-ARM (Medtronic Sofamor Danek, Inc., Memphis, TN, USA) with Stealth Station TREON System (Medtronic Sofamor Danek). (A,B, Images provided by Medtronic.) (Adapted from Drazin D, Liu JC, Acosta Jr FL. CT navigated lateral interbody fusion. *Journal of Clinical Neuroscience: Official Journal of the Neurosurgical Society of Australasia.* 2013;20(10):1438–1441.)

Interestingly, study authors noted that the lowest accuracy was observed at the L1-2 level, which was located the farthest from the dynamic reference frame affixed to the anterior superior iliac spine. Apart from accuracy, the study also investigated the time needed to successfully position interbody cages. Although significantly more time was needed during the initial setup of the navigation system, subsequent steps required less time with navigation, resulting in similar overall operative time.[13]

Pedicle Screw Placement

When initially developed, navigation for pedicle screw placement was severely limited by poor image quality and underdeveloped computational software. However, over the years, navigation for pedicle screw placement has been explored extensively in the context of open procedures. Studies have generally demonstrated improved accuracy when comparing navigated techniques with images registered through fluoroscopy, conventional CT scans, or O-arm technology (Fig. 5.3).[14] In particular, Kosmopoulos and Schizas demonstrated that when pooling 130 studies of over 35,000 pedicle screws, median screw placement accuracy was 95.2% in navigated cases as compared to 90.3% in non-navigated cases,[15] a conclusion supported by other reviews.[16–18] Most of these studies have investigated non-minimally invasive surgery, where even freehand pedicle screw technique can be utilized. Many minimally invasive interbody fusion cases, however, rely on percutaneous pedicle screw placement for posterior stabilization.

Percutaneous pedicle screw placement is an important adjunct to minimally invasive interbody fusion as it allows for posterior stabilization without extensive paraspinal muscle dissection, as would be observed in open fusion cases. This can significantly reduce postoperative wound pain, particularly when considering the reduced morbidity from avoiding muscle dissection from transverse processes, as would be performed for traditional posterolateral lumbar spine fusion surgery. One drawback however, of percutaneous pedicle screw placement is facet violation, which is more likely in this instance because the facet joint is not directly

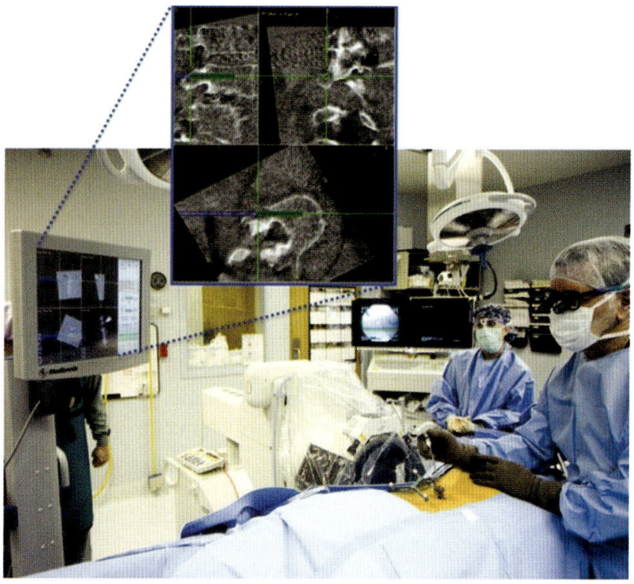

• **Fig. 5.3** Intraoperative use of 3D computed tomography guidance system. (Images provided by Medtronic.) (Adapted from Bourgeois AC, Faulkner AR, Pasciak AS, Bradley YC. The evolution of image-guided lumbosacral spine surgery. *Annals of Translational Medicine.* 2015;3(5):69.)

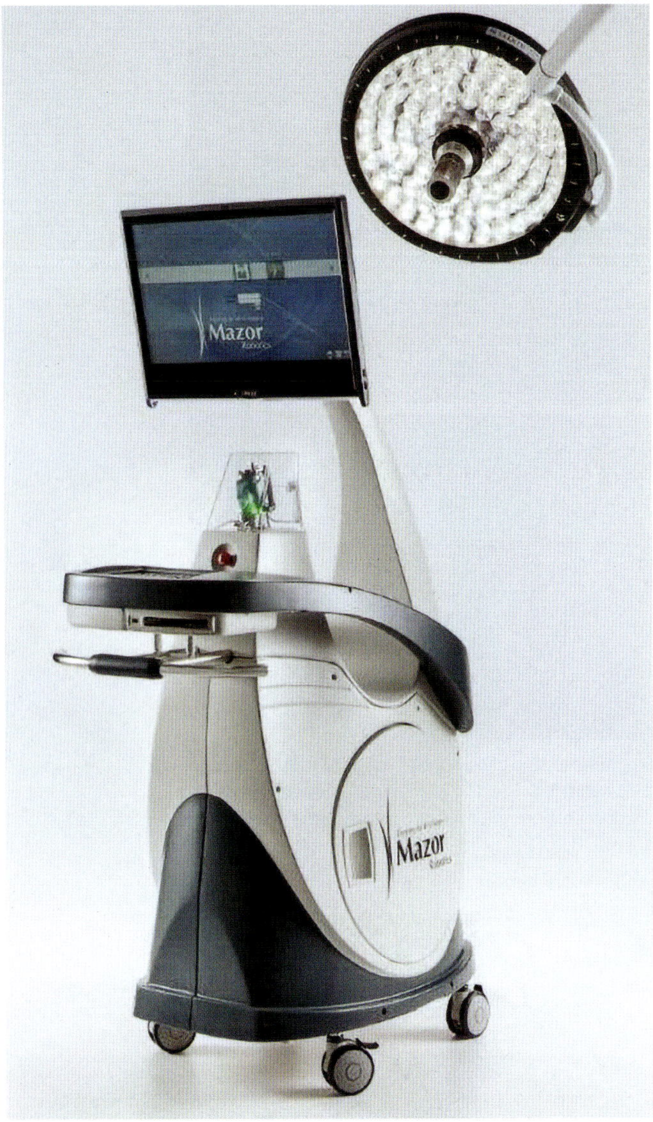

• **Fig. 5.4** Mazor Robotics Renaissance guidance system.

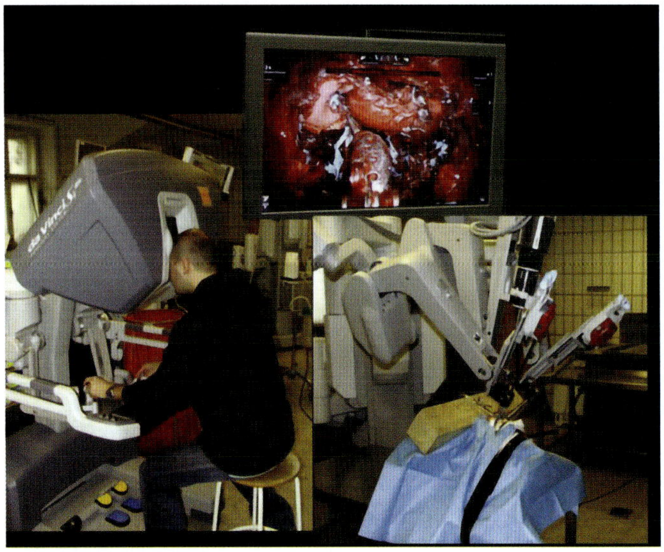

• **Fig. 5.5** Exemplary application of robotics and endoscopy. The da Vinci Surgical System is used for pituitary surgery in a cadaver specimen at the Centre for Anatomy and Cell Biology, Medical University of Vienna, Vienna, Austria. (From Di Leva A. et al. A journey into the technical evolution of neuroendoscopy. *World Neurosurg*. 2014;82(6):e777–e789, Figure 10.)

visualized.[4] Additionally, there is an increase in future risk of symptomatic adjacent segment degeneration and a resultant need for further revision surgery. Other concerns include the risk of anterior guide wire migration through the vertebral body, particularly in severely osteoporotic patients, which may increase the risk of intestinal or great vessel injury.

To address these concerns, navigation techniques have been developed for use in minimally invasive lumbar spine surgery. Robotic innovations, such as the Mazor Robotics Renaissance guidance system, uses preoperative CT images as guides to plan for the surgical procedure with much more precision before beginning the surgery (Fig. 5.4). Intraoperatively, the robotic system can be placed in a specific location and can achieve a specified trajectory, allowing instrument placement by the surgeon with more precision (Fig. 5.5).[19] The Renaissance Guidance System has been studied in spinal instrumentation procedures. Percutaneous pedical screw placement, for example, was examined, illustrating higher accuracy of placement with much lower radiation exposure. Kantelhardt et al.[20] demonstrated a mean decrease of 43 seconds of intraoperative x-ray exposure in robotic-guided procedures as compared with the conventional imaging methods as well. Additionally, using the robotic system for minimally invasive cases can decrease damage to the surrounding healthy tissue and lead to faster recovery.[20]

The Envision 3DTM: Image Guidance System (7D Surgical Inc.) is another image-guided navigation system that does not utilize any x-ray radiation to generate images, effectively eliminating the radiation risk, increasing accuracy, and streamlining the surgical setup. It functions to create a 3D image of the exposed patient anatomy by manipulating the surgical lights into a special pattern. This pattern, in turn, is read by the Envision system to generate an image used as a reference surface. The patient's anatomy can be superimposed with the placement of surgical tools, increasing accuracy without excess radiation (Fig. 5.6).[21]

During MIS-TLIF procedures, overall significant improvements in pedicle screw accuracy have been reported. Tian et al.[1] observed higher pedicle screw accuracy rates (93.3 vs. 73.4%) when comparing patients treated with computer-assisted MIS-TLIF to those treated with fluoroscopy and open TLIF, with the accuracy judged as overt pedicle perforation. Notably, this study found no significant differences in either radiographic or clinical outcomes as postoperative pain and Oswestry Disability Index (ODI) scores were similar between the two cohorts from three months onwards.[1] Similar results were obtained by Fraser et al.[8] and Nakashima et al.[10] who demonstrated significantly improved pedicle screw accuracy when using navigation during MIS-TLIF procedures (90.9 vs. 73.7% and 92.7 vs. 84.7%, respectively).[8,10]

In contrast to minimally invasive spine surgery from a posterior approach, pedicle screw placement during LLIF is not as well studied. When posterior instrumentation is utilized to support an interbody cage placed through either a direct or extreme lateral approach, the surgery can be staged to allow for full access to the posterior elements through a conventional percutaneous approach. However, some surgeons will opt for unilateral percutaneous pedicle screw placement to obviate the necessity for staging or for adjusting the patient's position on the operating table. At this time, however, there are no studies evaluating the use of

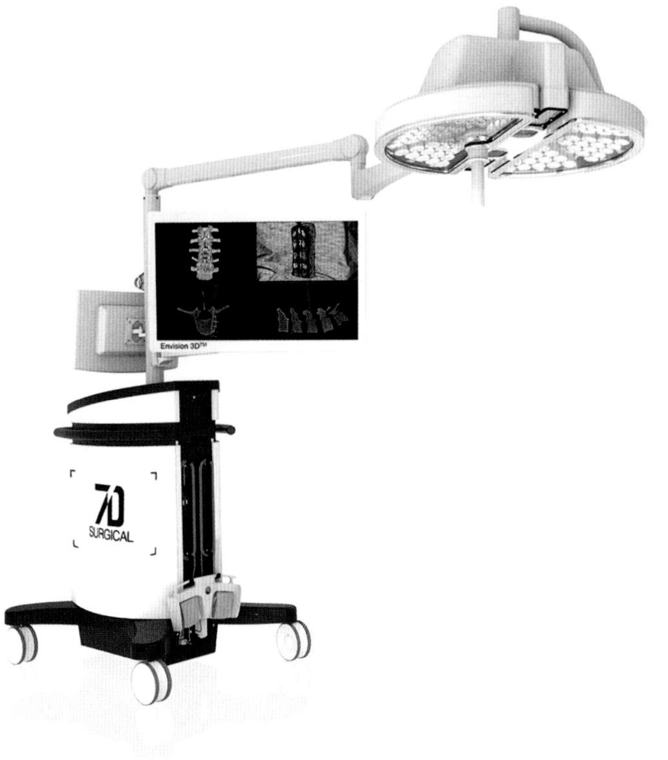

• **Fig. 5.6** The Envision 3DTM: Image Guidance System. (Courtesy 7D Surgical Inc., Toronto, ON, Canada).

navigation for unilateral pedicle screw placement following interbody screw placement by a true transpsoas approach.

Minimally invasive approaches to the spine can be challenging, and there are multiple nuances of which surgeons should be aware. Many of these matters stem from the general lack of access as the entry path is often limited to a narrow channel, a significant detriment, particularly in comparison to arthroscopic approaches to large joints. When considering diskectomies, a larger working space often must be created within the disk to allow for its effective removal. An issue which may arise from a limited workspace is that specific pathology, often times, can only be accessed when instruments are placed in a particular trajectory. To combat this problem, variable angle scopes can allow for improved visualization in cases of challenging access. Recent improvements in wireless high-definition image transmission have further improved visualization, marking many of these concerns as invalid. With many trained surgeons, the visualization in these minimally invasive techniques can approach the level of an open procedure.

Conclusion

Minimally invasive spine surgery has the capacity to reduce patient morbidity and length of stay without detrimental effects to long-term outcomes. Given the lack of full visualization, as is afforded in traditional open approaches, minimally invasive spine surgery relies heavily on imaging. In the past, fluoroscopy has been the mainstay in terms of guiding both interbody cages and percutaneous pedicle screw placement. However, owing to concerns of radiation exposure to the spine surgeons and potential issues with accuracy, recent research has focused on the development of navigation-based techniques that allow computer-aided visualization of cage and screw orientation relative to bony structures.

The accuracy of navigation-based techniques for open pedicle screw placement is known to improve on that of both freehand and conventional fluoroscopy. Less information is available concerning how navigation influences the accuracy of both cage and percutaneous screw placement. And, although similar accuracy has been demonstrated concerning the lateral approach to interbody screw placement via either conventional fluoroscopy or navigation, the literature has demonstrated substantial improvements in accuracy when considering navigation of percutaneous pedicle screws by a posterior approach. Unfortunately, there is little information regarding navigated percutaneous screw placement when the patient remains in a lateral decubitus position.

Further research is needed to improve navigation technology and to further explore how it influences interbody cage placement accuracy. Although this topic is out of the scope of the present chapter, future studies will also be needed to fully evaluate the cost-effectiveness[22] of using navigation technology during interbody fusion cases, as this will have marked weight on clinical decision making. Ultimately, despite potential workflow variations and associated costs, the use of navigation-based techniques will become an important part of every minimally invasive spine surgeon's clinical practice.

References

1. Tian W, Xu YF, Liu B, et al. Computer-assisted minimally invasive transforaminal lumbar interbody fusion may be better than open surgery for treating degenerative lumbar disease. *J Spinal Disorders Tech*. 2017;30(6):237–242.
2. Funao H, Ishii K, Momoshima S, et al. Surgeons' exposure to radiation in single- and multi-level minimally invasive transforaminal lumbar interbody fusion; a prospective study. *PLoS One*. 2014;9(4):e95233.
3. Bindal RK, Glaze S, Ognoskie M, et al. Surgeon and patient radiation exposure in minimally invasive transforaminal lumbar interbody fusion. *Journal of neurosurgery. Spine*. 2008;9(6):570–573.
4. Cho JY, Chan CK, Lee SH, et al. The accuracy of 3D image navigation with a cutaneously fixed dynamic reference frame in minimally invasive transforaminal lumbar interbody fusion. *Comput Aided Surg*. 2012;17(6):300–309.
5. Taher F, Hughes AP, Sama AA, et al. 2013 Young Investigator Award winner: how safe is lateral lumbar interbody fusion for the surgeon? A prospective in vivo radiation exposure study. *Spine*. 2013;38(16):1386–1392.
6. Clark JC, Jasmer G, Marciano FF, et al. Minimally invasive transforaminal lumbar interbody fusions and fluoroscopy: a low-dose protocol to minimize ionizing radiation. *Neurosurg Focus*. 2013;35(2):E8.
7. Strong EB TT. Intraoperative use of CT Imaging. *Otolaryngol Clinic North Am*. 2013;46(5):719–732.
8. Fraser J, Gebhard H, Irie D, Parikh K, Hartl R. Iso-C/3-dimensional neuronavigation versus conventional fluoroscopy for minimally invasive pedicle screw placement in lumbar fusion. *Minim Invas Neurosurg*. 2010;53(4):184–190.
9. Wang Y, Le DQ, Li H, et al. Navigated percutaneous lumbosacral interbody fusion: a feasibility study with three-dimensional surgical simulation and cadaveric experiment. *Spine*. 2011;36(16):E1105–1111.
10. Nakashima H, Sato K, Ando T, et al. Comparison of the percutaneous screw placement precision of isocentric C-arm 3-dimensional fluoroscopy-navigated pedicle screw implantation and conventional fluoroscopy method with minimally invasive surgery. *J Spinal Disorders Tech*. 2009;22(7):468–472.
11. Drazin D, Liu JC, Acosta Jr FL. CT navigated lateral interbody fusion. *J Clin Neurosci*. 2013;20(10):1438–1441.

12. Park P. Three-dimensional computed tomography-based spinal navigation in minimally invasive lateral lumbar interbody fusion: feasibility, technique, and initial results. *Neurosurgery.* 2015;11(suppl 2):259–267.
13. Webb JE, Regev GJ, Garfin SR, et al. Navigation-assisted fluoroscopy in minimally invasive direct lateral interbody fusion: a cadaveric study. *SAS J.* 2010;4(4):115–121.
14. Bourgeois AC, Faulkner AR, Pasciak AS, Bradley YC. The evolution of image-guided lumbosacral spne surgery. *Ann Transl Med.* 2015;3(5):69.
15. Kosmopoulos V, Schizas C. Pedicle screw placement accuracy: a meta-analysis. *Spine.* 2007;32(3):E111–E120.
16. Gelalis ID, Paschos NK, Pakos EE, et al. Accuracy of pedicle screw placement: a systematic review of prospective in vivo studies comparing free hand, fluoroscopy guidance and navigation techniques. *Eur Spine J.* 2012;21(2):247–255.
17. Puvanesarajah V, Liauw JA, Lo SF, et al. Techniques and accuracy of thoracolumbar pedicle screw placement. *World J Orthop.* 2014; 5(2):112–123.
18. Tian NF, Huang QS, Zhou P, et al. Pedicle screw insertion accuracy with different assisted methods: a systematic review and meta-analysis of comparative studies. *Eur Spine J.* 2011;20(6):846–859.
19. Di Ieva A, Tam M, Tschabitscher M, et al. A journey into the technical evolution of neuroendoscopy. *World Neurosurg.* 2014;82(6): e777–e789.
20. Kantelhardt SR, Martinez R, Baerwinkel S, et al. Perioperative course and accuracy of screw positioning in conventional, open robotic-guided and percutaneous robotic-guided, pedicle screw placement. *Eur Spine J.* 2011;20(6):860–868.
21. Jones DB, Sung R, Weinberg C, Korelitz T, Andrews R. Three-dimensional modeling may improve surgical education and clinical practice. *Surg Innov.* 2016;23(2):189–195.
22. Al-Khouja L, Shweikeh F, Pashman R, et al. Economics of image guidance and navigation in spine surgery. *Surg Neurol Int.* 2015;6 (suppl 10):S323–S326.

6 Mini-Open Anterior Lumbar Interbody Fusion (ALIF)

R. DOUGLAS ORR

Introduction

The anterior lumbar interbody fusion (ALIF) is a powerful and versatile tool for obtaining interbody fusion for a variety of conditions. Anterior fusion for disk disease was first described by Burns,[1] and Harmon[2] first described a retroperitoneal approach in 1950. The current mini-open perirectus approach was first described by Crock.[3] Since that time many studies have been released using this approach for a variety of indications.[4–8] Although used predominantly to obtain fusion, it is also excellent for restoring lumbar lordosis[9] and can be used for indirect decompression, especially in the setting of foraminal stenosis.[10] The technique is used predominantly at L4-5 and L5-S1, but can be used at L3-4 and, in rare cases in the author's experience, at L2-3. It can be used for one-, two-, and, in slender patients, three-level procedures.

This surgery is most commonly done as a team approach with a vascular or general surgeon, but can be done safely by a properly trained spinal surgeon without a vascular surgeon.[11,12]

Indications

The mini-open ALIF can be used in almost any indication for lumbar fusion from L3 to the sacrum. It was initially described for fusion for back pain in disk degeneration.[3] It has been shown to provide good results in isthmic spondylolisthesis when combined with posterior instrumentation.[4] The author has also used the ALIF extensively in the setting of degenerative spondylolisthesis without central stenosis and iatrogenic spondylolisthesis after previous laminectomy. With the high failure rates seen in long fusions to the sacrum for adult deformity, it has become common to use the ALIF at the L5-S1 level to improve fusion rate.[6] The ability to release the anterior longitudinal ligament and place a trapezoidal cage or graft in the disk space makes it a powerful tool for restoration of lordosis.[9] The procedure can have very high fusion rates especially with the use of recombinant human bone morphogenetic protein (rhBMP2)[5] and, as a result, is often used in the treatment of symptomatic pseudarthrosis.[8] This is the author's preferred method of treating pseudarthrosis after posterolateral or posterior-based interbody fusions (PLIF and TLIF). It has also been used in the treatment of septic discitis.[7] This is a difficult indication because of the presence of significant lymphatic and inflammatory tissues around the vascular bifurcation (my experience). In patients with symptomatic foraminal stenosis who have failed direct decompression owing to the lack of vertical height in the foramen, an ALIF can significantly increase foraminal volume[10] and be a good treatment option.

Limitations

The limitations to the mini ALIF approach are generally either anatomic, approach, or diagnosis related. The anatomic plane used for this approach is prerenal. As a result, when trying to reach the upper lumbar levels the renal artery and kidney prevent access to the disk. As a result, the upper limit is generally the L3-4 level. The approach corridor should be collinear to the disk to allow appropriate disk preparation and implant placement. In patients with a high sacral slope, a collinear approach is blocked by the symphysis pubis and is anatomically not possible. The vascular anatomy of the lumbosacral junction is quite variable. In some cases the location of the bifurcation can make access to the disk difficult or impossible.[13]

Obesity is a relative contraindication to the ALIF approach. The width of the access corridor is limited by the width of the rectus sheath. In obese patients, particularly those with higher retroperitoneal or intraperitoneal fat deposits, the distance to the spine and the narrow corridor make the approach very difficult. In an obese patient with mostly prefascial fat, a longer skin incision can be used to reach the rectus sheath, and the approach may be possible. The author tends to use a body mass index of more than 35 as a cut-off for the ALIF approach.

Although it has been shown that increasing disk height with an ALIF can increase central canal diameter,[10] use of the ALIF approach for the treatment of severe central stenosis is probably not warranted. Similarly, the treatment of central stenosis in a patient with no listhesis and normal disk height would not be effective.

As mentioned previously, this approach can be used for the treatment of discitis and osteomyelitis. The limiting factor here is how much thickening of the perivascular tissues around the bifurcation exists. This thickened tissue makes identifying and mobilizing the great vessels difficult. Careful study of the preoperative imaging is necessary to see if the approach would be safe in this setting.

The ability to develop the retroperitoneal plane and mobilize the vessels is the key to safely reaching the disk space. In patients who have had previous retroperitoneal surgery or radiation, the planes no longer exist and the ALIF is not an option. Previous abdominal surgery is generally not a limitation. The exception to this is in patients with pelvic floor reconstructions where a sling has been tacked up to the sacrum. It may be necessary to obtain previous operative notes to see if this was done. The necessity of mobilizing the left common iliac vein and location of the inferior vena cave makes a left-sided retroperitoneal approach mandatory for L3-4 and L4-5. In the author's experience, in some patients with previous left-sided ALIF where the left common iliac is relatively lateral, a right-sided approach can be used to access L5-S1 and is sometimes also used in an isolated L5-S1 fusion to preserve the left-sided retroperitoneum for potential future surgery.

Technique

Preoperative Assessment

When assessing patients for possible anterior interbody fusion several factors need to be considered. The first consideration is whether the disk can be accessed successfully. In morbidly obese individuals the mini-open ALIF approach is sometimes impossible owing to the distance from skin to spine. In the author's practice those with a body mass index of greater than 35 are usually not candidates. Previous retroperitoneal surgery or radiation are also contraindications. One exception to this in the author's practice is a previous left-sided ALIF surgery if attempting to access L5-S1. In many cases it possible to do these through a right-sided approach.

Careful review of the preoperative imaging will also identify patients unsuited to this approach. A standing lateral x-ray study, including the symphysis pubis, should always be performed. If a projected line from the superior endplate of S1 does not pass above the symphysis, the disk space will be inaccessible and an alternate fusion technique should be used (Fig. 6.1). In addition, the x-ray study will show the relationship of the spinal levels to superficial bony landmarks to guide incision placement (Fig. 6.2).

Careful review of a computed tomography scan or magnetic resonance image will usually give a good view of the vascular anatomy and will, in some cases, reveal anatomy unfavorable to the procedure.[13] Computed tomography and magnetic resonance imaging are also very useful in patients where a surgeon is considering an ALIF for infection. The dense concentration of lymphatic tissue related to the periaortic lymphatics can make this approach very difficult in these patients.

Operative Technique

Anesthesia and Positioning

Mini ALIF is performed under general anesthesia with neuromuscular blockade. Not having skeletal relaxation makes the approach much more difficult. A Foley catheter should be placed because a full bladder can interfere with the approach. The patient is positioned supine on the surgeon's table of choice. A flexible table

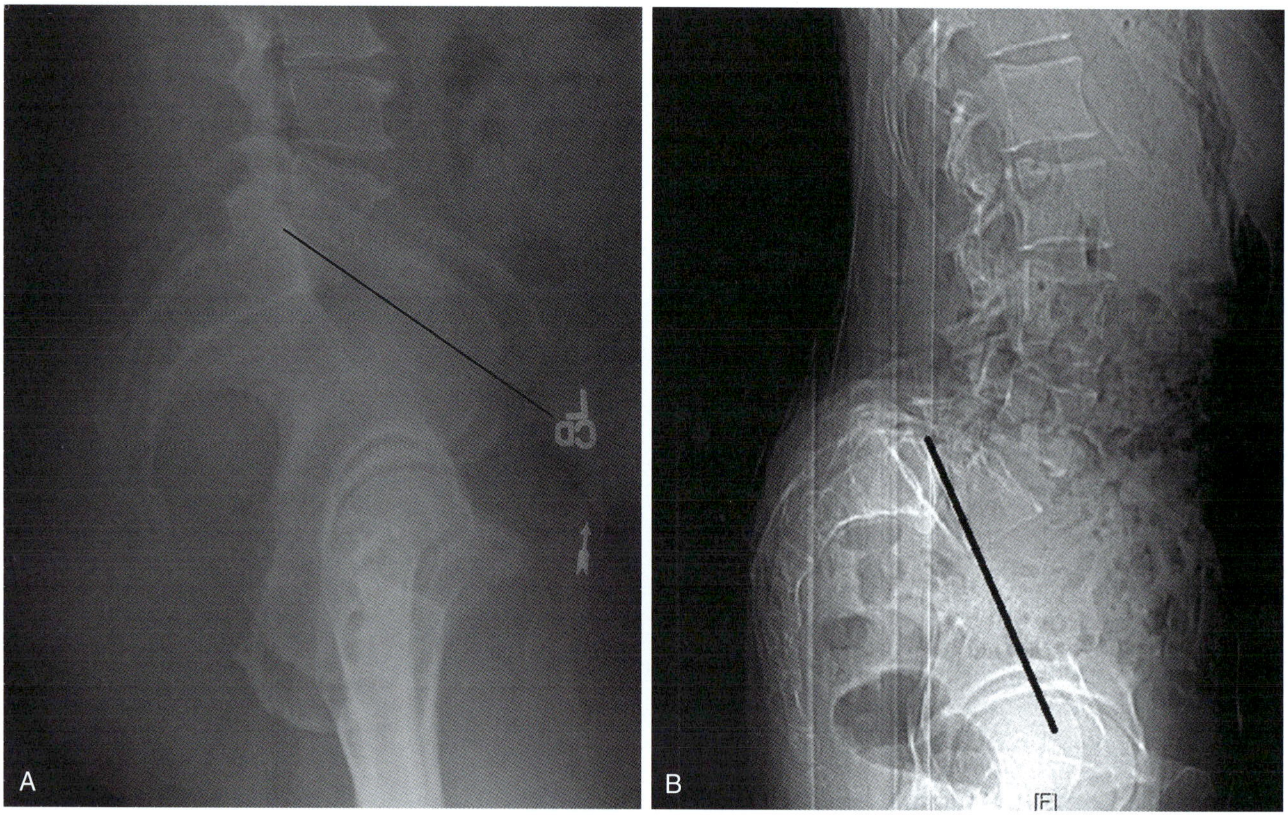

• **Fig. 6.1** **A.** The line projected from the S1 endplate is above the pubic symphysis and an anterior lumbar interbody fusion (ALIF) approach is possible. **B.** A line projected from the S1 endplate passes below the symphysis and an ALIF approach would not be possible.

with a kidney rest placed under the level of interest can be used to increase lumbar lordosis. The author's preference is a flat radiolucent table with an inflatable arterial line bag placed under the level of interest to be inflated or deflated as necessary during the procedure. In three-level procedures, increasing the lumbar lordosis will often make access to L3-4 very difficult so the author do not inflate the bag until this level is done. In addition, if the incision has been made too low to access the upper of two disks, reducing any applied lordosis can ease exposure.

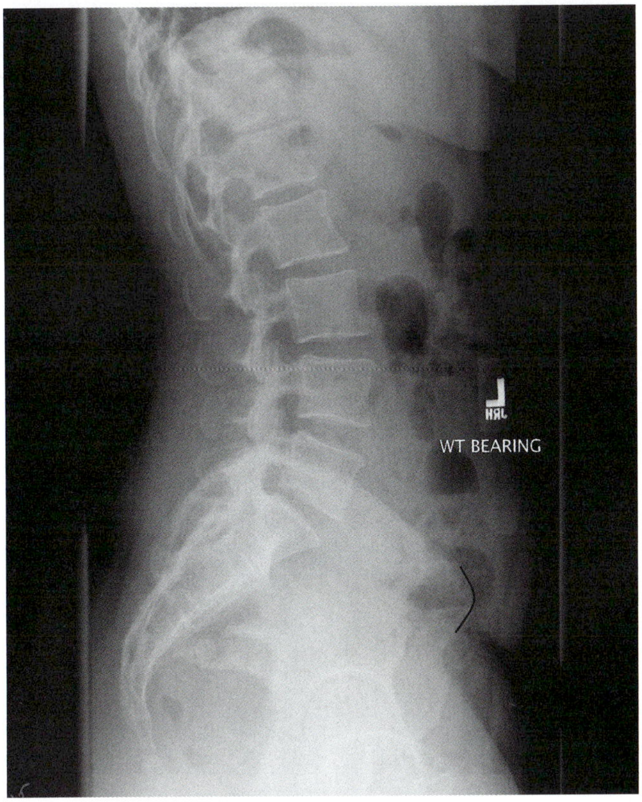

• **Fig. 6.2** The anterior superior iliac spine is outlined. In this patient an incision for an L5-S1 anterior lumbar interbody fusion would be at the level of the ASIS. L4-5 would be reached through an incision above the iliac crest. *ASIS*, anterior superior iliac spine.

Incision

Some authors advocate using the umbilicus as a guide to placing the incision.[14] In the author's experience this is a highly mobile and unreliable landmark. In many patients' once anesthetized, the sacral promontory can be directly palpated and used as a landmark. The preoperative x-ray can be used to compare the location of the anterior superior iliac spine to the level of interest (Fig. 6.3). The top of the iliac crest can also be used, but it is less reliable in obese patients. When in doubt, fluoroscopy may be utilized to identify the level. Incision should be colinear with the inferior endplate for single level procedures; midpoint of the intervening vertebral body for two levels and colinear with the middle disk in three levels. A transverse skin incision can be used in single or multilevel procedures. The rectus is divided transversely in single level procedures and obliquely inferomedial to superolateral for a multilevel procedure.

Steps of the Surgical Procedure

The incision is carried down to the rectus fascia, which is then divided (Fig. 6.4). It is generally easier to enter the preperitoneal and retroperitoneal intervals lateral to the rectus muscle, but going lateral to the rectus can make it difficult to get across the midline once on the disk space. Rectus innervation comes from lateral to medial direction, so an approach medial to the rectus has a lower risk of denervating the muscle. The author's preference is to go lateral to the rectus for all single-level procedures and selectively go medially in multilevels. Often the musculotendinous insertions of the rectus muscle to the fascia are encountered. These are sharply

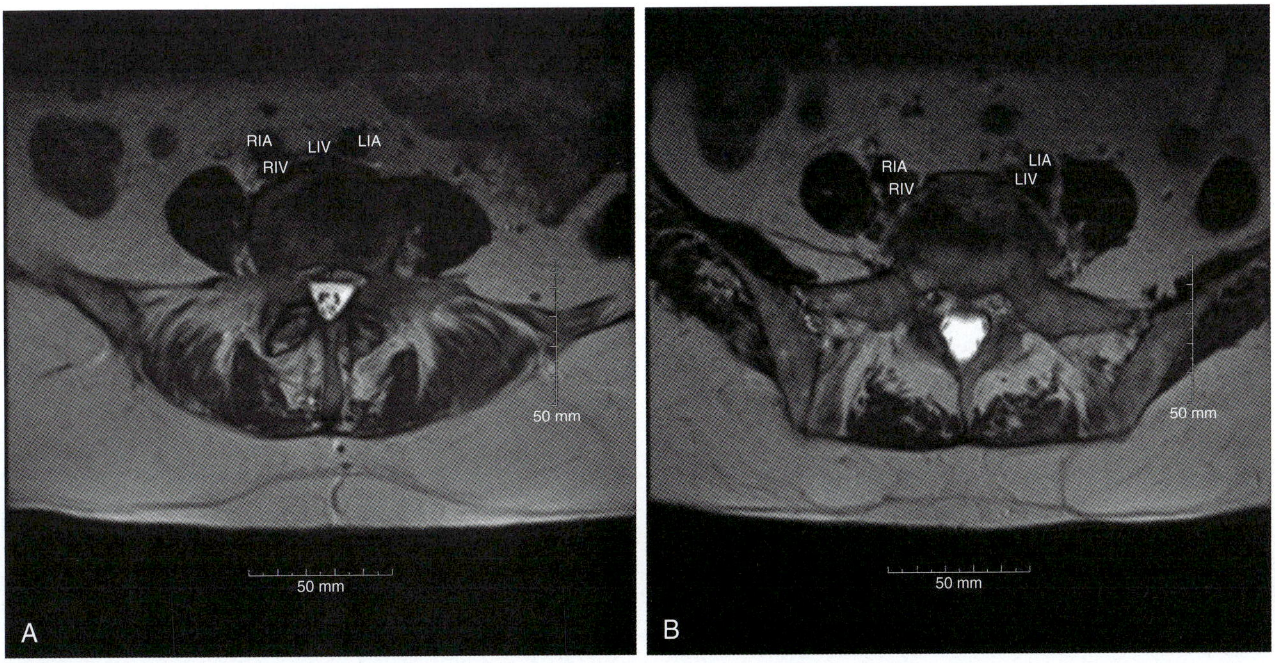

• **Fig. 6.3 A.** An axial magnetic resonance image (MRI) through the L4-5 disk space identifying the right iliac artery *(RIA)*, right iliac vein *(RIV)*, left iliac vein *(LIV)*, and left iliac artery *(LIA)*. **B.** An axial MRI through the L5-S1 disk space in the same patient.

dissected off the posterior aspect of the anterior sheath to mobilize the muscle.

Blunt dissection with finger or sponge stick in an inferolateral direction is used to start to develop the intervals. Once the interior aspect of the iliac wing and its overlying iliacus muscle are identified, begin to sweep the peritoneum medially and sweep up to identify the arcuate line that is the inferior margin of the posterior rectus sheath. This is usually more palpable than visible (Fig. 6.5). Peritoneum is then swept medially off of the posterior sheath and the sheath is divided longitudinally as far laterally as possible. In some cases the arcuate line cannot be identified. In this case, elevate the posterior sheath with toothed forceps and sharply divide the sheath for 3 to 5 mm. Then use a Kittner dissector to sweep peritoneum off the sheath and then divide it. If a peritonectomy occurs it should be repaired as soon as possible to prevent herniation of abdominal contents.

Blunt dissection is used to sweep the peritoneum medially; the next structure to be exposed should be the psoas muscle. This is directly visualized and carried medially until either the left common iliac artery or the sulcus between the psoas and the spine is visualized. Ureter will often be seen on the posterior aspect of the peritoneum and should be mobilized medially still adherent to the sac (Fig. 6.6).

Retractor Systems

Numerous retractor systems are available in the market. Some are designed specifically for this procedure and some are general vascular retractors. Some attach to the table and some to the spine directly through screws in the blade. Which one to use is a very personal decision. The author's preference is a system that attaches to the table on both sides of the patient bccausc this is more stable (Fig. 6.7). Retractor blades that can be pivoted are useful. Occasionally a small sharp Hohman retractor impacted into the bone and secured to the retractor frame or a Steinman pin can also be useful to maintain exposure.

Exposure of the L4-5 Level

The L4-5 is typically the most difficult level to expose. Begin by palpating the disk space. Assemble the retractor system and place one blade medially holding the iliac artery and aorta. One blade superior and one inferior are then placed. The level should be confirmed with x-ray before proceeding. Using a kittner dissector, bisect bluntly until annulus is visualized and sweep as much tissue medially as possible. Visualize the lateral edge of the left common iliac vein. It is important to carefully explore for the iliolumbar vein

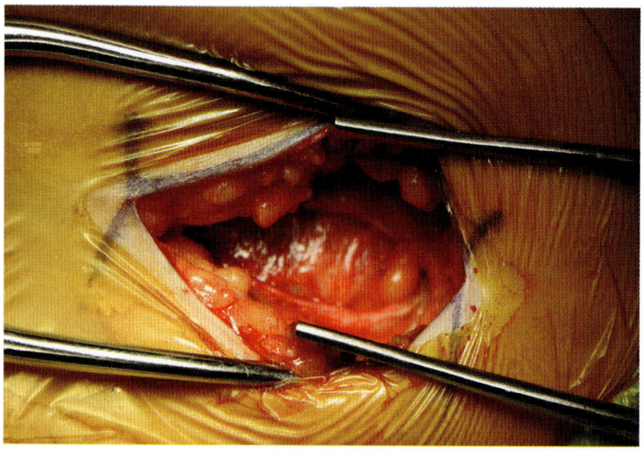

• **Fig. 6.4** Skin incision has been made and the fascia of the anterior rectus sheath has been divided revealing the fibers of the rectus sheath underneath.

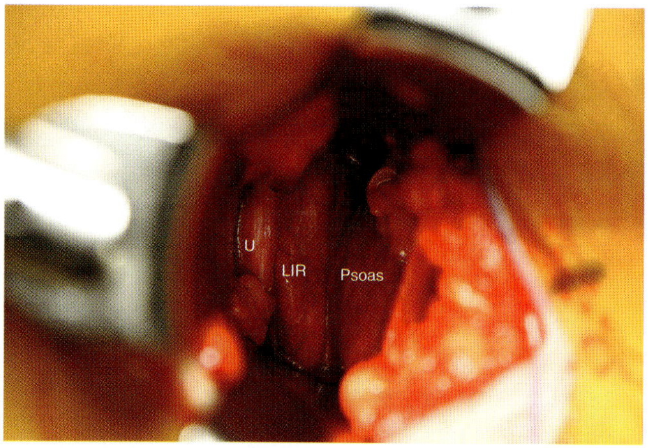

• **Fig. 6.6** The deep layer prior to exposing the spine showing the psoas (Psoas), left iliac artery (LIA), and ureter (U).

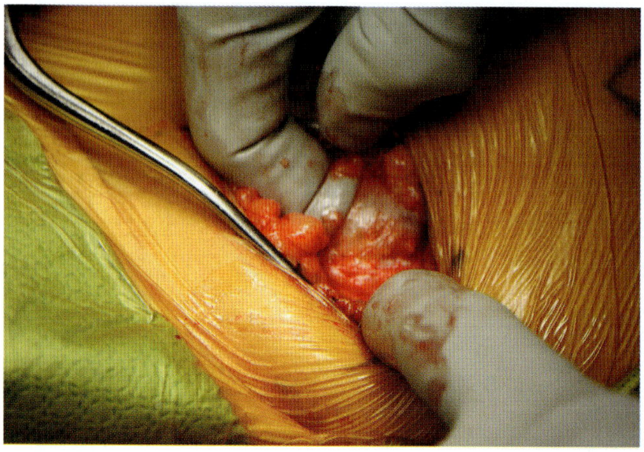

• **Fig. 6.5** A finger has been placed under the inferior margin of the posterior rectus sheath demonstrating the arcuate line that would then be divided longitudinally.

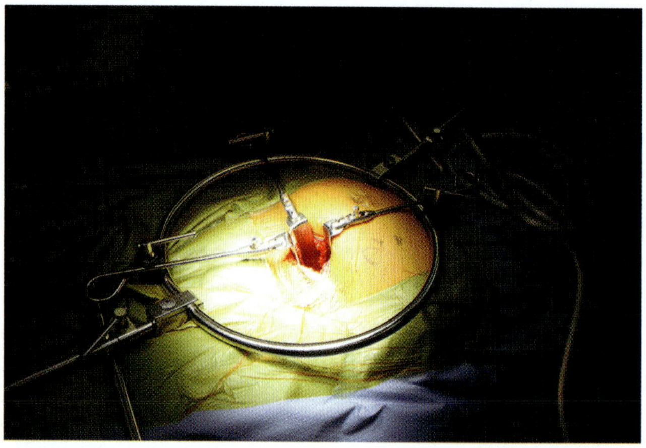

• **Fig. 6.7** A table-mounted retractor system designed for the anterior lumbar interbody fusion (ALIF) procedure that can be mounted to both sides of the table.

at this point. This vein can be quite variable in its occurrence and location.[15] It arises off the posterolateral aspect of the left common iliac vein. It is usually easiest to visualize by applying gentle retraction to the vein medially and then following the lateral aspect of the vein until a structural tether appears preventing the vein from being moved. It generally runs posterosuperiorly toward the L5 foramen. If found, it should be tied off and divided. Vascular clips can be used, but in the author's experience, they have a tendency to come off while manipulating the vein. Always look for a second and even a third before moving on as multiple veins can occur (Fig. 6.8).

Once the iliolumbar vein has been divided, use blunt dissection directly on the annulus to mobilize the left common iliac inferiorly and laterally until the disk is visualized and retractors are secured.

In some patients the vein can be tightly adherent to the disk and difficult to mobilize. In the author's experience patients being operated for pseudarthrosis of a previous posterior interbody fusion are a particular problem as are those with a previous infection.

Exposure of the L5-S1 Level

To expose the L5-S1 level, work in the interval just medial to the left common iliac vein. Palpate the disk. Place the right side retractor blade and a superior one holding the aortic bifurcation. Use a kittner dissector to dissect tissue bluntly off the annulus. Look for the midline sacral vessels. There are typically two veins and one artery but, as with the iliolumbar vein, the vessels can be quite variable.[16] If the vessels are small they can be taken with bipolar cautery and divided. Larger veins, up to 1 cm, can be found and should be ligated. Often working in the bed posterior to the divided vessels provides the easiest way to remove tissue from the disk annulus.

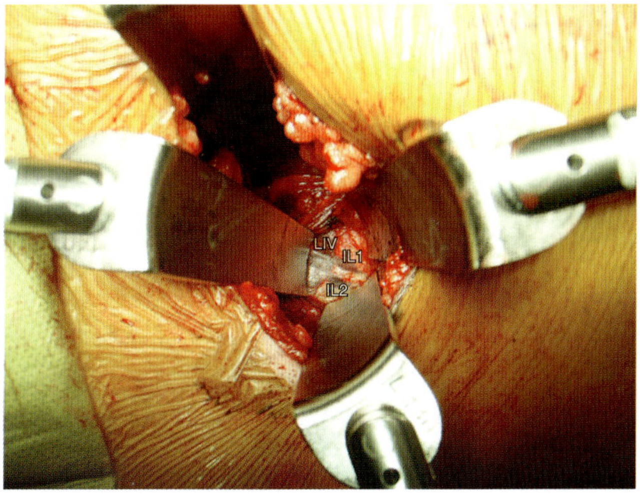

• **Fig. 6.8** During an approach to L4-5, the left iliac vein has been identified as having two iliolumbar veins.

The left common iliac vein will often overlay the superolateral aspect of the disk and should be bluntly swept off the disk and held under a retractor blade (Fig. 6.9).

Exposure of the L3-4 Level

It is often difficult to get below the inferior margin of the posterior sheath when approaching the L3-4 level. In this case, elevate and divide the posterior sheath through a small incision, then sweep peritoneum off the sheath and divide it longitudinally. The remainder of the initial approach is the same.

Look at the preoperative axial images and, in most cases, the inferior vena cava will be found on the right side of the disk space and is usually not seen once the disk is exposed.

Once the disk is palpated, retractor blades are placed. The author prefers to place one blade medially, one superior and lastly one inferior to maintain exposure. These should be ligated and divided. The L4 segmental vein is relatively more tethered and less mobile owing to its proximity to the bifurcation, and it is more susceptible to avulsion. In the author's experience, the L3 segmental vessel does not usually need to be divided. Once the vessel has been divided, bluntly sweep the anterior tissues across the annulus to expose the disk.

Diskectomy and Endplate Preparation

The amount of the disk needing to be exposed depends on the size of implant intended for the space. A wider exposure allows an easier diskectomy but involves more risk to the iliac vein and vena cava, especially at L4-5. At a minimum, the exposure should be slightly more than the width of the intended implant.

Once the disk is exposed, the annulus is incised. The author's preference is to perform a box annulotomy with resection of the annulus. A Cobb elevator can then be used to separate the endplate cartilage from the subchondral bone. Currettes are then used

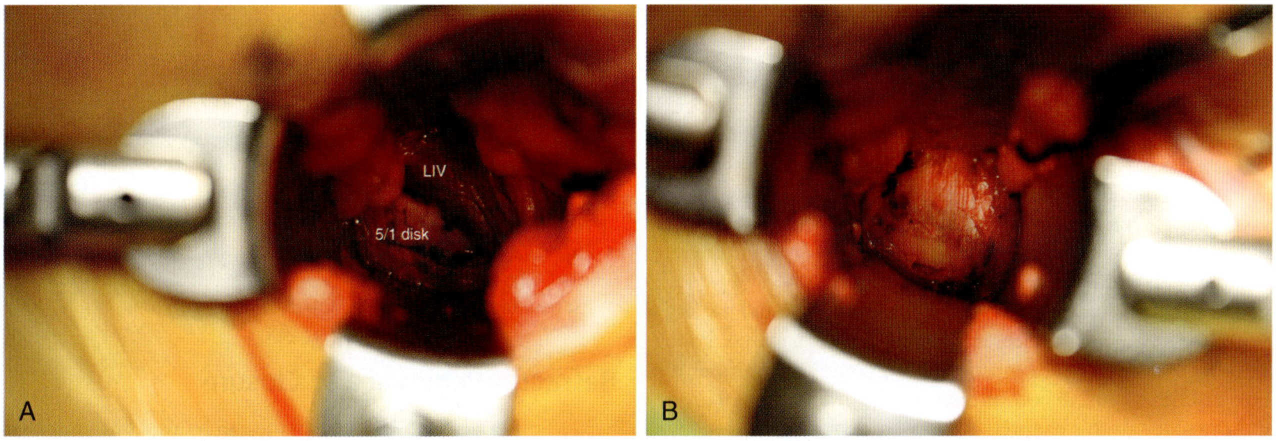

• **Fig. 6.9** **A.** An exposure of the L5-S1 disk showing an overlying left iliac vein. **B.** The left iliac vein and bifurcation of the iliac veins have now been placed under the retractor blades exposing the L5-S1 disk.

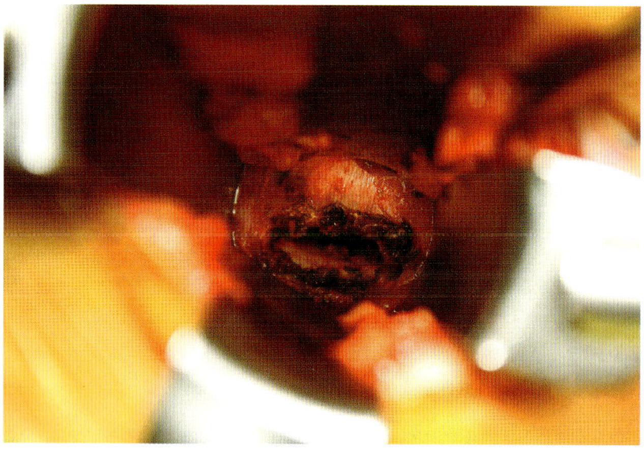

• **Fig. 6.10** An annulotomy has been made and a diskectomy carried out. Cautery has been used to remove superfluous annular fibers.

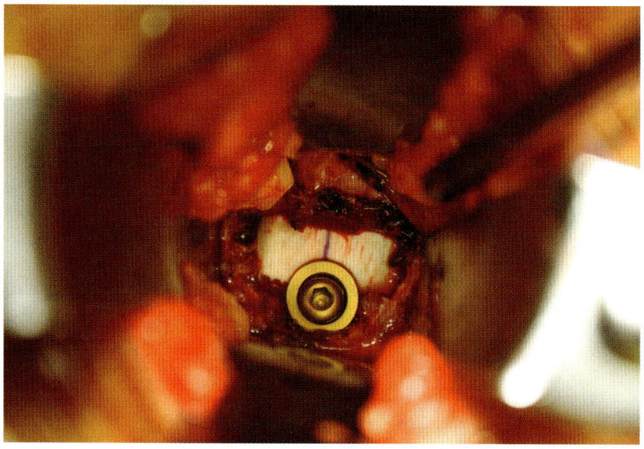

• **Fig. 6.11** After completing the diskectomy, a femoral ring allograft implant has been placed. A screw with a washer has been placed to prevent the graft dislodging while the patient is transferred prone for posterior instrumentation.

to remove the nucleus pulposus and endplate cartilages. All disk material, other than the lateral and posterior annulus, should be removed and the endplates should be curetted down to the point of visualizing punctate-bleeding bone to adequately prepare the fusion bed (Fig. 6.10).

Implant Placement

Numerous implant options are available, including allograft, autograft (Fig. 6.11), threaded cages, and impacted cages. Some cages also have integrated screws or spikes for stability. No good comparative studies suggest any one has significant clinical advantages and surgeon preference guides most implant choices. One caveat is the use of structural allograft with rhBMP-2 as a stand-alone, which has been shown to have a high failure rate.[17] This effect can be obviated with rigid posterior instrumentation.[18]

One of the goals of ALIF surgery is to restore disk height and lordosis. The height of the nearest normal disk is usually a good guide to implant height and most implants come in a number of lordotic profiles. A discussion of how much lordosis to obtain is beyond the scope of this chapter, but a good rule is to aim for sufficient increased lordosis so that the superior endplate of L4 would be parallel to the floor on the *standing film* (Fig 6.12).

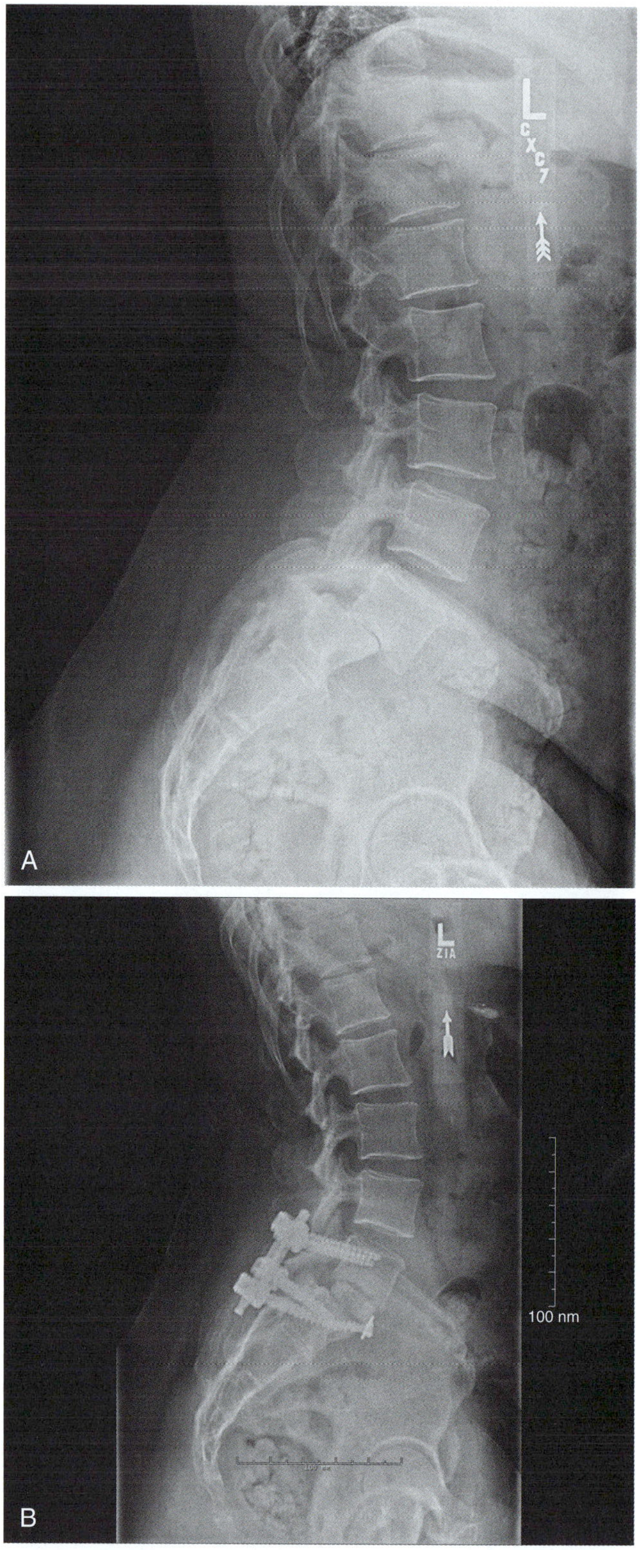

• **Fig. 6.12** Pre- (A) and postoperative (B) lateral x-rays of a 42-year-old woman who underwent anterior lumbar interbody fusion and posterior instrumentation for a grade 2 degenerative spondylolisthesis.

Retractor Removal and Closure

When removing the retractor blades after implantation, extreme caution must be exercised to remove them because of the potential for vascular injury; the dictum is to remove the most risky blade first. This would be the right-sided blade at L3-4 and L4-5; the left-sided blade at L5-S1 followed by the inferior blade at L4-5 and the superior blade at L5-S1. That way, if significant bleeding does occur, you have better retraction to obtain control and directly repair the torn vessels. Once the blades are removed the anterior sheath is repaired and the skin closed. The posterior sheath does not need to be repaired.

Postoperative Care

In general, patients can begin drinking clear fluids immediately and rapidly progress their diet. Activity restrictions postoperative are based more on the status of the posterior spine. If done as a stand-alone, activity can be resumed fairly quickly. More extensive posterior surgery will necessitate a more gradual return to activity.

Presacral Parasympathetic Plexus and Retrograde Ejaculation

One of the known risks of the ALIF approach is retrograde ejaculation.[15] This is caused by damage to the presacral parasympathetic plexus.[15] It is less common in the retroperitoneal approach. Risk can be lessened with careful technique. Avoid the use of monopolar cautery on the disk space and bluntly dissect down on to the annulus and sweep the filmy tissues anterior to the annulus containing the plexus as one mass in the direction of exposure. Once the annular incision has been made, monopolar cautery can be used within the disk space.

Conclusion

The anterior mini-open ALIF approach is a valuable tool in the treatment of many pathologies of the lower lumbar spine. It is relatively minimally invasive and well-tolerated. It provides for high fusion rates and excellent restoration of lordosis compared to TLIF or lateral LIF. It does have limitations and is difficult to perform in obese patients, revision patients and those with difficult vascular anatomy. Although usually done with an approach/access surgeon (i.e., vascular or general surgeon), it can be also safely done by appropriately trained spine surgeon without such assistance with exposure. Overall, anterior mini-open ALIF is a valuable tool in a surgeon's armamentarium.

References

1. Burns B. An operation for spondylolisthesis. *Lancet*. 1933;19:1223.
2. Harmon P. Anterior disc excision and vertebral body fusion for intervertebral disc syndromes of the lower lumbar spine: three- to five-year results in 244 cases. *Clin Orthop*. 1963;26:107–127.
3. Crock H. Anterior lumbar interbody fusion. *Clin Orthop*. 1982;165:157–163.
4. Swan J. Surgical treatment for unstable low-grade isthmic spondylolisthesis in adults: a prospective controlled study of posterior instrumented fusion compared with combined anterior-posterior fusion. *Spine J*. 2006;6(6):606–614.
5. Burkus JK. Six-year outcomes of anterior lumbar interbody arthrodesis with use of interbody fusion cages and recombinant human bone morphogenetic protein-2. *J Bone Joint Surg Am*. 2009;91(5):1181–1189.
6. Dorward IG. Transforaminal versus anterior lumbar interbody fusion in long deformity constructs: a matched cohort analysis. *Spine (Phila Pa 1976)*. 2013;38(12):E755–E762.
7. Lin Y. Single level lumbar pyogenic spondylodiscitis treated with mini-open anterior debridement and fusion in combination with posterior percutaneous fixation via a modified anterior lumbar interbody fusion approach. *J Neurosurg Spine*. 2015;23(6):747–753.
8. Chun DS. Lumbar pseudarthrosis: a review of current diagnosis and treatment. *Neurosurg Focus*. 2015;39(4):E10.
9. Uribe JS. 'Preservation or restoration of segmental and regional spinal lordosis using minimally invasive interbody fusion techniques in degenerative lumbar conditions: a literature review. *Spine (Phila Pa 1976)*. 2016;41(suppl 8):S50–S58.
10. Kim NH. A computed tomographic analysis of the changes in the spinal canal after anterior lumbar interbody fusion. *Clin Orthop Relat Res*. 1993;286:180–191.
11. Jarrett CD. Anterior exposure of the lumbar spine with and without an "access surgeon": morbidity analysis of 265 cases. *J Spine Disord Tech*. 2009;22(8):559–564.
12. Holt RT. The efficacy of anterior spine exposure by an orthopedic surgeon. *J Spine Disord Tech*. 2003;16(5):477–486.
13. Inamasu J. Three dimensional computed tomography of the abdominal great vessels pertinent to L4-L5 anterior lumbar interbody fusion. *Minim Invasive Neurosurg*. 2005;48(3):127–131.
14. Guyer RD. Perirectus retroperitoneal approach for anterior lumbar interbody fusion. In: TA Zdeblick TA, ed. *Anterior Approaches to the Spine*. St. Louis: Quality Medical Publishing; 1999:203–216.
15. Tiusanen H. Retrograde ejaculation after anterior lumbar interbody fusion. *Eur Spine J*. 1995;4(6):339–342.
16. Sasso RC. Retrograde ejaculation after anterior lumbar interbody fusion: transperitoneal versus retroperitoneal approach. *Spine (Phila PA 1976)*. 2003;28(10):1023–1026.
17. Nalbandian MM. Variations in the iliolumbar vein during the anterior approach for spinal procedures. *Spine (Phil Pa 1976)*. 2013;38(8):E445–E4450.
18. Tribus CB. The vascular anatomy anterior to the L5/S1 disc space. *Spine (Phila PA 1976)*. 2001;26(11):1205–1208.

7

Posterior Lumbar Interbody Fusion (PLIF)

ANDRE M. JAKOI, NEIL N. PATEL, MARTIN H. PHAM, AND JEFFREY C. WANG

Introduction

The technique of posterior lumbar interbody fusion (PLIF) is an important technique in the current spine surgeon's armamentarium. That being said, the surgery is still defined by its level of technical difficulty and controversy exists regarding the safety of PLIF compared with other approaches to the intervertebral space.[1,2]

The first in-depth description of a PLIF was described by Cloward, as an operation where the disk space is exposed from a posterior approach and a fusion is performed by directly grafting the intervertebral space.[3] Classically, PLIF is performed via bilateral MEDIAL facet resection and exposure of the disk space; with retraction of the dura, the disk is visualized. Initially, some advocated that the procedure be maintained at the height of the neural foramen after diskectomy, preventing collapse and keeping the nerve root free of bony compression. The procedure also has the advantage of potentially increasing the fusion rate by direct graft-to-bone contact with compressive force (i.e., by placing the bone graft in the intervertebral space).

Posterior lumbar interbody fusion added extensively to the procedure of lumbar fusion, but it is not without its downsides. The procedure (see below) requires resection of the medial facet and retraction of the dura and traversing nerve root to visualize the disk space in order to perform the interbody fusion. At times, this retraction may be significant. As compared with transforaminal lumbar interbody fusion and posterior lateral fusion, there has been greater reports of dural tear, epidural fibrosis, nerve root injury, and chronic arachnoiditis.

Although more recent advances, such as transforaminal and direct lateral approaches to the disk space, have decreased the frequency in which PLIF is performed, PLIF remains an important staple for spine surgeons.

Surgical Indications

The literature still supports surgeon preference in regard to interbody fusion and its indication whenever a lumbar fusion is performed. The argument that the intervertebral space is biologically and mechanically superior for fusion compared with the intertransverse space because of its larger surface area of highly vascular bony endplate and because the interbody bone graft is subject to compressive forces, is a controversial one. Despite those theoretic advantages and the avoidance of large amounts of muscle damage that occur from exposure for posterolateral fusion, it has been difficult to show clinical superiority of interbody fusions over posterolateral fusions for most lumbar degenerative pathology. Most published studies comparing the techniques reveal similar outcomes regardless of what fusion technique is performed.[4-6] That being said however, there are certain circumstances when interbody fusion offers definite advantages, such as adding an interbody fusion to a posterolateral fusion which has been shown to increase the rate of achieving successful arthrodesis.[7] Additionally, placement of an interbody graft at the anterior column allows for restoration of optimal disk height and therefore maintenance or improvement of segmental lordosis and optimal sagittal balance.

Some authors have argued that interbody fusion should be combined with posterolateral fusion in patients at high risk for failed fusion, such as smokers.[8] For patients with pseudoarthrosis after failed posterolateral fusion, an interbody technique is a good salvage operation to augment revision procedures. In patients with isthmic spondylolisthesis who undergo deformity reduction, it has been well documented that an interbody graft offers a biomechanical advantage, which protects pedicle screw instrumentation with an anterior load sharing graft and aiding in maintenance of alignment.[4,8,9] Controversially, the procedure may be used in augmenting the ablation of the disk space in patients with discogenic pain with the thought process being only interbody fusion can completely remove motion at a painful disk and the nuclear material resection may eliminate the anatomic source of pain.[9,10] It is known that the outer annulus is richly innervated with nociceptive fibers and that mechanical deformation or inflammation caused by a damaged nucleus can stimulate these nociceptors. One thought is that although posterolateral fusion can increase axial stiffness by 40%, interbody fusion can increase axial stiffness by 80% to minimize any micromotion even further and reduce any nociceptive stimulation of sensitized painful disks. Lastly, interbody fusion by technique allows for removal of much disk tissue along with any nociceptors involved in the generation of pain.

Open vs. Minimally Invasive

Open Technique

The patient is positioned in hyperextension to help create lumbar lordosis (Fig. 7.1). The abdomen should hang free for unimpeded venous return, which will decompress the epidural venous plexus and help reduce bleeding. A radiolucent positioning frame is useful so that intraoperative fluoroscopic imaging can be obtained to

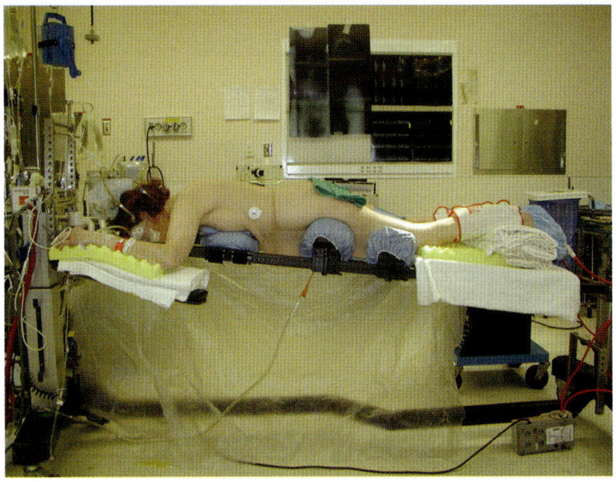

• **Fig. 7.1** Patient in the prone position on a Jackson table illustrating hyperextension of the lumbar spine. (Adapted from Benzel E. *Spine Surgery: Techniques, Complication Avoidance, & Management*. 3rd ed. Philadelphia: Elsevier Saunders; 2012: Fig. 53-2b.)

confirm correct placement of screws and grafts. Attention should also be directed to the proper position of chest support, which will help to ensure adequate ventilation. Orbital pressure should always be avoided to prevent mechanical damage to the cornea or globe, which may ultimately cause visual loss. Some surgeons may choose to place the patient in a slightly reversed Trendelenburg position to help reduce the heightened intraocular pressure incurred by the prone position. Arms may be positioned outstretched or tucked next to the patient but done so as to prevent brachial plexus injury and allow for easy access to intravenous lines. If positioning the arms outstretched, they should be placed with shoulder abduction and elbow flexion to 90 degrees.

Using a combination of external landmarks, palpation of the spinous processes if possible, and/or the use of preoperative fluoroscopy, a midline incision should be planned over the levels of interest. A standard approach to the posterior lumbar spine is performed with dissection through subcutaneous tissue to the lumbosacral fascia. This is usually done with electrocautery as to provide hemostasis but may be done with sharp dissection of a scalpel. Sharp dissection is continued through the fascia. Once the correct levels are then identified using intraoperative fluoroscopy, exposure of the laminae above and below the level to be fused is completed using a subperiosteal technique. Further dissection is continued to the transverse processes of each level. It is important to remember which facet joint capsules may be sacrificed and which joint capsules should be preserved in order not to incur a potential for early adjacent segment disease by destabilizing the level above or below your proposed fusion construct. Once subperiosteal dissection is completed in regard to the laminae and transverse processes of each level, dissection is complete and laminectomy may be initiated (Fig. 7.2).

Pedicle screws may be placed before or after beginning the interbody fusion based on surgeon preference. The surgeon should be aware, however, that PLIF destabilizes the motion segment and should require adequate pedicle fixation.

A wide laminectomy and resection of the medial portion of the facet joints are essential to minimize retraction of the dura and nerve roots. A large amount of variation exists in regard to surgeon preference for the amount of bony resection; however, commonly it is carried laterally as far as the pedicle, removing at least half of the superior and inferior facets. The wide exposure will help avoid traction injury to the lumbar roots which may cause neuropathic pain and weakness (Figs. 7.3 and 7.4). In general, the exposure of

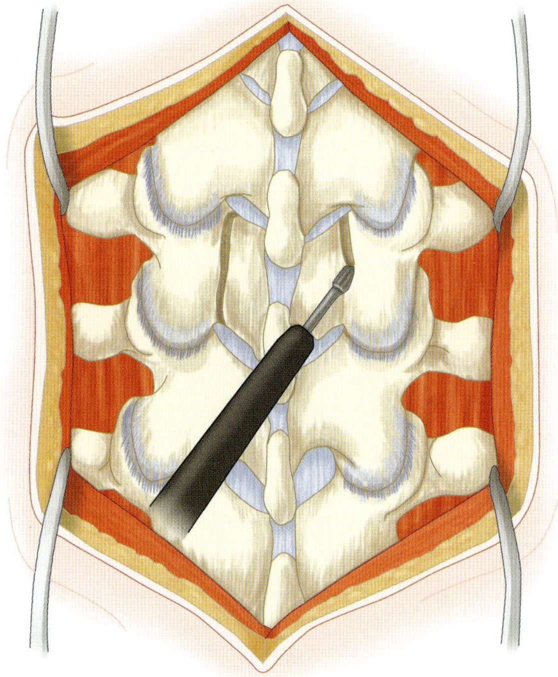

• **Fig. 7.2** Operative view of the surgical anatomy and exposure just prior to laminectomy, with transverse processes visualized. (Adapted from Benzel E. *Spine Surgery: Techniques, Complication Avoidance, & Management*. 3rd ed. Philadelphia: Elsevier Saunders; 2012: Fig. 53-4.)

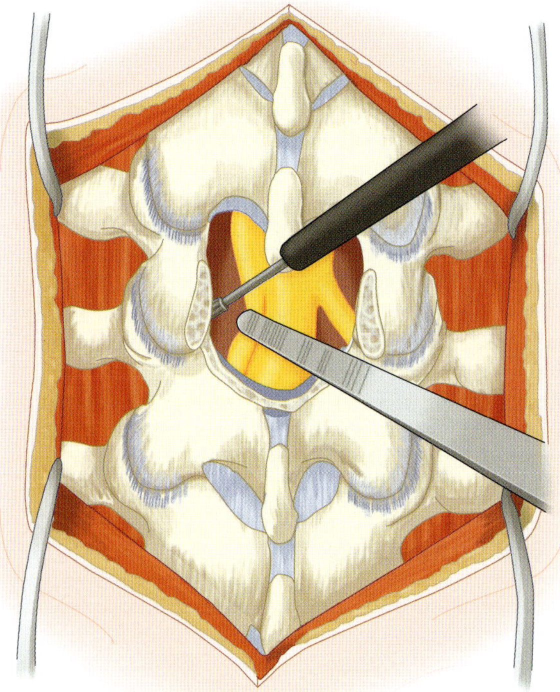

• **Fig. 7.3** Operative view of the surgical anatomy and exposure post laminectomy. (Adapted from Benzel E. *Spine Surgery: Techniques, Complication Avoidance, & Management*. 3rd ed. Philadelphia: Elsevier Saunders; 2012: Fig. 53-7.)

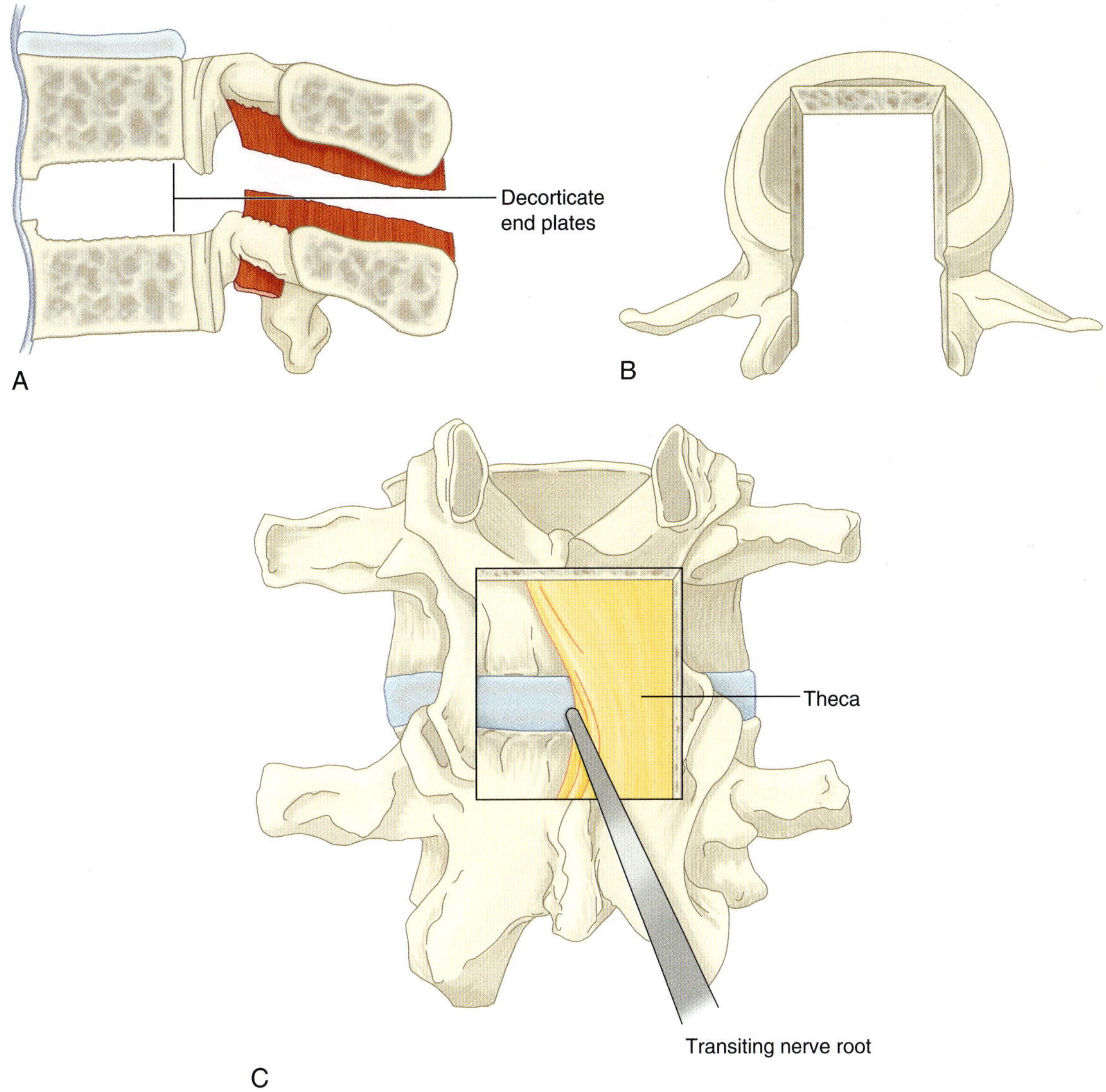

• **Fig. 7.4** Operative view of the surgical anatomy. (A) Sagittal view (B) axial view (C) coronal view with exposure and dura retracted to visualize the disk space. (Adapted from Benzel E. *Spine Surgery: Techniques, Complication Avoidance, & Management*. 3rd ed. Philadelphia: Elsevier Saunders; 2012: Fig. 54-1b/c.)

the disk space should extend lateral to the medial border of the pedicle below. Adequate exposure may require sacrifice of the facet joints, particularly in the upper lumbar spine, which will not destabilize the spine once pedicle screw fixation is implemented. The facet joints should always be removed when correcting deformity because this facilitates correction at that particular level. The superior edge of the upper lamina should be preserved to maintain the posterior ligamentous attachments to the vertebra above the fusion.

An abundant epidural plexus is usually encountered at the lateral border of the spinal canal. Bipolar electrocautery and packing with cottoned patties can prevent the excessive bleeding that may accompany an interbody fusion technique. Following cauterization, the venous plexus should be sharply divided to facilitate mobilization of the nerve roots and dura. A nerve root retractor is used to retract the dura and provide a degree of protection. The dura should not be retracted past the midline of the spinal canal in an attempt to limit nerve injury (personal experience). Additional cauterization may be required to clear the epidural tissue from the disk space. Once clearly identified and with assurance that the dura and nerve are protected, a rectangular opening is cut in the annulus with a scalpel. When extending the annular opening laterally, care is taken to protect the exiting nerve root. This is done by sweeping any soft tissue toward the root and then leaving the retractor in place to protect the root while working laterally.

The annular opening is then repeated in exactly the same fashion on the contralateral side. Intervertebral disk space spreaders are then used to distract the intervertebral space sequentially. These spreaders, which are flat bars of increasing width with rounded edges, are inserted into the disk space horizontally and rotated 90 degrees, which will distract the disk space. If the disk space is initially too narrow, sometimes it may be helpful to insert an elevator or curette to identify the path. It is vital not to use force so as to avoid inadvertent penetration into the vertebral body. Lateral fluoroscopy can be helpful to confirm

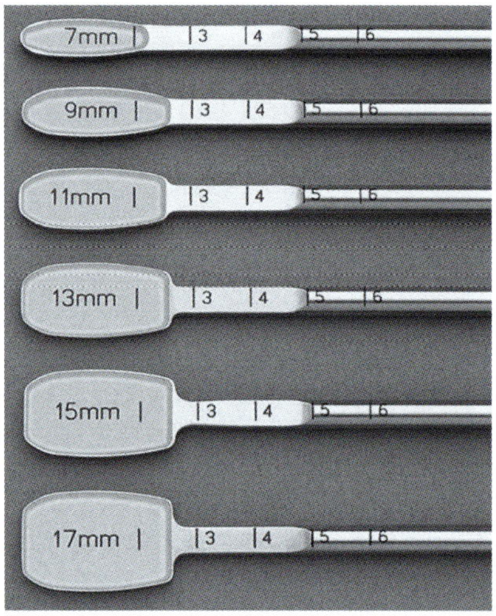

• **Fig. 7.5** Examples of intervertebral shavers that will facilitate disk and cartilaginous endplate removal in preparation of the disk space for interbody placement. (Adapted from Benzel E. *Spine Surgery: Techniques, Complication Avoidance, & Management*. 3rd ed. Philadelphia: Elsevier Saunders; 2012: Fig. 54-2a.)

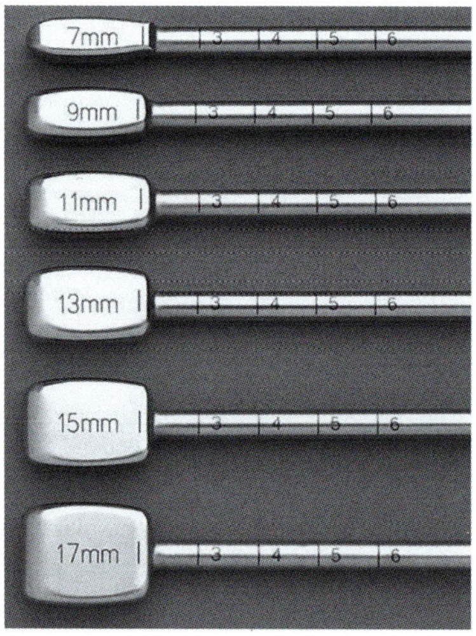

• **Fig. 7.6** Examples of intervertebral body graft sizer trials. (Adapted from Benzel E. *Spine Surgery: Techniques, Complication Avoidance, & Management*. 3rd ed. Philadelphia: Elsevier Saunders; 2012: Fig. 54-2b.)

that the starting tools are correctly placed in the interspace. The disk is then gradually distracted, working from side to side with increasingly large spreaders until resistance is met. The interspace should not be over distracted, or the endplates may collapse. It is not necessary to maximize distraction to achieve lordosis and decompression of the nerve roots should be accomplished by foraminotomy, not overzealous distraction. Placing a maximally tapered graft is the best way to increase lordosis. Placing a tall graft has many disadvantages; it increases the amount of dural retraction necessary, it increases the volume of bone graft needed to fill the interspace, and it increases the distance over which the fusion must occur.

After distracting the space to a comfortable working distance, usually 11 or 12 mm in the author's experience, one of the spreaders is removed and a four-sided Collis curette 1 or 2 mm smaller than the largest spreader used is inserted horizontally, then rotated clockwise and counterclockwise to separate the cartilage from the bony endplate (Fig. 7.5). This maneuver shaves the cartilaginous endplate from the bony endplate, which will permit rapid and complete removal of disk material and prepare the interspace for fusion. This step is repeated at various depths and angles to clean as much of the endplate as possible. The curettes can be sharp, and it is important not to violate the endplates. One may use a Kerrison rongeur to resect loosened annulus on the endplates.

The diskectomy is completed with standard curettes and pituitary rongeurs. A reverse curette is very effective in removing any remaining cartilage from the endplates. It is important not to go too deep when using curettes because the anterior annulus is sometimes deficient, particularly in patients with spondylolisthesis. This will avoid both visceral injury as well as the potentially catastrophic occurrence of a great vessel vascular injury. After cleaning the interspace of disk material, the intervertebral spreader is reinserted, sometimes one size larger than previously used before removing the disk and cartilaginous endplate. The opposite side of the disk is now prepared in the same routine.

The interspace has now been grossly destabilized. Graft trials are then used sequentially to fit into the interspace (Figs. 7.6 and 7.7). The graft should not be taller than the largest spreader

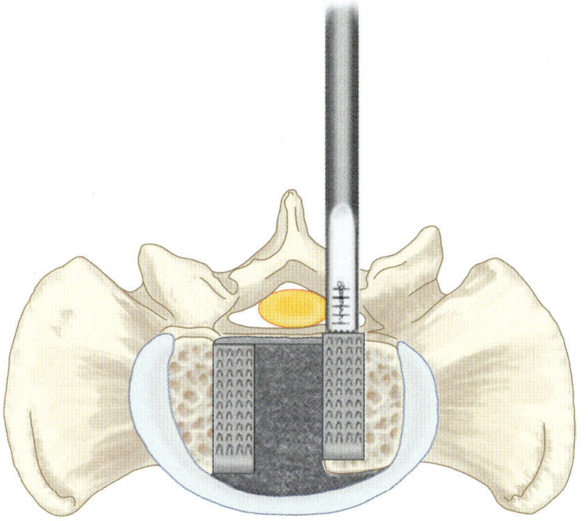

• **Fig. 7.7** Image of two posterior lumbar interbody fusion cages within the disk space. (Adapted from Benzel E. *Spine Surgery: Techniques, Complication Avoidance, & Management*. 3rd ed. Philadelphia: Elsevier Saunders; 2012: Fig. 54-2c.)

used. It can be tapered to achieve the desired lordosis. Fluoroscopy is often utilized while placing graft trials. This will ensure adequate size and segmental angulation. After ensuring that the dura and exiting nerve root are protected, the trapezoidal graft packed with graft material is inserted horizontally in the disk space and then rotated into its final lordotic position (if a lordotic graft is used) (Fig. 7.8). The intervertebral spreader is removed from the opposite side of the disk space.

Cancellous bone graft is packed from the opposite side into the middle of the interspace. Finally, the second trapezoidal graft is inserted into position. Additional graft may be packed around the wedges to fill the disk space maximally with bone. The foramina and the midline under the dura are inspected to ensure no cancellous bone or disk material was displaced into the spinal canal or neural foramen.

Following placement of the intervertebral grafts, the pedicle screw instrumentation must be placed if not already done so. These screws are very easy to place following graft placement in that the

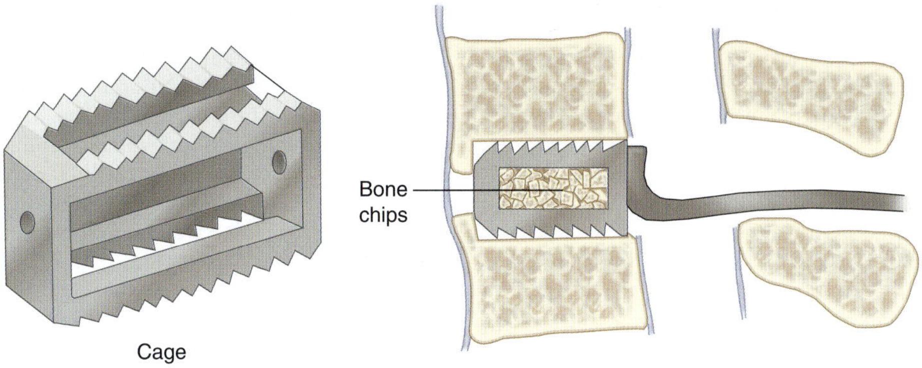

• **Fig. 7.8** Sagittal view of a carbon fiber cage appropriately positioned after successful preparation of the intervertebral body endplates. (Adapted from Benzel E. *Spine Surgery: Techniques, Complication Avoidance, & Management*. 3rd ed. Philadelphia: Elsevier Saunders; 2012: Fig. 54-3a.)

rostral and caudal pedicles to be instrumented may be palpated with any angled instrument such as the Woodson elevator. Standard landmarks may be utilized. The entry point for the pedicle screw is at the junction of the transverse process, pars interarticularis, and superior articulating facet joint. Often the mammillary process is located at this junction. A pilot hole may be drilled with a high-speed burr to expose the cancellous bone of the pedicle. A pedicle probe (gear shift) may then be used to advance slowly through the pedicle and into the vertebral body. The medial, superior, and inferior walls may palpated during insertion to ensure there is no breech. The probe is advanced to the desired depth, often 40 mm. This hole may then be probed with a pedicle probe to ensure there are four walls and a floor of the pedicle hole. If a breech is palpated, the pedicle probe may then be redirected to enter the pedicle and vertebral body correctly. If difficult, fluoroscopy may be utilized to ensure correct trajectory.

Following placement of screws, rods are placed between screws and compression applied across each rod. Compression helps ensure a proper fit of the interbody graft and bony endplate and will also effect segmental lordosis.

Minimally Invasive Technique

Recently, there has been interest in developing surgical techniques to minimize the amount of dissection of the paraspinal musculature. As the paraspinal muscles are sacrificed, there is subsequent atrophy and possibly poorer outcome. Development of minimally invasive techniques (MIS) for PLIF have lagged somewhat behind other interbody techniques, mostly because of the requirement for a central decompression and bilateral placement of cages within the intervertebral space. However, the introduction of cortical bone screw trajectories for pedicle screw fixation from a medial-to-lateral trajectory has allowed for the development of these MIS approaches specifically for PLIF surgery.[11]

The patient is positioned on a radiolucent operating table in conventional fashion (similar to an open PLIF technique). Once the correct operative level is confirmed, using anteroposterior (AP) and lateral fluoroscopy, a single posterior incision is made over the level of interest. Centering the tube over the facet and transverse process interface is usually preferred, as this will allow for optimal positioning when decompression and pedicle screw insertion are later required. The posterior musculature is then retracted down a muscle-splitting corridor that is extended to the lateral borders of the facet joints. Tubular retractor systems or stands can be used. Dissection can be limited with the use of the

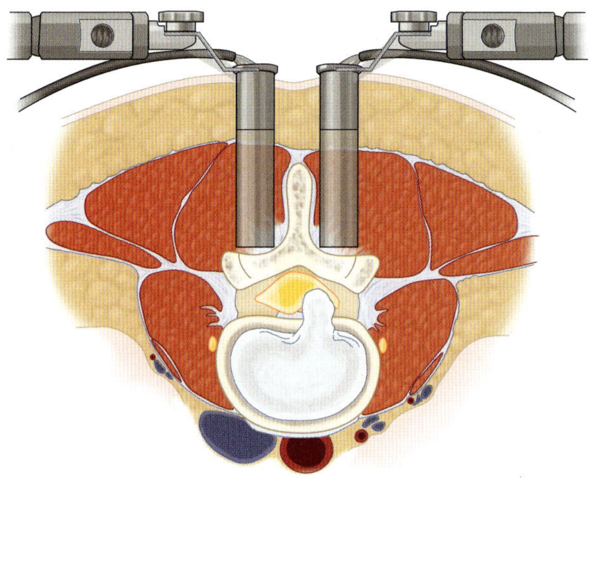

• **Fig. 7.9** Minimally invasive posterior lumbar interbody fusion (PLIF) dilation/tubular retraction. (Adapted from Benzel E. *Spine Surgery: Techniques, Complication Avoidance, & Management*. 3rd ed. Philadelphia: Elsevier Saunders; 2012: Fig. 60-1.)

tube because it can be directed to access the appropriate anatomy for each step of the procedure (Fig. 7.9). Laminectomies and partial or complete facetectomies are then completed with high speed burr and/or Kerrison rongeurs to allow for both access to the disk space and intended decompression of the neural elements. These steps are identical to that of the open procedure, but within the allotted space of the tube or stand used. As with the open procedure, it is imperative to perform proper decompression of the neural structures, as well as prepare adequate disk space with thorough removal of disk material, leaving bony endplates exposed on both sides. Bilateral interbody grafts are then placed on the lateral border of the apophyseal ring to allow for better load sharing on cortical bone as well as to obviate much of the need for dural sac retraction. As with the open technique, sagittally tapered lordotic cages can be placed using an insert and rotate technique. The insert and rotate technique involves preparing the endplates as previously discussed in the open technique section. The difference is this technique usually does not require overdistraction or cutting of any channel through the posterior endplates. The implant is inserted and then rotated into place, facilitating restoration of lordosis. Bone graft may then be afterloaded and placed to either side of the implants to help facilitate fusion. The main benefit is that this technique requires minimal neural retraction compared to that of an impacted cage technique, which involves over-distraction of the posterior disk space and usually far more neural retraction.

Medial-to-lateral cortical bone screws are then placed for pedicle screw fixation under fluoroscopic guidance. The technique for placement involves first identifying the superior most lateral edge of the pars; the entry point is 3 to 5 mm medial to this landmark. The trajectory is typically 15 degrees medial-to-lateral and 30 degrees inferior-to-superior. This trajectory may be less steep for the caudal screw to allow for a limited surgical exposure. Because of the medial entry point of these cortical bone pedicle screws, the size of the incision for MIS-PLIF can be limited to as little as 3 to 3.5 cm in length. If available, navigation may also be used to place cortical screws.

Traditional pedicle screws can also be used with the same landmarks as with the open technique. Biplanar fluoroscopy can be used to confirm both the proper starting point and that the pedicle screw is contained within the pedicle. A Jamshidi needle can be used with biplanar fluoroscopy to obtain the appropriate trajectory and place a guidewire. The tap and then subsequent pedicle screw may be inserted over the guidewire. If available, navigation may also be used to insert the pedicle screw.

PLIF vs TLIF

Although Cloward[3] and others have emphasized the importance of a wide exposure to minimize dural retraction and nerve root injuries during PLIF, other authors described a more medial approach, which was often associated with a higher incidence of nerve root injuries. In 1997, Harms and colleagues[12,13] reported a technique for performing a posterior interbody fusion through a more lateral approach than previously described. These surgeons advocated a unilateral approach to the disk space through the neural foramen by removing the facet joint. This approach allowed access to the disk space through a "triangular safe zone" between the exiting nerve root and the lateral dural edge.[14] In this way, an interbody fusion could be performed with minimal or no retraction of the dura. The technique has been adopted by many surgeons and has been shown to have a reduction of nerve root injuries when compared with PLIF.[15,16]

One theoretic disadvantage of the transforaminal lumbar interbody fusion (TLIF) technique is that because only a unilateral approach to the disk space is done, it is impossible to remove the disk material completely. Javernick et al.[17] showed that an average of 31% more disk material could be removed when a bilateral approach was done. This finding led to the concern that fusion rate may not be satisfactory with a unilateral approach. In an animal model, the inclusion of disk material with autologous bone in cages led to a significant impairment of fusion.[18] Despite the concerns, although no prospective randomized comparison has been done, the unilateral approach to the disk space may result in adequate fusion rates. A meta-analysis on reported fusion rates after open TLIF found a mean fusion rate of 90.9% across 716 patients from 16 studies.[19] Current trends have found surgeons moving toward minimally invasive techniques for placement of TLIF grafts. A recent meta-analysis on specifically MIS-TLIF surgeries similarly found high fusion rates of 92% to 99% across 40 series with a total of 1320 patients.[20] Comparison of series using bone morphogenetic protein with those that did not revealed average fusion rates of 96.6% vs. 92.5%, respectively.

Outcomes and Complications of PLIF

The outcome of PLIF surgery depends on several factors. Probably the most important, as with all spine surgery, is the proper patient selection. Lumbar fusion done for the wrong reasons or on the wrong patient will yield unfavorable results. A careful review of the literature on the outcomes of PLIF makes it clear that it is a technically demanding procedure. Variations in technique, experience, and skill will all have a significant influence on the rate of fusion and frequency of complications occurring.

In large series, fusion rates greater than 95% have routinely been reported, regardless of cage material used.[4,21–23] In contrast, Rivet et al.[24] reported only 77% of patients achieving solid arthrodesis despite the use of cancellous iliac graft and supplementary pedicle fixation. Fuji et al.[25] reported a nonunion rate of 72% in their series with the use of threaded cages placed posteriorly without supplemental fixation. It is difficult, therefore, to determine whether poor technique or other factors are responsible for the poor fusion results reported in those series.

Outcomes between conventional open versus minimally invasive PLIF techniques have not shown long-term significant differences. Sidhu et al.[26] performed a systematic review analyzing open versus MIS-PLIF studies and noted that MIS techniques did have longer operative time, but overall shorter hospital stay and less blood loss. Also, two studies showed better short-term outcomes with the MIS technique; however, the majority of studies reviewed showed no difference in short- or long-term outcomes. Complication rates and reoperation rates were also similar.[26] Fusion rates have also been similar. However, randomized, controlled studies have not been performed.

Nerve root injury is the most devastating injury that may occur during a PLIF. The reported incidence of this complication varies widely, which further adds to the notion that surgical experience and technical skill are important factors affecting complications with this procedure. Hosono et al.[27] reviewed 240 patients operated on by four different surgeons and correlated complications rates with surgeon experience. Forty-one patients had some kind of nerve injury, although mostly transient.[27] Davne and Myers[28] reported only a 0.4% rate of traction root injury in their series of 384 PLIF procedures. Krishna et al.[29] reported postoperative neuralgia in 7.1% of their patients, but they were able to reduce the incidence of this complication by half when modifying their technique and removing the superior facet to widen the exposure. Barnes et al.[30] reported a 13.6% incidence of permanent nerve root injury when using threaded fusion cages but no nerve root injury when using much smaller allograft wedges. These results further reinforce the principle that wide exposure, careful technique, and avoidance of oversized grafts can minimize the risk of neurologic injury in PLIF.

Graft displacement and loosening is another complication that was associated with PLIF when the technique was initially described. This is a rare complication with the addition of pedicle screw stabilization. However, subsidence of the implants can more frequently occur. This phenomenon has been poorly documented in the literature. Factors predisposing to subsidence include inadequate graft technique and sizing as well as endplate injury during preparation. Patient factors, such as weight and osteoporosis, are also very important.[31] Pedicle screws alone do not prevent subsidence after PLIF and implant type has yet to be clearly associated with subsidence rates.[32–34] Other complications seen in PLIF are similar to that of all lumbar surgeries. Epidural hematoma, wound infections, other nonimplant-related complications occur as frequently with PLIF as they do in other reconstructive operations on the lumbar spine.

Conclusion

Posterior lumbar interbody fusion is a technically challenging operation, whether open or MIS, that has an important role in the modern management of lumbar spine pathology. Careful surgical technique that emphasizes wide exposure and avoidance of oversized implants can lead to excellent results with low complication rates and high fusion rates. Excellent results have been reported with a myriad of commercially available cages and grafts with no one clear advantage seen in one over another. PLIF is a useful way to provide anterior column support without the need for an anterior incision and may be an additional tool for the correction of spinal deformity.

The PLIF procedure offers some theoretic advantages over traditional posterolateral fusion techniques. Clinical studies have failed to show superiority of PLIF convincingly over other techniques, however. In clinical situations involving degenerative conditions of the lumbar spine, the role of PLIF as a part of treatment of the patient is more dependent on surgeon experience than any other factor.

References

1. White AH. Editorial commentary. In: White AH, Rothman RH, Ray CD, eds. *Lumbar Spine Surgery Techniques and Complications*. St. Louis: CV Mosby; 1987:294–295.
2. Verlooy J, Smedt KD, Selosse P. Failure of a modified posterior lumbar interbody fusion technique to produce adequate pain relief in isthmic spondylolytic grade I spondylolisthesis patients. *Spine (Phila Pa 1976)*. 1993;18:1491–1491.
3. Cloward RB. The treatment of ruptured intervertebral discs by vertebral body fusion: Indications, operative technique, after care. *J Neurosurg*. 1953;10:154–168.
4. Kim KT, Lee SH, Lee YH, et al. Clinical outcomes of 3 fusion methods through the posterior approach in the lumbar spine. *Spine (Phila Pa 1976)*. 2006;31:1351–1357.
5. Fritzell P, Hagg O, Wessberg P, et al. Chronic low back pain and fusion: a comparison of three surgical techniques: a prospective multicenter randomized study from the Swedish Lumbar Spine Study Group. *Spine (Phila Pa 1976)*. 2002;27:1131–1141.
6. Jacobs WC, Vreeling A, DeKleuver M. Fusion for low-grade adult isthmic spondylolisthesis: a systematic review of the literature. *Eur Spine J*. 2006;15:391–402.
7. Byrd 3rd JA, Scoles PV, Winter RB, et al. Adult idiopathic scoliosis treated by anterior and posterior spinal fusion. *J Bone Joint Surg Am*. 1987;69:843–850.
8. DiPaola CP, Molinari RW. Posterior lumbar interbody fusion. *J Am Acad Orthop Surg*. 2008;16:130–139.
9. Barrick WT, Schofferman JA, Reynolds JB, et al. Anterior lumbar fusion improves discogenic pain at levels of prior posterolateral fusion. *Spine (Phila Pa 1976)*. 2000;25:853–857.
10. Nachemson A, Zdeblick TA, O'Brien JP. Lumbar disc disease with discogenic pain. What surgical treatment is most effective? *Spine (Phila Pa 1976)*. 1996;21:1835–1838.
11. Khanna N, Deol G, Poulter G, Ahuja A. Medialized, muscle-splitting approach for posterior lumbar interbody fusion technique and multicenter perioperative results. *Spine (Phila Pa 1976)*. 2016;41(suppl 8):S90–S96.
12. Harms J, Jeszenszky D, Stoltze D, et al. True spondylolisthesis reduction and monosegmental fusion in spondylolisthesis. In: Bridwell KH, Dewald RL, eds. *The Textbook of Spine Surgery*. 2nd ed. Philadelphia: Lippincott-Raven; 1997:1337–1347.
13. Harms JG, Jeszenszky D. Die posterior, lumbale, interkorporelle Fusion in unilateraler transforminaler Technik. *Oper Orthop Traumatol*. 1998;10:90–102. [in German].
14. Kambin P. Arthroscopic microdiskectomy. *Mt Sinai J Med*. 1991;58:159–164.
15. Humphreys SC, Hodges SD, Patwardhan AG, et al. Comparison of posterior and transforaminal approaches to lumbar interbody fusion. *Spine (Phila Pa 1976)*. 2001;26:567–571.
16. Cole CD, McCall TD, Schmidt MH, et al. Comparison of low back fusion techniques: transforaminal lumbar interbody fusion (TLIF) or posterior lumbar interbody fusion (PLIF) approaches. *Curr Rev Musculoskeletal Med*. 2009;2:118–126.
17. Javernick MA, Kuklo TR, Polly Jr DW. Transforaminal lumbar interbody fusion: unilateral versus bilateral disk removal—an in vivo study. *Am J Orthop*. 2003;32:344–348.
18. Li H, Zou X, Laursen M, et al. The influence of intervertebral disc tissue on anterior spinal interbody fusion: an experimental study on pigs. *Eur Spine J*. 2002;11:476–481.
19. Wu RH, Fraser FJ, Hartl R. Minimal access versus open transforaminal lumbar interbody fusion: meta-analysis of fusion rates. *Spine (Phila Pa 1976)*. 2010;35:2273–2281.
20. Parajón A, Alimi M, Christos P, et al. Minimally invasive transforaminal lumbar interbody fusion: meta-analyses of the fusion rates. What is the optimal graft material? *Global Spine J*. 2015;05:A307.
21. Brantigan JW, Steffee AD, Lewis ML, et al. Lumbar interbody fusion using the Brantigan I/F cage for posterior lumbar interbody fusion and the variable pedicle screw placement system: two-year results from a Food and Drug Administration investigational device exemption clinical trial. *Spine (Phila Pa 1976)*. 2000;25:1437–1446.
22. Arnold PM, Robbins S, Paullus W, et al. Clinical outcomes of lumbar degenerative disc disease treated with posterior lumbar interbody fusion allograft spacer: a prospective, multicenter trial with 2-year follow-up. *Am J Orthop*. 2009;38:E115–E122.
23. Kuslich SD, Danielson G, Dowdel JD, et al. Four-year follow-up results of lumbar spine arthrodesis using the Bagby and Kuslich lumbar fusion cage. *Spine (Phila Pa 1976)*. 2000;25:2656–2662.
24. Rivet DJ, Jeck D, Brennan J, et al. Clinical outcomes and complications associated with pedicle screw fixation-augmented lumbar interbody fusion. *J Neurosurg Spine*. 2004;1:261–266.
25. Fuji T, Oda T, Kato Y, et al. Posterior lumbar interbody fusion using titanium cylindrical threaded cages: is optimal interbody fusion possible without other instrumentation? *J Orthop Sci*. 2003;8:142–147.
26. Sidhu GS, Henkelman E, Vaccaro AR, et al. Minimally invasive versus open posterior lumbar interbody fusion: a systematic review. *Clin Orthop Relat Res*. 2014;472:1792–1799.
27. Hosono N, Namekata M, Makino T, et al. Perioperative complications of primary posterior lumbar interbody fusion for nonisthmic spondylolisthesis: analysis of risk factors. *J Neurosurg. Spine*. 2008;9:403–407.
28. Davne SH, Myers DL. Complications of lumbar spinal fusion with transpedicular instrumentation. *Spine (Phila Pa 1976)*. 1992;17(suppl 6):S184–S189.
29. Krishna M, Pollock RD, Bhatia C. Incidence, etiology, classification and management of neuralgia after posterior lumbar interbody fusion surgery in 226 patients. *Spine J*. 2008;8:374–379.
30. Barnes B, Rodts Jr GE, Haid Jr HW, et al. Allograft implants for posterior lumbar interbody fusion: Results comparing cylindrical dowels and impacted wedges. *Neurosurgery*. 2002;51:1191–1198.
31. Okuda S, Oda T, Miyauchi A, et al. Surgical outcomes of posterior lumbar interbody fusion in elderly patients. *J Bone Joint Surg Am*. 2006;88:2714–2720.
32. Brantigan JW. Pseudoarthrosis rate after allograft posterior lumbar interbody fusion with pedicle screw and plate fixation. *Spine (Phila Pa 1976)*. 2004;19:1271–1279.
33. Abbushi A, Cabraja M, Thomale UW, et al. The influence of cage positioning and cage type on cage migration and fusion rates in patients with monosegmental posterior lumbar interbody fusion and posterior fixation. *Eur Spine J*. 2009;18:1621–1628.
34. Tokuhashi Y, Ajiro Y, Umezawa N. Subsidence of metal interbody cage after posterior lumbar interbody fusion with pedicle screw fixation. *Orthopedics*. 2009;32:259.

8

Transformaminal Lumbar Interbody Fusion (TLIF)

MAURICIO J. AVILA, ALI A. BAAJ, RODRIGO NAVARRO-RAMIREZ, AND ROGER HÄRTL

Introduction

Posterior lumbar interbody fusion techniques have been popular since the 1950.[1] Specifically, posterior lumbar interbody fusion (PLIF) was a very popular technique; however, it required removal of both facets in order to achieve adequate graft positioning.[2] To surpass the inherent limitations of the PLIF, Harms and Rollinger,[3] in 1982, described the placement of the interbody bone graft via a transforaminal approach. In the transforaminal lumbar interbody fusion (TLIF) procedure, bone graft and an interbody spacer are placed via a posterolateral transforaminal route into a distracted disk space in conjunction with a supplemental pedicle screw construct.[4] This TLIF approach allows less retraction of the thecal sac and neural structures; it spared the contralateral lamina and facet (vs. PLIF) providing a bigger surface for fusion.[2,3] Additionally, advantages of the TLIF over PLIF are fewer complications, elimination of epidural scarring, and less intraoperative bleeding.[5] Furthermore, given TLIF's unilateral approach, preservation of the lumbar spine musculoligamentous complex is obtained.[6] Recently some variations of the open TLIF have been described, such as the mini-open TLIF for a single-level approach.[4] Despite the introduction of the minimally invasive TLIF (MIS TLIF), open TLIF is still routinely used in many centers owing to the high bony fusion achieved (>90%) and similar complications rate when compared with MIS TLIF.[7]

Surgical Indications and Technique

Indications

The primary objective of any interbody fusion is to stabilize the spine. Table 8.1 shows the indications for lumbar interbody fusions. Table 8.2 presents the relative contraindications for the procedure.

Technique

The patient is first placed under general anesthesia, intubated, and then positioned prone on a radiolucent surgical table (Fig. 8.1). Intravenous antibiotics should be administered prior to performing the skin incision. The surgeon must avoid placing the patient in a flat-back or kyphotic position before performing the TLIF, because the patient may be fused into that nonphysiologic position.[4] Positioning the patient in optional lordosis is accomplished by providing maximal hip extension during positioning. Pressure points are appropriately padded, and the surgical field is prepared and draped in a sterile fashion. Biplanar fluoroscopy may then be used to localize the indexed level accurately. A vertical incision (5–7 cm) is performed and the muscles and soft tissues are retracted laterally to expose the spinous processes, lamina, facet joints, and transverse process (Fig. 8.2). A laminectomy, facetectomy, or both are performed, depending on the clinical presentation. Minimally, a unilateral laminotomy and partial facetectomy are performed on the more symptomatic side.[5] The exiting nerve root is identified and carefully preserved.

Once the neural elements are adequately decompressed, pedicle screws are placed in a standard fashion. The disk space is then identified and a standard diskectomy is performed. Adequate removal of the cartilaginous endplate is necessary; however, preservation of the bony endplates is required to prevent graft subsidence.[8] With the use of a combination of interspace wedges and serial distraction of the pedicle screws, an increase in disk height is accomplished and maintained (Fig. 8.3).

An interbody graft of the adequate size is prepared and packed with autograft or other fusion substrate. A nerve retractor is placed against the traversing nerve root to protect it during graft placement while always trying to minimize the retraction of the thecal

TABLE 8.1 Indications for Lumbar Interbody Fusion

- Spondylolisthesis (Grade I or II)
- Degenerative disk disease causing discogenic back pain
- Recurrent lumbar disk herniation with significant mechanical back pain
- Postdiskectomy collapse with neural foraminal stenosis and radiculopathy
- Recurrent (third time or more) lumbar disk herniation with radiculopathy (with or without back pain)
- Pseudoarthrosis
- Postlaminectomy kyphosis
- Traumatic instability
- Lumbar deformity (with coronal and/or sagittal plane imbalance)

Adapted from Winn HR, Kliot M, Brem H. *Youmans Neurological Surgery.* Philadelphia, Elsevier Saunders; 2003

TABLE 8.2 Relative Contraindications for Lumbar Interbody Fusion

- Multilevel (>3 levels) degenerative disk disease (except in deformity cases)
- Single-level disk disease causing radiculopathy without symptoms of mechanical low back pain or instability
- Severe osteoporosis

Adapted from Mummaneni PV, Rodts GE, Jr. The mini-open transforaminal lumbar interbody fusion. *Neurosurgery.* 2005;57(4 Suppl):256–261; discussion 261; and Mummaneni PV, Haid RW, Rodts GE. Lumbar interbody fusion: state-of-the-art technical advances. Invited submission from the Joint Section Meeting on Disorders of the Spine and Peripheral Nerves, March 2004. *J Neurosur Spine.* 2004;1(1):24–30.)

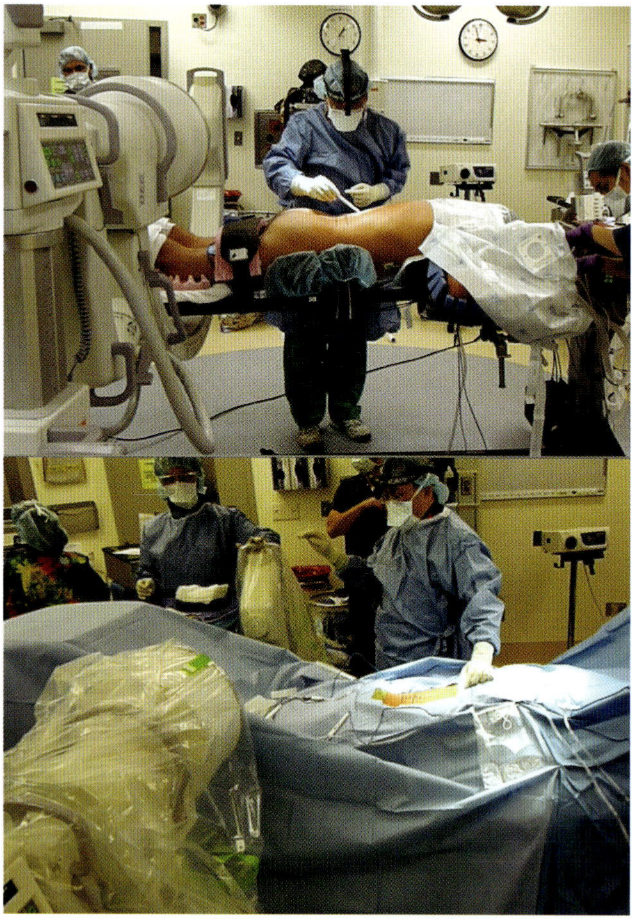

• **Fig. 8.1** The patient is placed prone on a radiolucent table; bony prominences are properly padded. Fluoroscopy is suggested for localization to avoid wrong level surgery at three different time points: (1) previous to the incision and confirmation; (2) after bone exposure; and (3) before the diskectomy.

sac. The first cage is impacted until it is just under the posterior edge of the vertebral body. It is important to begin moving the cage medially just as it sinks within the disk space. This allows the mesh to be placed across the vertebral body, making room for the second cage on the ipsilateral side (Figs. 8.4 and 8.5).

After the interbody construct is placed, the pedicle screws are attached to and compressed on the rod, thereby restoring lumbar lordosis while maintaining the restored disk height. This restores

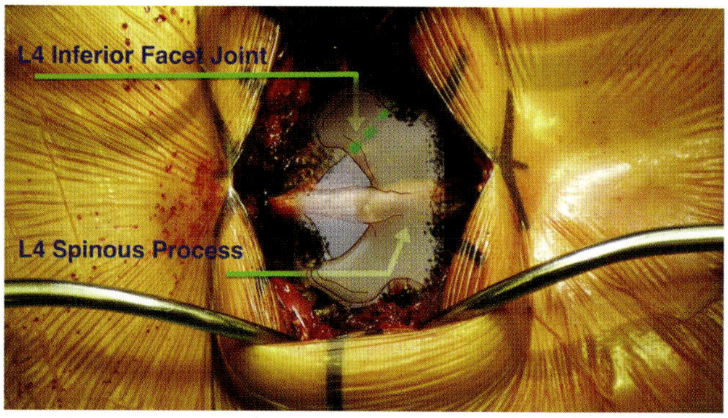

• **Fig. 8.2** During a transforaminal lumbar interbody fusion open approach, proper identification of the index level should include the following: the superior and inferior spinous processes, lamina, articulating processes, and transverse processes. An angled curate can be inserted below the spinous process immediate to the indexed level to be used as a marker while taking x-rays for adequate localization.

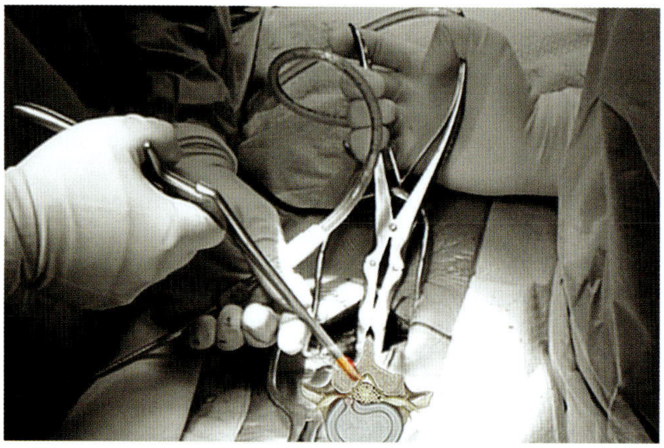

• **Fig. 8.3** Yellow ligament resection and lateral recess bony decompression can be performed under interlaminar manual distraction. This is especially helpful for those cases with severe degeneration. Automatic interlaminar retractors can be used as well. Once the nerve root of interest or both nerve roots have been decompressed, disk identification and diskectomy are performed.

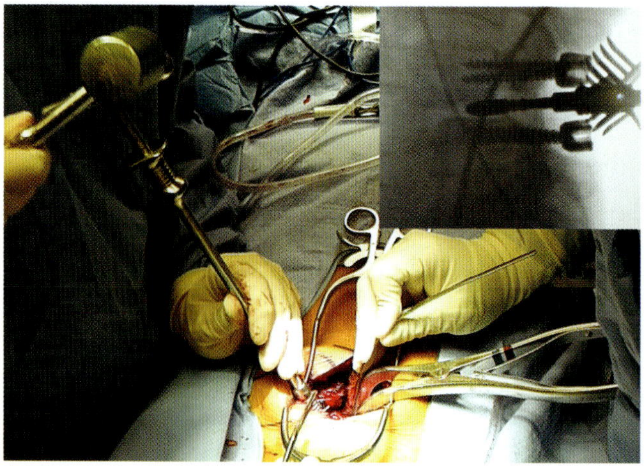

• **Fig. 8.4** After diskectomy, the cage trial is inserted. Special attention while impacting the cage trial must be taken because excessive force may cause endplate fractures that may lead to subsequent subsidence and pseudoarthrosis.

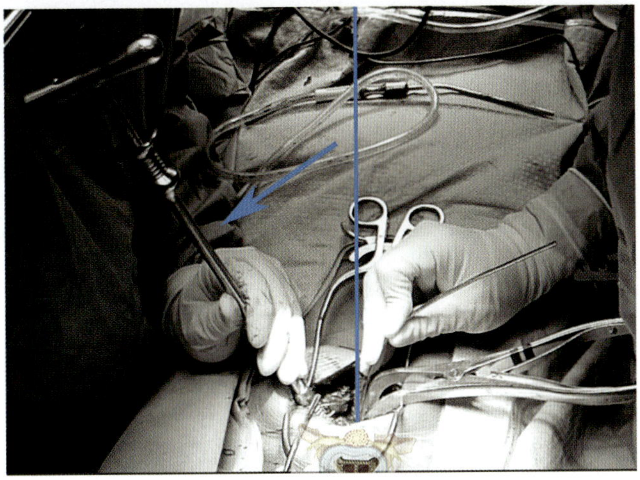

• **Fig. 8.5** The cage is inserted first, in an almost perpendicular direction to the floor/patient, and then the handle is tilted outward to direct the cage medially and anteriorly. Bone chips can be used as graft before the cage is inserted to promote fusion.

lordosis and compresses the interbody graft to prevent graft migration and facilitate fusion.

A multilayer closure is performed using absorbable sutures in the lumbodorsal fascia and subdermis. Staples or nylon sutures are used to close the skin.

Limitations

As opposed to other types of interbody fusion, open TLIF is versatile. The main limitations of the procedure are on the number of levels applied and the greater risk of failure in the osteoporotic spine. Although a TLIF may be applied at all levels of the lumbar spine, it is generally indicated for one to three levels. At more than this number of levels, the time to perform such a procedure may be excessive. Moreover, care must be taken when performing TLIF at the upper lumbar levels. As one approaches the conus medullaris, there is less retraction of the thecal sac (i.e., dura), thus limiting TLIF at L1-2 and potentially L2-3.

The chance of endplate damage is greater in the osteoporotic spine. If this occurs during endplate preparation or cage placement, subsidence may occur and hence construct failure. If TLIF is used in the setting of osteoporosis, significant care must be utilized during endplate preparation and implant placement.

Surgical Technique (Video 8.1)

Step 1, Exposure

- A subperiosteal dissection is suggested. Exposure of the adjacent segments above and below the indexed levels is performed (spinous processes, facet joints, transverse process).
- The ligamentum flavum is first released medially just under the spinous process and then proceeding laterally to facilitate its subsequent resection.
- The limits of the TLIF working zone are medially the dural sac and traversing nerve, superiorly the exiting nerve root, inferiorly the pedicle of the inferior vertebra below the disk space, and laterally the extraforaminal space.
- The inferior facet of the superior vertebra adjacent to the indexed disk space is removed. The superior facet surface of the inferior vertebra to the indexed disk will be visible and it has to be removed with the aid of Kerrison rongeours, high-speed drill, or osteotome according to the surgeon's preference. However, extra care should be taken during this part of the procedure not to push down the facet because it could damage the exiting nerve root down below.
- Proper identification of the exiting nerve root, traversing nerve root, thecal sac, and disk may be possible at this time.

Step 2, Disk Identification and Diskectomy

- Once the disk has been identified, dissection of the annulus fibrous has to be done; sometimes bipolar cauterization of the epidural veins may be necessary to avoid excessive bleeding.
- The annulotomy is performed using an #11 blade and the first cut is recommended to be done parallel the exiting nerve root. A radical diskectomy is performed.
- Endplate preparation is key and care not to violate the endplate must be taken.
- If the disk space is collapsed, sequential insertion of rotating dilators is recommended.
- Interbody cage trials are sequentially inserted until the trial fits very snugly.
- Bone chips are inserted and directed anteriorly using bayoneted forceps. Then the appropriate size cage is advanced anteriorly and medially by tilting the handle laterally.

Step 3, Cage Choice Rationale

Regardless of the type of cage (C-shape/banana, straight/PLIF cage, expandable cage), it must sit as anteriorly and medially as possible, without violating the endplates; try to make the cage sit on a bone-to-bone surface to promote fusion and stability.

Step 4, Screw Placement

- Ipsilateral or contralateral screw placement under fluoroscopic guidance and/or navigation, as well as utilization of distraction or compression of the screws while performing the diskectomy, depends on the surgeon's preference.
- Lateral and anteroposterior fluoroscopy is used to confirm adequate screw and cage placement.

Step 5, Posterolateral Fusion

- Decorticating the facets, remaining lamina and transverse processes and applying BMP or bone chips on top is also surgeon's preference.

Closure

- Layer by layer closure is recommended; the fascia and fat pad should be approximated and then the skin has to be closed without tension for better cosmetic results.
- Usually for a single-level TLIF with no excessive bleeding, leaving a lumbar drain may not be necessary nor recommended.

Postoperative Care

- Early mobilization is recommended after surgery.
- Consider DVT prophylaxis if patient is not ambulating after day 1.
- Adequate pain management.

Complications/Side Effects

- Use of nonsteroidal antiinflammatory drugs can compromise fusion.
- Early return to exercise or physical activity may promote cage loosening and pseudoarthrosis.

Outcomes in a Nutshell

- Endplate preparation is key.
- Use of expandable cages provides contralateral decompression.[9]
- Perform the direct approach from the symptomatic side.
- Do not over distract the expandable cages to avoid endplate violation.
- Navigation can eliminate the need for fluoroscopy.[10]
- Intraoperative neuromonitoring to confirm the pedicle integrity after screw placement is always recommended.
- Facet joint bone removal is preformed using an osteotome rather than a high-speed drill to preserve as much bone as possible to be used as a graft and filling the intervertebral cage.

Conclusion

Open-TLIF has proved to be an effective direct decompression technique and, when compared with MIS-TLIF, the latest report has not shown significant difference in clinical and/or radiologic outcomes in terms of postoperative clinical outcomes and infection or fusion rates. If the goal is sagittal balance restoration, ALIF or extraforaminal lumbar interbody fusion (ELIF) should be considered. In addition, open-TLIF has been associated with lower costs compared with MIS-TLIF.[11]

References

1. Cloward RB. The treatment of ruptured lumbar intervertebral discs by vertebral body fusion. I. Indications, operative technique, after care. *J Neurosurg*. 1953;10(2):154–168.
2. Winn HR. *Youmans Neurological Surgery*. 5th ed. Philadelphia: Elsevier Saunders; 2004.
3. Harms J, Rolinger H. [A one-stager procedure in operative treatment of spondylolistheses: dorsal traction-reposition and anterior fusion ([author's transl)]. *Z Orthop Grenzgeb*. 1982;120(3):343–347. [in German].
4. Mummaneni PV, Rodts Jr GE. The mini-open transforaminal lumbar interbody fusion. *Neurosurgery*. 2005;57(suppl 4):256–261; discussion 61.
5. Rosenberg WS, Mummaneni PV. Transforaminal lumbar interbody fusion: technique, complications, and early results. *Neurosurgery*. 2001;48(3):569–574; discussion 574–575.
6. Mura PP, Costaglioli M, Piredda M, et al. TLIF for symptomatic disc degeneration: a retrospective study of 100 patients. *Eur Spine J*. 2011;20(suppl 1):S57–60.
7. Wu RH, Fraser JF, Hartl R. Minimal access versus open transforaminal lumbar interbody fusion: meta-analysis of fusion rates. *Spine*. 2010;35(26):2273–2281.
8. Baaj AA, Mummaneni PV, Uribe JS, et al., eds. *Handbook of Spine Surgery*. 2nd ed. New York: Thieme; 2012.
9. Alimi M, Shin B, Macielak M, et al. Expandable polyaryl-ether-ether-ketone spacers for interbody distraction in the lumbar spine. *Global Spine J*. 2015;5(3):169–178.
10. Lian X, Navarro-Ramirez R, Berlin C, et al. Total 3D Airo navigation for minimally invasive transforaminal lumbar interbody fusion. *Bio Med Res Int*. 2016, article 5027340.
11. Sulaiman WA, Singh M. Minimally invasive versus open transforaminal lumbar interbody fusion for degenerative spondylolisthesis grades 1-2: patient-reported clinical outcomes and cost-utility analysis. *Ochsner J*. 2014;14(1):32–37.

9

Minimally Invasive Transforaminal Lumbar Interbody Fusion (MITLIF)

ABHISHEK KUMAR, SAMUEL C. OVERLEY, AND SHEERAZ QURESHI

Introduction

Minimally invasive transforaminal lumbar interbody fusion (MITLIF) allows a surgeon to restore intervertebral disk height, lumbar lordosis, and achieve an indirect decompression of the spinal canal and neural foramen while preserving vital posterior soft tissues. Adequate exposure of anatomic landmarks in open transforaminal lumbar interbody fusion (OTLIF) mandates a longer muscle-splitting incision and use of large self-retaining retractors at high tension that can generate pressures in the erector spinae musculature from 61 to 158 mm Hg.[1] The resultant prolonged retraction induces ischemic changes resulting in reduced muscle fiber diameter, fibrosis, and fatty infiltration.[2] These degenerative changes, in combination with disruption of stabilizing ligamentous structures, have been implicated as a major source of chronic back pain, failed back syndrome, and reductions in patient-reported functional outcome scores following open lumbar spine surgery.[3]

Foley et al.[4] introduced MITLIF in 2003 as a means of achieving the same objectives as OTLIF while minimizing iatrogenic soft tissue injury. Use of a tubular retractor placed via sequential dilation maintains continuity of muscle fibers and allows equal distribution of pressure around the wound edges. Critics of the MITLIF will cite technical limitations including loss of surface area for fusion, as the posterolateral recess is typically not exposed, and a heavy reliance on fluoroscopic imaging that increases radiation exposure to the surgeon, patient, and operating room staff. Lack of exposure of anatomic landmarks and limited working space also contribute to a significant learning curve for a surgeon looking to adopt MITLIF.[5] To limit exposing the patient and surgical staff to risk, it is imperative that the surgeon follows a reproducible process of patient evaluation and perioperative care. The goal of this chapter is to describe in detail the MITLIF focusing on preoperative evaluation, intraoperative technical pearls, patient outcomes, and complication avoidance.

Surgical Indication

The MITLIF carries the same indications as OTLIF; both allow restoration of disk height with a structural interbody graft resting in the anterior column, which is responsible for bearing 80% of the load transmitted through the spine. This recreates the normal sagittal alignment between the two vertebrae and opens the facet joints to their native apposition, thereby achieving an indirect decompression of the spinal canal and contralateral nerve root. An MITLIF is an effective treatment for symptomatic spondylolisthesis, lumbar stenosis with instability, recurrent disk herniations, as well as instability secondary to trauma, pseudarthrosis, or iatrogenic sources.

Limitations

Contraindications and limitations with respect to MITLIF can be divided into those that are absolute and those that are relative. Absolute contraindications to both OTLIF and MITLIF include conjoined nerve roots, acute trauma, or active infection. Aberrant location and connections seen with conjoined roots make safe performance of a TLIF nearly impossible, as limited mobility of the nerve root restricts access to the intervertebral disk (Fig. 9.1). With acute trauma to the vertebral endplate there is no stable foundation to distract upon or to support the interbody cage, greatly increasing the risk of nonunion or cage migration. Active systemic infection is a contraindication to TLIF as well as other elective orthopedic surgeries where metal hardware is implanted into the body. However, it should be noted that implantation of titanium interbody cages with posterior spinal fixation has been shown to be safe and effective in the treatment of discitis or vertebral osteomyelitis as it provides the necessary stability for healing to occur. Treatment includes focused antibiotic therapy, typically for 12 weeks, and radical debridement of infected tissue mandating an open approach.[6] Relative contraindications would include severe epidural scarring, severe osteoporosis, or grade III and IV spondylolisthesis. MITLIF may be preferable to OTLIF in the setting of morbid obesity or soft tissue compromise owing to burns, trauma, or cutaneous lesions.

Perceived complexity of the MITLIF increases when there is severe collapse of the disk space or significant osteophyte formation, especially over the posterior edge of the disk space (Fig. 9.2). When encountering these cases, the preoperative images should be scrutinized for the presence of a mobile spondylolisthesis or vacuum phenomenon within the disk. Both of these signs indicate laxity of the soft tissues around the disk space, which should allow for distraction and restoration of height. When osteophyte overgrowth covers the disk, the experienced surgeon can use an osteotome or bur to debride the lip and gain entry to the disk space.

In general, no specific situations exist in which OTLIF is overtly better suited than MITLIF; however, this depends on the surgeon's experience with each technique. Notably, the progressive narrowing of the interpedicular distance at each cranial level in

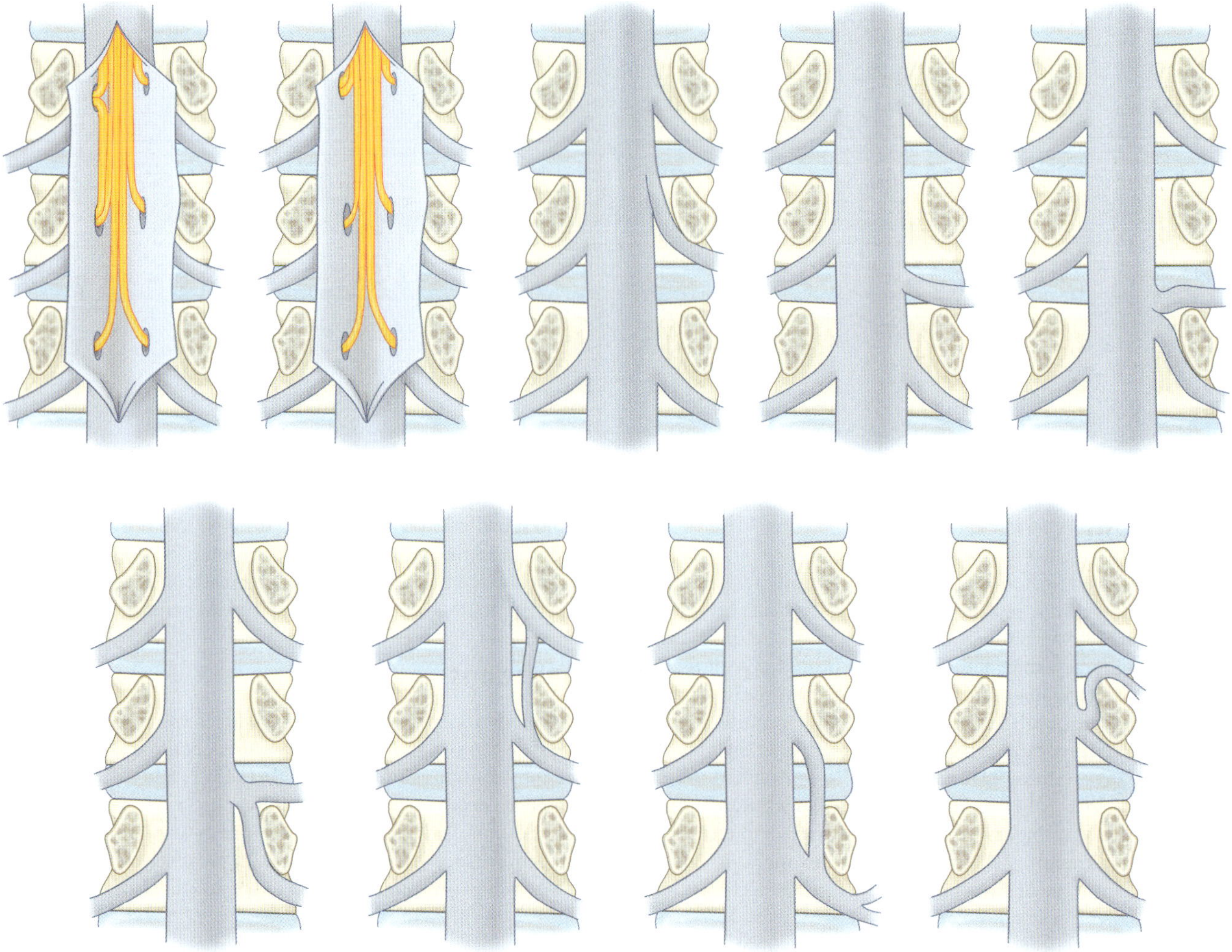

• **Fig. 9.1** Visual representation of the conjoined nerve root variants.

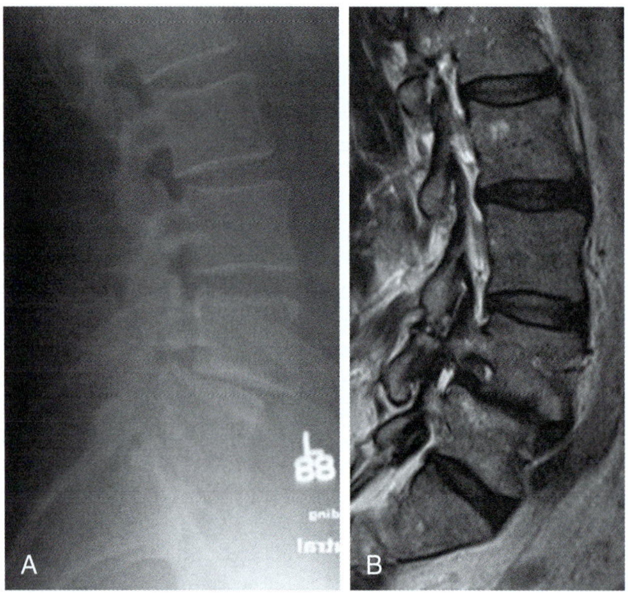

• **Fig. 9.2** Collapsed disk space with posterosuperior osteophyte of L5 overlying the disk space. (A) X-ray. (B) MRI.

the lumbar spine makes performing an MITLIF much more difficult above the L3-4 disk. Performing a facetectomy in this region reveals the dural sac and a small Kambin's triangle, which increases the risk of dural tear or postoperative radiculopathy from retraction of neural structures.

Surgical Technique

Preoperative Planning

Patient History

Laterality of radicular symptoms should be noted and, in the setting of bilateral symptoms, it should be determined which side is more symptomatic via focused questioning and provocative maneuvers. Typically, the facetectomy is performed on the more symptomatic side, whereas the contralateral side may be addressed via indirect decompression or direct decompression by undercutting the spinous process and contralateral facet. Laterality of a previous decompression or diskectomy should be taken into account especially when first gaining experience with the procedure.

When using a minimally invasive approach, the posterolateral recesses are not exposed and, as a result, the surface area available for fusion is reduced compared with the open procedure. Therefore, the surgeon may elect to use bone morphogenetic protein (BMP-2) anterior to or within the interbody cage to help achieve a solid fusion. It should be noted that use of BMP-2 in this fashion is considered off-label and therefore consideration of patient-related risk factors is necessary along with informed patient consent. Any history of previous or active cancer should be explored; in women of childbearing age, a pregnancy test should be conducted if indicated. These patients should also be advised to avoid becoming pregnant for one year following surgery. The BMP-2 is typically delivered in an absorbable collagen sponge and may be deployed anterior to the cage or as a strip of sponge placed inside the center of the cage. When utilizing BMP-2, the author prefers to place a strip inside the cage, in order to limit contact with the neural structures, which may cause a postoperative radiculitis. Some surgeons also utilize fibrin glue or other barriers to seal the annulotomy site to prevent egress of BMP-2 into the neural foramen where it may lead to heterotopic ossification.[7]

Imaging

Baseline preoperative anteroposterior (AP) and lateral radiographs allow for the evaluation of disk height, sagittal alignment, and presence of osteophytes, whereas flexion-extension films will reveal the presence of instability. In the absence of neurologic symptoms, preoperative magnetic resonance imaging (MRI) may not be necessary. If the patient has contraindications to MRI or previous hardware that would obscure visualization, then computed tomography (CT) myelography should be considered. These examinations allow the surgeon to identify central, lateral recess, or foraminal stenosis to be correlated with patient symptomatology and physical examination findings. Facet hypertrophy can be assessed on AP radiographs; however, a CT scan can be helpful in surgical planning as severe osteophyte formation from either facet may obscure visualization of the joint space, which is an important intraoperative landmark. Compressive osteophytes from the contralateral joint may demand the use of a foraminotomy rongeur to aid in undercutting the superior facet when performing contralateral decompression. Computed tomography may also be compared with MR images to determine if the source of compression is primarily caused by bony or soft tissue structures. Ultimately, selection of which side to approach and how much of a decompression to perform is made based on patient symptomatology rather than CT/MRI findings. These scans are primarily used to evaluate for the presence of aberrant anatomy and create a safe plan for execution of the surgical procedure.

Bone mineral density testing is not routinely ordered; however, it should be considered in patients at risk because the incidence of subsidence or cage migration is far greater in osteopenic and osteoporotic patients. In patients with poor bone quality, opting for a posterolateral fusion may provide a more equitable risk-to-benefit ratio.

Patient Positioning

The procedure begins with the induction of general anesthesia and turning the patient onto the operating table. Two commonly used table options are available to the surgeon. A Jackson table with radiolucent posts and a chest pad is appropriate; however, in the authors' opinion, this conformation may create lumbar lordosis in excess of the typical anatomic alignment. The authors prefer to use a Wilson frame with the pads lowered down completely and with the pelvis and the knees well supported. This results in a more anatomic lumbar lordosis, which facilitates access to the disk space under the exiting nerve root. Care must be taken, however, when using a Wilson frame. Failure to position as outlined above may result in loss of lordosis and the patient fused in a relative flat back.

Ideally, the stand of the C-arm and monitor should be placed opposite the surgeon for easy visualization and to afford working space. A T-bar attachment should also be fixed to the table opposite the surgeon to support the flexible arm that will hold the tubular retractor in place (Figs. 9.3 and 9.4). Neuromonitoring remains controversial in routine degenerative spine operations. The authors do utilize somatosensory-evoked potentials as well as free-running electromyography (EMG). These modalities alert the surgeon to excessive nerve root retraction during diskectomy or cage implantation. If used, it is crucial that the appropriate dermatomes and myotomes are monitored corresponding to the instrumented levels. Motor-evoked potentials may also be monitored; however, the authors do not routinely use this modality.

Percutaneous Pedicle Screws

Depending on surgeon preference, percutaneous instrumentation of the spine may be conducted with a single or double C-arm technique. In the double C-arm technique, the major hurdle is proper preoperative positioning. First, a C-arm should be moved into position perpendicular to the table for a lateral image and then the 'C' should be tilted toward the head of the bed so that the arm sits close to the undersurface of the table. The second C-arm for AP fluoroscopy will sit at an angle to the table and should approach from distally (Fig. 9.5). In the single C-arm technique, the critical step is to align the image intensifier perpendicular to the superior endplate with the vertebral body in neutral rotation, identified by the spinous process in the middle of the body and pedicles equal in size and relationship to the lateral walls (Fig. 9.6).

Some surgeons prefer to draw out the incisions for each pedicle screw before starting the procedure by first identifying the center of each pedicle then making a mark 1 cm lateral to this point. In the authors' experience, these skin markings will tend to deviate as each k-wire is inserted, which may result in suboptimal placement of the incisions. Rather, the entry points should be identified and marked sequentially for each Jamshidi needle (Fig. 9.7). Skin should be incised using a #10 scalpel, with the incision carried down through the fascia. Fluoroscopic guidance and tactile feedback from the needle tip should be utilized to align the Jamshidi needle at the junction of the transverse process and superior articular process. The Jamshidi needle should then be advanced under fluoroscopic guidance so that the tip of the needle reaches the pedicle–vertebral body junction on the lateral image before it reaches the medial border of the pedicle on the AP (Figs. 9.8–9.10). This typically corresponds to depth of insertion of approximately 2.0 cm. A guidewire may then be passed, feeling for impaction of cancellous bone. The authors prefer the use of nitinol wires as opposed to stainless steel. Nitinol allows the wires to be bent and held away from the operative field without the formation of a permanent kink. Such a kink may create difficulty when placing instruments over the wire and may even result in driving the wire deeper into or beyond the vertebral body during tapping or screw placement. Once all wires have been placed, they may be held out of the way using a towel clamp to create room for placement of the tubular retractor. Alternatively

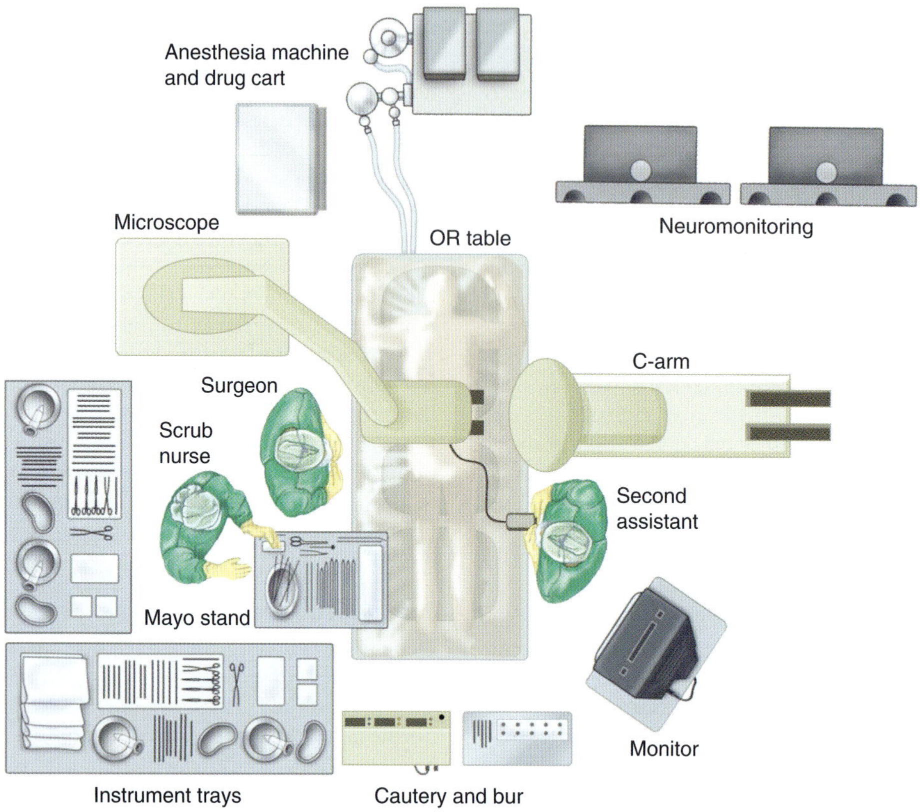

• **Fig. 9.3** Operating room setup with a single fluoroscopy machine.

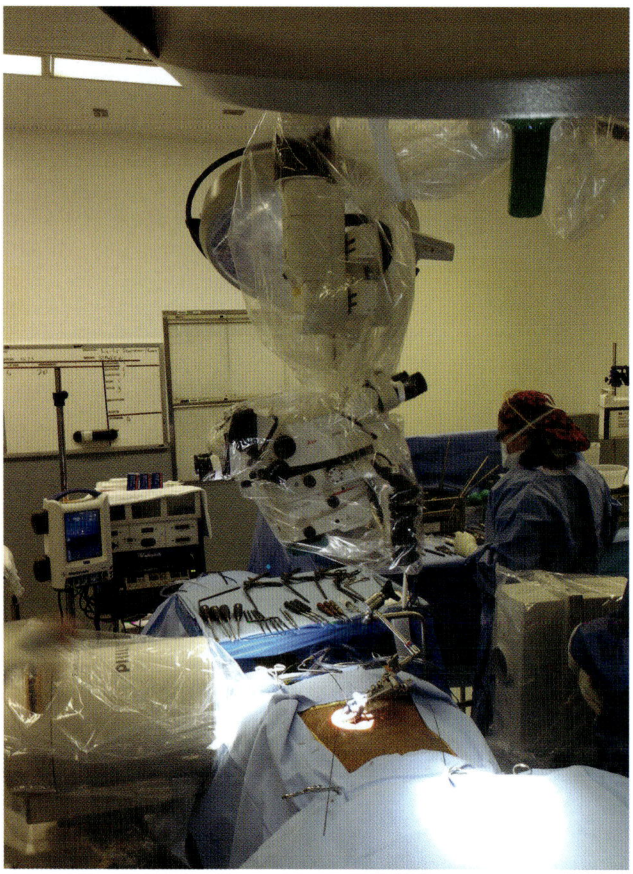

• **Fig. 9.4** Image of authors' preferred operating room setup.

at this point, screws may be placed on the side contralateral of the planned TLIF (see below). If utilized in this manner, a rod may be placed and used to aid in distraction of the intervertebral space.

Tubular Access and Decompression

Tubular access and decompression begins with extension of one of the pedicle screw incisions to allow sequential dilation and placement of an 18- to 26-mm diameter tubular retractor. Selection of retractor size depends on the size of the patient, surgeon preference, and magnitude of facet hypertrophy. In a large patient, or a patient with significant facet hypertrophy, a larger tubular retractor makes localization and performance of the TLIF much easier. In smaller patients, a large tube may impinge on the spinous process or lamina, limiting depth of insertion, which can compromise visualization owing to muscle creep. Access may be achieved through either the superior or inferior incision; however, typically the inferior incision provides easier access owing to its proximity. The authors prefer to use an 18-mm tube and press this retractor into the skin at the time of cannulation of the inferior pedicle to ensure an appropriately sized incision from the outset of the procedure. Sequential dilation splits the erector spinae musculature so that minimal tissue remains overlying the facet; however, any remaining tissue can be cauterized and removed with a pituitary rongeur.

The capsule of the facet joint is then peeled back with monopolar cautery to reveal the joint space (Fig. 9.11, Video 9.1). Inferior facetectomy may then be conducted using a high-speed burr or, alternatively, an osteotome and mallet to preserve some autologous bone graft (Fig. 9.12). The process is then repeated for the superior facet, resecting it in a plane parallel to the endplate of the vertebral body. Edges of the facetectomy can then be revised using a Kerrison

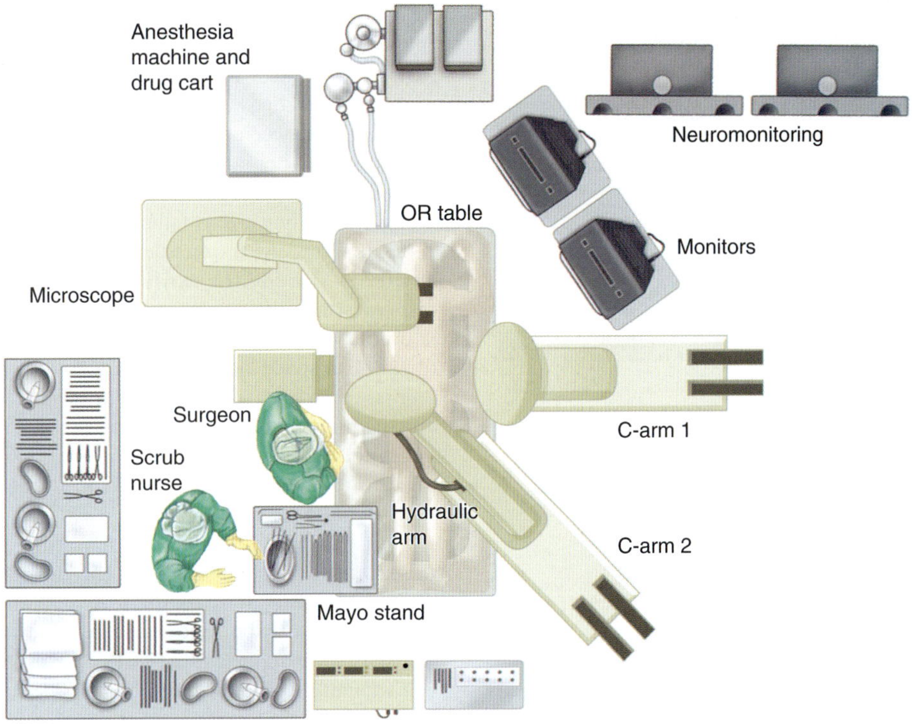

• **Fig. 9.5** Operating room setup with a biplanar fluoroscopy.

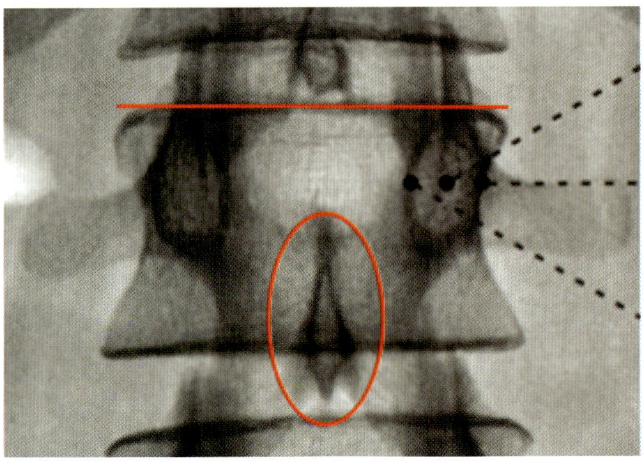

• **Fig. 9.6** A true anteroposterior fluoroscopic image showing an isodense superior endplate and spinous process without obliquity *(oval)*. The pedicles should appear as clearly defined ovals.

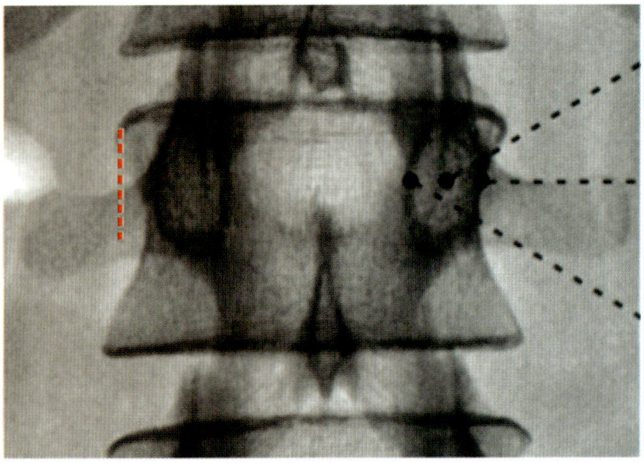

• **Fig. 9.7** Planned incision for pedicle screw cannulation.

rongeur to ensure that the resection of the inferior facet reaches the pars interarticularis and resection of the superior facet is carried down to its base where it meets the pedicle. Medially, the Kerrison rongeur may be carried across the ipsilateral lamina to perform a hemilaminectomy. In patients with bilateral symptoms, rotation of the table away from the surgeon and tilting the tube allow the spinous process, contralateral lamina and contralateral superior facet to be undercut using the bur and Kerrison rongeur (Figs. 9.13 and 9.14). When performing this contralateral decompression, the ligamentum flavum should be preserved until all bony work is completed in order to protect the dural sac. Contralateral decompression may be performed either before or after placement of the interbody cage.

Disk Space Preparation and Interbody Grafting

Identification of the disk space can sometimes prove challenging. The authors' preferred technique is to utilize a combination of number-4 Penfield and bipolar cautery to sweep tissue up and away from the pedicle-body junction of the inferior vertebra (Fig. 9.15). Hemostatic agents are helpful during this step to stem bleeding from epidural veins. Once the disk has been appropriately identified, a box-shaped annulotomy is performed using either a number 11 or 15 scalpel blade on a long bayonetted handle. Removal of this annular flap with a pituitary rongeur affords access to the disk space for preparation using distractors, shavers, curettes, and rasps. The authors' preferred method is to

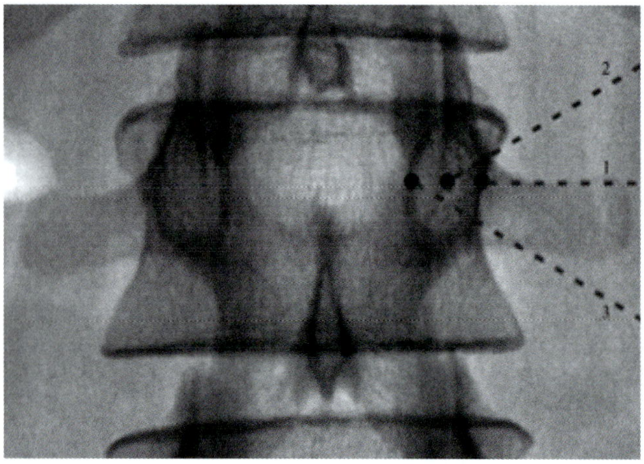

• **Fig. 9.8** The starting point *(1)* should be at the lateral cortical margin of the pedicle. After advancing 1.5 cm, the tip should be in the center of the pedicle *(2)*, finally ending at point *3* after >2 cm have been inserted.

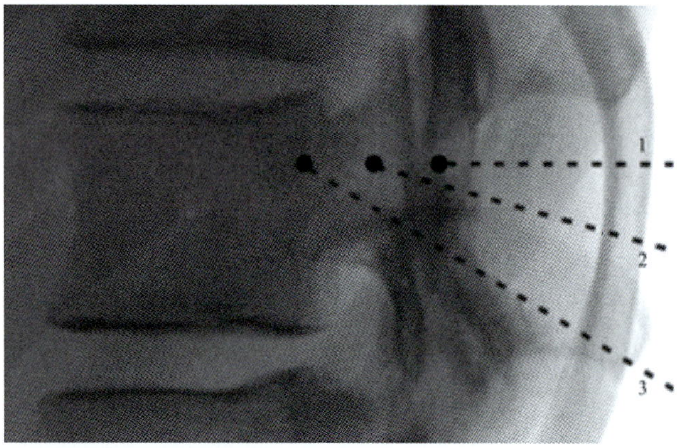

• **Fig. 9.9** Point 1 is the starting point, point 2 is where the tip has been inserted about 1.5 cm, and point 3 corresponds to >2 cm (into the posterior vertebral body).

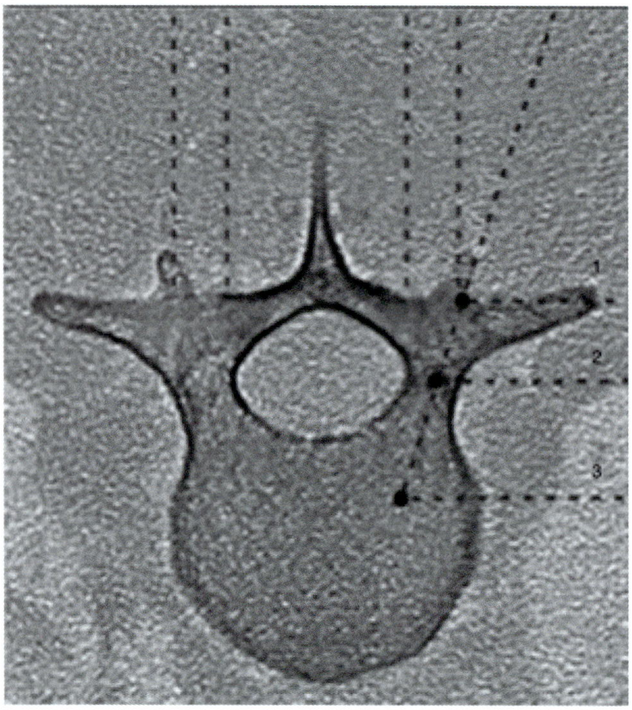

• **Fig. 9.10** An axial representation of the progression of the Jamshidi needle.

begin with sequential distraction of the disk space starting with the smallest distractor (usually a 6 or 7 mm). In the setting of significant disk collapse, it is helpful to leave each distractor in place for a short period of time to allow progressive stretching of the soft tissues. This allows subsequent distractors to pass more easily and reduces the risk of violating the endplates. The optimal size is reached when a moderate amount of force is required to distract between the bodies; the size of this distractor corresponds to the height of the desired cage. Once the optimal trial size has been identified and confirmed with lateral fluoroscopy, a disk shaver one size smaller is introduced and turned multiple times in different trajectories. This is followed by use of a ring curette to debride the cartilaginous endplate thoroughly and a rasp to stimulate punctate bleeding. A long pituitary rongeur is used throughout to remove loose pieces of disk. Saline flush of the disk space also aids in releasing any remaining disk fragments. Thorough diskectomy to clean the vertebral endplates and stimulate punctate bleeding is important to maximize the potential for fusion. At the same time, one must avoid disrupting the endplate, which may compromise stability, increasing the risk of cage subsidence.

During these steps, the scrub nurse should be preparing the interbody cage by packing the interstices with either autograft or allograft bone. A small strip of BMP-2 soaked collagen sponge may also be used; however, the possibility of inducing transient postoperative radiculitis or excessive bone formation in the neural foramen must be considered. Of note, the use of BMP-2 in this manner is considered off-label. Insertion of the cage into the disk space should then be conducted under direct visualization to avoid traction or injury to the exiting nerve root and dural sac.

Pedicle Screw Instrumentation

A cannulated tap sized 1 mm below the desired screw diameter is passed over each guidewire and advanced to the level of the pedicle–vertebral body junction under fluoroscopic guidance. Care must be taken to ensure that the guidewire does not displace posteriorly as the tap is removed. Extended tab screws are then inserted and utilized to facilitate passage of a rod underneath the fascial layer. Prior to placement of the rod, the intervening fascial layer between screw heads should be incised with a scalpel blade. Sweeping a finger along this gap will confirm that the fascia is split and the rod has room to pass. Grasping the extended tabs between the fingers and thumb provides vibrational feedback to whether the rod is in place or not. To confirm placement, the tulip head may be twisted; if it does not rotate, the rod must be between the tabs. Set screws may then be placed through the provided alignment guide. Fluoroscopic guidance should be used at this stage to ensure the guide is perpendicular to the screw head. Failure to perform this step may result in cross-threading of the set screw. This predisposes to loosening of the rod and potential failure of the hardware construct. Prior to final tightening of the set screw, compression may be applied to load the cage and restore segmental lordosis. Note that this maneuver may result in a small loss of foraminal height, which may be relevant to the contralateral nerve root, especially when a thorough contralateral decompression is not performed.

In the setting of a spondylolisthesis, the magnitude and ease with which a reduction is achieved depends on multiple factors, including duration of symptoms, type of spondylolisthesis, and patient body habitus. Often, the spondylolisthesis may partially reduce simply with patient positioning. Diskectomy and insertion of the interbody cage have the effect of re-tensioning the soft

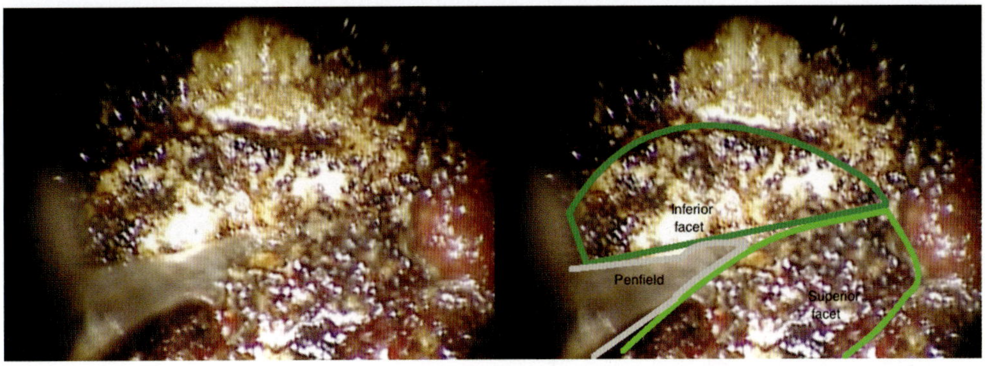

• **Fig. 9.11** Facet joint space probed with a number 4 Penfield dissector.

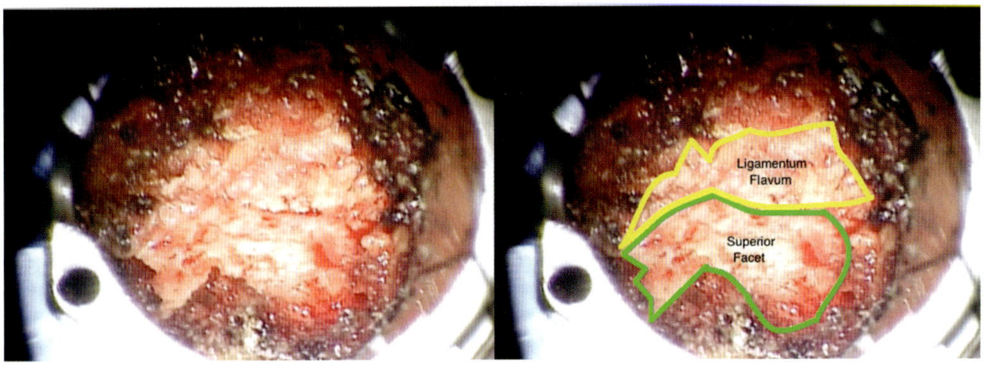

• **Fig. 9.12** Superior facet and part of ligamentum flavum exposed following inferior facetectomy.

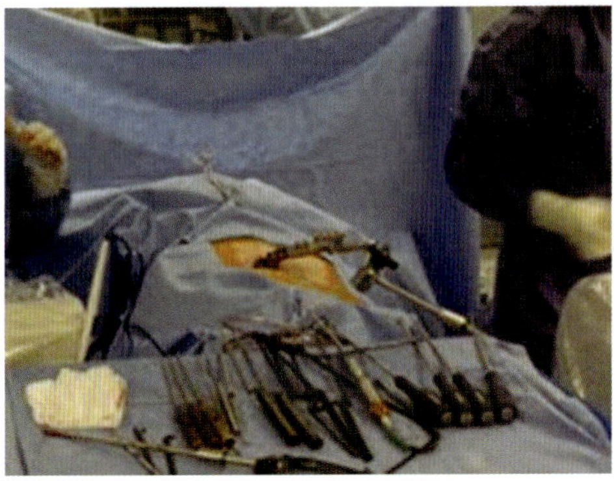

• **Fig. 9.13** Table rotated toward the surgeon and tube angled more acutely to look across the dura to perform contralateral decompression.

tissues, which also helps in restoring alignment. Finally, reduction can be achieved during rod insertion by tightening the set screws of the anterolisthesed vertebra last (Fig. 9.16). In this maneuver, the interbody cage acts as a fulcrum for the vertebral body to slide back upon as the rod is tightened down by the set screw. Care must be taken with this technique as the application of excessive force, especially in the setting of poor screw purchase in osteoporotic bone, may cause the pedicle screw to back out. As stated earlier, the MITLIF is typically used in the treatment of grade I or grade II spondylolisthesis, with higher grade slips considered a relative contraindication for most surgeons. Typically, as long as a proper decompression is performed, the magnitude of reduction of the spondylolisthesis is inconsequential from the perspective of patient outcome. Persistence of a grade I slip following these three reduction maneuvers should be accepted because pursuit of a complete reduction may do more harm than good.

Wound Closure

Meticulous hemostasis should be performed, followed by copious irrigation, especially when utilizing BMP-2. Sweeping a finger along each screw head can help release tethered muscle fibers, which may be a cause of discomfort postoperatively. Local anesthetic is injected under the fascia after closure as well as in the subcutaneous tissue. The incision should be closed in layers and covered with liquid adhesive dressing.

Postoperative Care

Dutiful postoperative care begins during the initial clinic visit at which time the patient should be educated about the typical postoperative course. Establishing accurate patient expectations is critical to achieve reproducible outcomes and maintain high levels of patient satisfaction. Pain and soreness of the lower back are to be expected and infrequent sharp pains caused by muscle spasm may occur. The authors attempt to avoid use of patient-controlled analgesic regimens in favor of oral narcotics in concert with muscle relaxants. Use of a lumbosacral orthosis (LSO) in the postoperative phase may provide relief from muscle spasms when ambulating; however, in the authors' practice, LSOs are not routinely prescribed. Supervised physiotherapy should include training and education regarding a home physiotherapy plan. By minimizing soft tissue trauma, the MITLIF significantly reduces postoperative pain and morbidity, which means that patients can often be discharged home on the first postoperative day.

Complications

The overall complication profile for MITLIF is similar to OTLIF and may be divided into technical, systemic, and infectious etiologies. Technical complications encountered include dural tears, screw

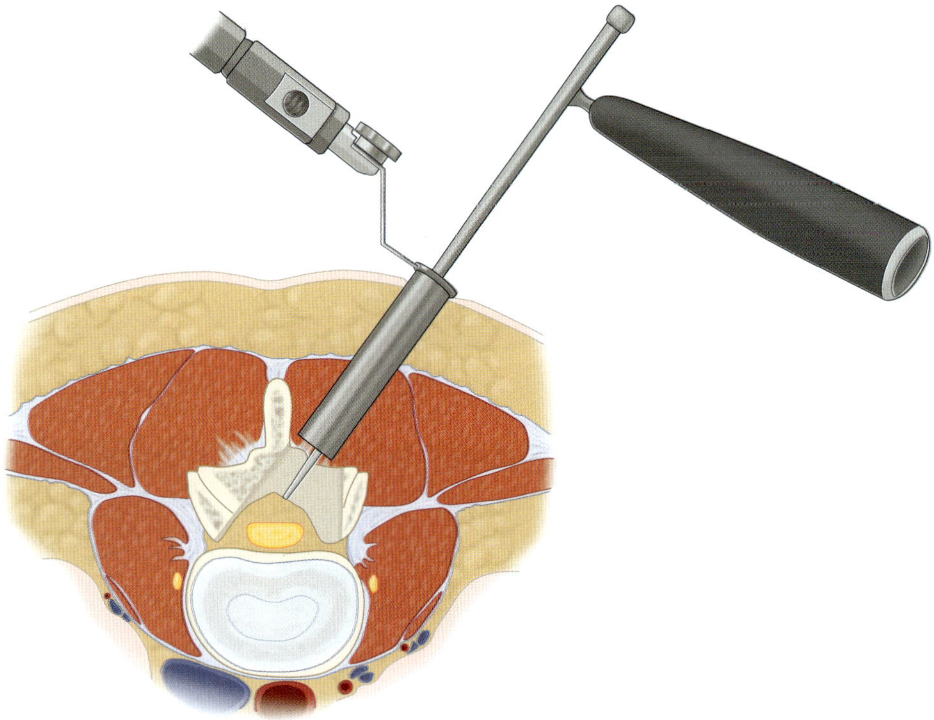

• **Fig. 9.14** Bilateral decompression achieved by undercutting the spinous process, contralateral lamina, and superior facet.

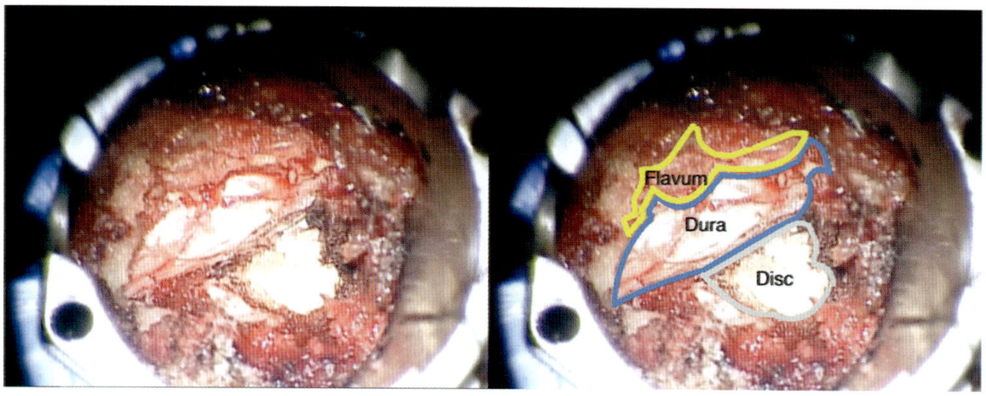

• **Fig. 9.15** The intervertebral disk is now visualized along with the dura and some remaining ligamentum flavum.

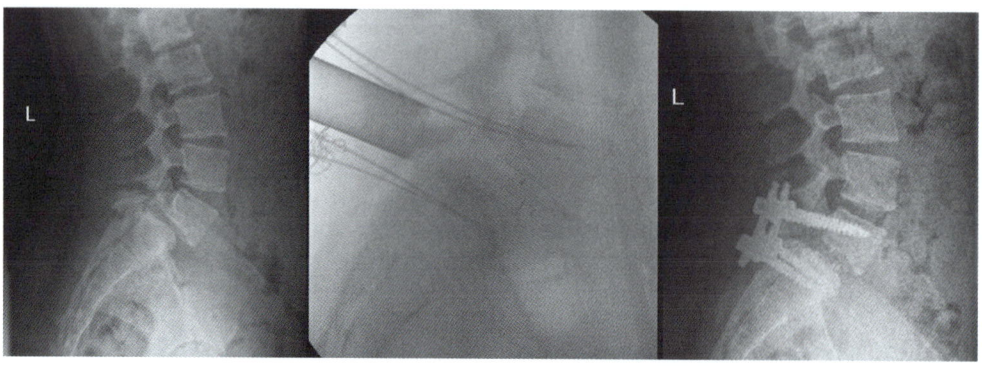

• **Fig. 9.16** Progressive reduction of a spondylolisthesis following positioning, diskectomy, and instrumentation.

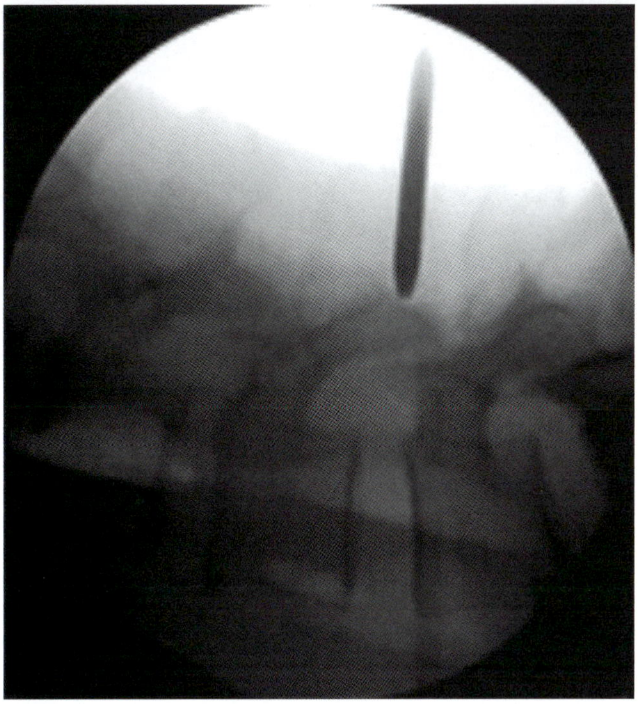

• **Fig. 9.17** First dilator tube placed in line with the disk space on lateral fluoroscopy.

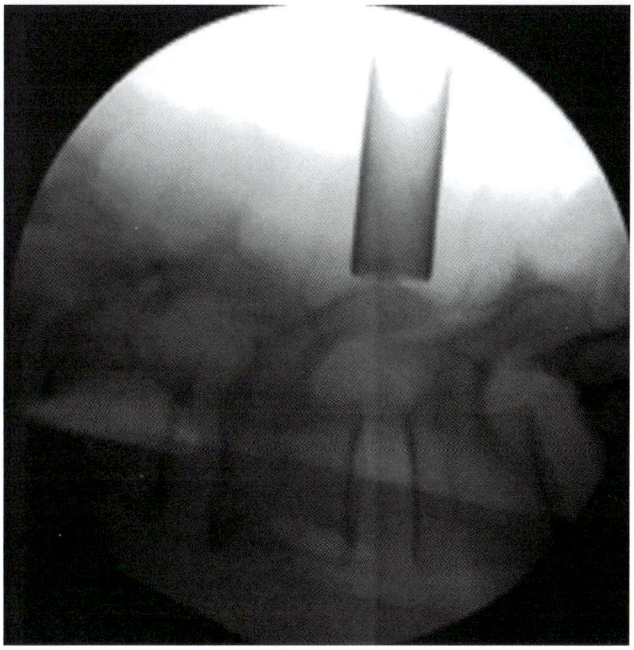

• **Fig. 9.18** Working tube in line with disk space on lateral fluoroscopy.

malposition, neural element injury, and cage migration. Systemic complications primarily include pneumonia, urinary tract infection, and deep vein thrombosis. The risk of superficial or deep wound infection is reduced in MITLIF because the tubular retractor requires a much smaller incision and avoids creation of dead space. Recently, Wei et al.[8] conducted a systematic review of 14 studies comparing MITLIF with OTLIF with an emphasis on the rate of the complications. They found a pooled complication rate of 11.87% (54/455 cases) for the MITLIF group versus 14.35% (64/446 cases) for the OTLIF group. They also reported a significantly decreased rate of wound infections in the MITLIF group as compared with the OTLIF group (12% vs. 25%). The pooled technical errors reported were very similar for both groups (29 MITLIF vs. 28 OTLIF) despite popular opinion of MITLIF as a more technically demanding procedure with a steep learning curve.

Many of the technical complications related to MITLIF may be attributed to difficulty in visualization and identification of local structures. Whether the surgeon is performing the case via a pedicle-based retraction system or a static tubular retractor, a thorough understanding of the anatomy is necessary to compensate for the lack of observable landmarks. As with most spine surgeries, safe MITLIF begins with appropriate identification of the operative level and fluoroscopic confirmation of this after docking the retractor system. The dilator tube should be located directly in line with the disk space on true lateral fluoroscopy and just medial to the facet line on AP fluoroscopy (Figs. 9.17 and 9.18). Once the dilator tube is docked on the facet, the surgeon may begin to expose the joint with electrocautery, paying attention to identify the joint space between the two facets. This is a key landmark that orients and guides the surgeon when performing the facetectomy. Following bony resection, care must be taken to visualize both the exiting and traversing nerve roots in order to establish a safe working portal in Kambin's triangle (Fig. 9.19).

In cases of spondylolisthesis, the exiting root tends to rest in a more inferior position than usual and therefore may be confused

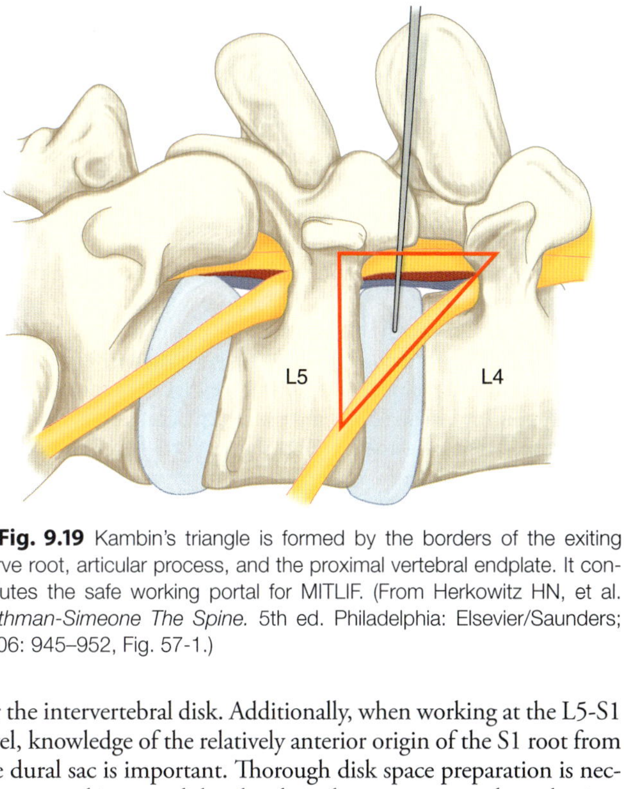

• **Fig. 9.19** Kambin's triangle is formed by the borders of the exiting nerve root, articular process, and the proximal vertebral endplate. It constitutes the safe working portal for MITLIF. (From Herkowitz HN, et al. *Rothman-Simeone The Spine.* 5th ed. Philadelphia: Elsevier/Saunders; 2006: 945–952, Fig. 57-1.)

for the intervertebral disk. Additionally, when working at the L5-S1 level, knowledge of the relatively anterior origin of the S1 root from the dural sac is important. Thorough disk space preparation is necessary to achieve a solid arthrodesis; however, overzealous shaving, distraction, or curettage may result in endplate violation, which is a contributing factor to vertebral body subsidence and cage migration. The surgeon must also be careful not to disrupt the anterior longitudinal ligament because this provides a protective layer for the great vessels, sympathetic ganglia, and peritoneum while also preventing postoperative anterior migration of the cage.

Nerve root damage is a feared complication in MITLIF, especially during the initial learning phase of the procedure. Pearls to help mitigate this complication primarily rely on proper tube position and spatial awareness. If the surgeon has difficulty identifying local landmarks, it may be a sign that the tubular retractor is not in the correct position. Any change in position of the tube should be followed by fluoroscopic confirmation of its location and angulation. If the tube is directed too medially, the traversing nerve root and dural sac are at risk for traction or direct injury. Conversely, if the tube is angled too laterally, the exiting nerve root may be directly in the field of view, placing it in danger. The nerve root is also placed at risk during cage implantation. This step should always be conducted under direct visualization to avoid compressing it or dragging it into the disk space. Nerve root injury may also occur secondary to pedicle screw malposition.

The first step of safe percutaneous pedicle screw instrumentation is the alignment of the vertebral body with the image intensifier. The spinous processes should be directly midline whereas the pedicles should be equal in size and should intersect the superior endplate and lateral walls of the vertebral body in a similar fashion. Finally, the superior endplate should be aligned with the beam, so that it appears as an isodense line. To avoid damage to the superior endplate, the needle entry point should be located at the 8 o'clock or 4 o'clock position with the trajectory of the Jamshidi needle heading to the center of the pedicle. This technique also prevents violation of the facet joint, which may potentially accelerate progression of adjacent segment disease.[9] Once located in an ideal position, the Jamshidi needle is advanced the length of the pedicle, approximately 2 cm, with the tip remaining inside the cortical density of the pedicle throughout (Fig. 9.20). If the tip of the Jamshidi needle crosses the medial cortical density of the pedicle prior to 2 cm of insertion, it has likely breached the medial wall and should be withdrawn and redirected. Depth markers along the Jamshidi needle are helpful to identify depth of insertion or, alternatively, once a proper starting point has been achieved, a ruler and marker may be used to create a line 2 cm above the skin.

To achieve fusion rates comparable to OTLIF, the surgeon must be diligent in removing the nucleus pulposus and denuding the vertebral body of endplate cartilage. With proper technique, it is possible to achieve a diskectomy through a minimally invasive approach that is equivalent to that achieved through open techniques.[10] Of note, the contralateral posterior zone of the disk is the most difficult to address in both situations and therefore deserves special attention. Proper cage placement is also important to prevent endplate subsidence, which is often associated with formation of a pseudarthrosis. For this reason, the authors prefer to use an articulating cage, which allows for placement of a longer cage compared with direct insertion of a "bullet" cage. During insertion, the cage is inserted until just past the midway point of the vertebral body after which it is rotated and impacted all of the way to the anterior margin of the vertebral body. With this technique, the cage rests up against the more stable cortical rim of the vertebral endplate. This conformation also allows for maximal restoration of disk height and segmental lordosis while minimizing the risk of subsidence. When disk preparation and cage placement are performed properly, fusion rates with MITLIF approach 90% and beyond.[11]

The use of BMP-2 has increased over the past decade and has become a popular fusion substrate for MITLIF. Major complications, such as cancer formation, osteolysis, postoperative radiculitis, and retrograde ejaculation, have been implicated in BMP-2 use, although the literature is rather divided on this topic.[12] Complications reported in the literature specific to utilization of BMP-2 in MITLIF include BMP-induced radiculitis and BMP-2-associated heterotopic neuroforaminal bone growth. The incidence of these complications ranges from 1.9% to 6.5% and is often associated with debilitating postoperative pain that frequently necessitates revision surgery. The etiology of BMP-2-related radiculitis is unclear; however, the prevailing theory is that it is related to the inflammatory-mediated response induced by BMP-2. This may occur as a result of physical contact of the BMP-2 soaked collagen sponge with the nerve root at some portion of the case, or a robust host inflammatory response within the disk space. Rihn et al.[13] found that the rate of BMP-2-related radiculitis was significantly reduced when a hydrogel sealant was applied to the annulotomy site after cage insertion. Theoretically, this sealant serves as a barrier to the disk space where the BMP resides and acts as a coating to protect the adjacent nerve roots and dural sac. Hydrogel sealants must be used judiciously in spine surgery because some are known to absorb water and expand, potentially causing compression of neurologic structures. The use of an insertion cannula to pack BMP-2 anterior to the cage may also prevent unwanted exposure of BMP-2 directly to the exiting or traversing roots.

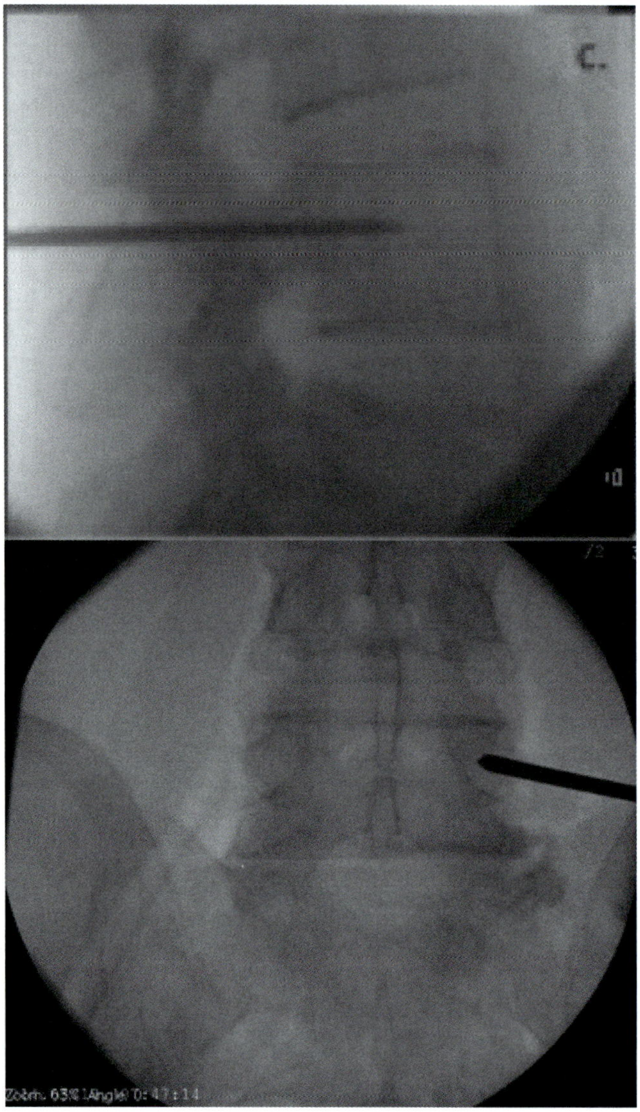

• **Fig. 9.20** Lateral view of Jamshidi needle shows it is inserted >2 cm through pedicle into vertebral body. Tip remains lateral to the medial border of the pedicle on anteroposterior view.

Heterotopic bone formation associated with BMP-2 use in MITLIF is also a significant concern. This space-occupying, newly formed bone has the potential to create new neuroforaminal stenosis that may necessitate a return to the operating room (Fig. 9.21). The mechanism for this process is poorly understood but is, at least

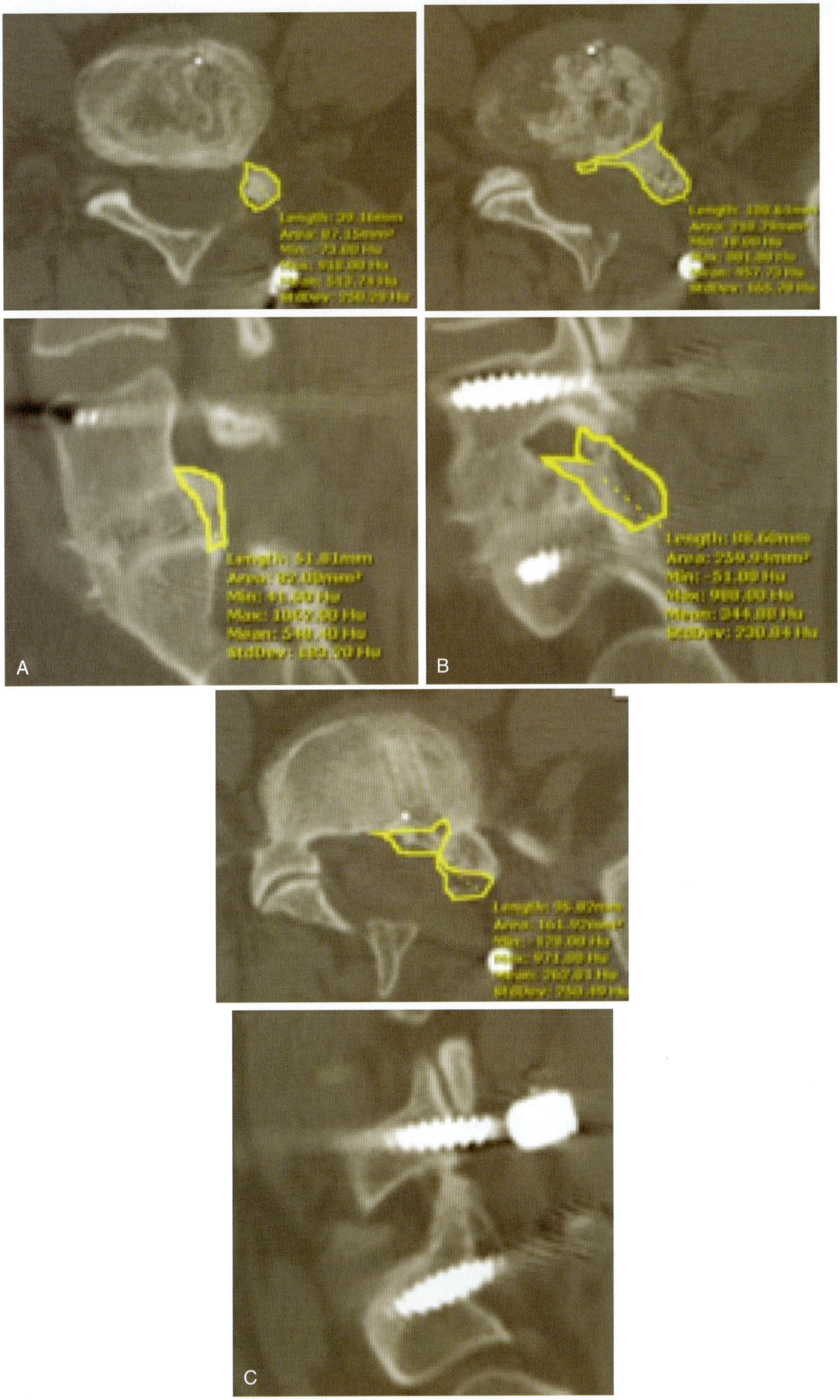

• **Fig. 9.21** Selected computed tomography slices showing heterotopic ossification extending from the intervertebral space to the neural foramen along the channel of cage insertion.

in part, owing to endplate bleeding that seeps through the annulotomy into the canal or neural foramen. This blood may serve as a conduit for osteoprogenitor cells and BMP molecules. Placement of the BMP ventral to the cage or inside a well-placed cage resting at the anterior rim of the vertebral body may help reduce the incidence of this complication. Again, the use of a hydrogel sealant may also prevent leakage of BMP into the neuroforamen. If heterotopic ossification is suspected, as in the case of new postoperative radiculitis, a CT scan is recommended to evaluate further. Revision surgery may be indicated; however, risk of dural tear or further injury to the nerve root must be recognized.

Outcomes

The last decade has seen multiple studies demonstrating the benefits of MITLIF in regard to the patient and hospital system as a whole. Skovrlj et al.[14] reported on these outcomes in a systematic review of 26 studies comparing MITLIF with open TLIF. After pooling the data, they found no difference in operative time (MISTLIF 150 min, OTLIF 143 min, $P = .09$) with significantly less blood loss (325 mL vs. 581 mL in open, $P < .0001$), and significantly shorter length of stay in the MITLIF group as compared to open (7.7 d vs. 10.4 d, $P < .0001$). Karikari and Isaacs[15] recently published a review that reiterated these findings, reporting significantly less blood loss in the MITLIF group (150 to 456 mL) as compared with the open group (366 to 1147 mL) and a significantly shorter LOS in the MITLIF group compared with OTLIF (3 to 10.6 d vs. 4.2 to 14.6 d). When accounting for this shorter length of stay, reduced narcotic use, and faster return to work associated with MITLIF, Adogwa et al.[16] concluded that the average cost of an MITLIF was $35,996 compared with $44,727 for OTLIF. This study, although underpowered ($n = 30$), demonstrated the economic favorability of MITLIF with a lower cost and a higher value for quality-adjusted life-years (QALY) at 2 years' follow-up, resulting in a total two-year cost savings of $8,731 in favor of the MITLIF.[16]

In addition to reducing patient morbidity and improving recovery, the smaller incision and reduced muscle dissection in MITLIF also results in a lower rate of surgical site infection (SSI). This was validated in a comparison review of 10 MITLIF studies (362 total patients) and 20 OTLIF studies (1133 total patients). The cumulative SSI rate for MITLIF was reported to be significantly lower at 0.6% compared with 4% for OTLIF ($P = .0005$). This 3.4% reduction in the rate of SSI culminated in a savings of $98,974 per 100 MI-TLIF cases compared with OTLIF.[17]

Critics of MITLIF often cite the lack of a posterolateral fusion as a problem that would likely result in a lower fusion rate for the procedure; however, this assumption is not supported by the literature. Wu et al.[11] conducted a meta-analysis on this topic and found no significant difference in pooled fusion rates for MITLIF (94.8%, confidence interval [CI] 86.4% to 94%) and open TLIF (90.9%, CI 85.4% to 98.3%). The majority of these studies used the criteria of bridging bone on CT to determine whether a fusion had occurred. It is also important to note that BMP-2 was utilized in 6 of the 8 MITLIF studies compared with just 4 of the 16 OTLIF studies. The authors also reported on pooled data for complication rates, revealing a rate of 7.5% for MITLIF versus 12.6% for OTLIF.[18]

Despite recent increases in studies focused on MITLIF, there remains a paucity of level I and II literature. To date, one randomized, controlled trial[19] and two incompletely randomized controlled trials exist comparing outcomes of OTLIF with MITLIF (Shunwu et al.[20] randomized by admission date and Wang J et al.[21] randomized by consecutive odd/even order).[12–14] Wang et al.[19] reported on the use of minimal access TLIF with an expandable tubular retractor compared to OTLIF showing that it required significantly longer fluoroscopy time but resulted in less trauma to the multifidus and sacrospinalis muscles as expressed by electrophysiologic indicators. This translated to significantly better functional outcomes in the MITLIF group at 3 and 6-months, however this was not sustained at the 12- or 24-month follow-up. Shunwu et al.[20] demonstrated significant benefit to MITLIF through a tubular retractor in regards to postoperative back pain, blood loss, need for transfusion, time to ambulation, length of hospital stay and functional outcome. Wang et al.[21] also reported on the use of an expandable tubular retractor and echoed the same findings of increased fluoroscopy time with less blood loss and improved short-term functional outcome.

Conclusion

Minimally invasive transforaminal lumbar interbody fusion is a safe and effective technique to address pain and instability of the lumbar spine. Compared with traditional open TLIF, there are significant benefits in terms of minimizing patient morbidity, promoting faster return to function, and reducing costs to the hospital system. However, the surgeon must be cognizant of the learning curve associated with the transition from open surgery to minimally invasive techniques and be able to manage the increased radiation exposure associated with the procedure.

References

1. Styf JR, Willén J. The effects of external compression by three different retractors on pressure in the erector spine muscles during and after posterior lumbar spine surgery in humans. *Spine*. 1998;23(3):354–358.
2. Kawaguchi Y, Matsui H, Tsuji H. Back muscle injury after posterior lumbar spine surgery. part 1: histologic and histochemical analyses in rats. *Spine*. 1994;19(22):2590–2597.
3. Sihvonen T, Herno A, Paljärvi L, et al. Local denervation atrophy of paraspinal muscles in postoperative failed back syndrome. *Spine*. 1993;18(5):575–581.
4. Foley KT, Holly LT, Schwender JD. Minimally invasive lumbar fusion. *Spine (Phila Pa 1976)*. 2003;1;28(suppl 15):S26–S35.
5. Nandyala SV, Fineberg SJ, Pelton M, et al. Minimally invasive transforaminal lumbar interbody fusion: one surgeon's learning curve. *Spine J*. 2014;14(8):1460–1465.
6. Ruf M, Stoltze D, Merk HR, et al. Treatment of vertebral osteomyelitis by radical debridement and stabilization using titanium mesh cages. *Spine (Phila Pa 1976)*. 2007;32(9):E275–E280.
7. Patel VV, Zhao L, Wong P, et al. Controlling bone morphogenetic protein diffusion and bone morphogenetic protein-stimulated bone growth using fibrin glue. *Spine (Phila Pa 1976)*. 2006;31(11):1201–1206.
8. Wei H, Jiandong T, Xianpei W, et al. Minimally invasive versus open transforaminal lumbar fusion: a systematic review of complications. *Int. Orthop*. 2016;40(10):1883–1890.
9. Lee CS, Hwang CJ, Lee SW, et al. Risk factors for adjacent segment disease after lumbar fusion. *Eur Spine J*. 2009;18(11):1637–1643.
10. Rihn JA, Gandhi SD, Sheehan P, et al. Disc space preparation in transforaminal lumbar interbody fusion: a comparison of minimally invasive and open approaches. *Clin Orthop Relat Res*. 2014;472(6):1800–1805.
11. Wu RH, Fraser JF, Härtl R. Minimal access versus open transforaminal lumbar interbody fusion: meta-analysis of fusion rates. *Spine (Phila Pa 1976)*. 2010;35(26):2273–2281.

12. Savage JW, Kelly MP, Ellison SA, et al. A population-based review of bone morphogenetic protein: associated complication and reoperation rates after lumbar spinal fusion. *Neurosurg Focus.* 2015;39(4):E13.
13. Rihn JA, Patel R, Makda J, et al. Complications associated with single-level transforaminal lumbar interbody fusion. *Spine J.* 2009;9(8):623–629.
14. Skovrlj B, Belton P, Zarzour H, et al. Perioperative outcomes in minimally invasive lumbar spine surgery: a systematic review. *World J Orthop.* 2015;6(11):996–1005.
15. Karikari IO, Isaacs RE. Minimally invasive transforaminal lumbar interbody fusion: a review of techniques and outcomes. *Spine (Phila Pa 1976).* 2010;35(suppl 26):S294–S301.
16. Adogwa O, Parker SL, Bydon A, et al. Comparative effectiveness of minimally invasive versus open transforaminal lumbar interbody fusion: 2-year assessment of narcotic use, return to work, disability, and quality of life. *Clin Spine Surg.* 2011;24(8):479–484.
17. Parker SL, Adogwa O, Witham TF, et al. Post-operative infection after minimally invasive versus open transforaminal lumbar interbody fusion (TLIF): literature review and cost analysis. *Minim Invasive Neurosurg.* 2011;54(1):33–37.
18. Wu RH, Fraser JF, Härtl R. Minimal access versus open transforaminal lumbar interbody fusion: meta-analysis of fusion rates. *Spine (Phila Pa 1976).* 2010;35(26):2273–2281.
19. Wang HL, Lü FZ, Jiang JY, et al. Minimally invasive lumbar interbody fusion via MAST Quadrant retractor versus open surgery: a prospective randomized clinical trial. *Chin Med J (Engl).* 2011;124:3868–3874.
20. Shunwu F, Xing Z, Fengdong Z, Xiangqian F. Minimally invasive transforaminal lumbar interbody fusion for the treatment of degenerative lumbar diseases. *Spine (Phila Pa 1976).* 2010;35:162–1615.
21. Wang J, Zhou Y, Zhang ZF, et al. Minimally invasive or open transforaminal lumbar interbody fusion as revision surgery for patients previously treated by open discectomy and decompression of the lumbar spine. *Eur Spine J.* 2011;20:623–628.

10

Minimally Invasive Midline Lumbar Fusion (MIDLIF)

JACLYN J. RENFROW, MARK B. FRENKEL, AND CHARLES L. BRANCH, JR.

Introduction

Each year in the United States more than 250,000 individuals undergo spinal fusions for degenerative lumbar spine pathology. Minimally invasive techniques for posterior lumbar interbody fusion offer the benefits of a smaller incision, minimization of injury to muscles and tendons, and shorter hospital stays over traditional open techniques.[1,2] With regard to patient outcomes, a meta-analysis of 770 patients reported minimally invasive techniques for lumbar fusion also demonstrate significantly lower rate of adjacent level disease.[3] The evolution of minimally invasive approaches is in parallel with technologies allowing safe and adequate surgical access to accomplishing the surgical goals of replacing the disk space with a fusion nidus and placing instrumentation to ensure stability during this process. The MAST MIDLIF procedure, which was developed and introduced in 2011, uses a proprietary retractor and cortical bone screw fixation along with the interbody fusion technique.[4] This technique is unique in offering a midline bilateral minimally invasive alternative without the need for a tubular retractor. This allows for recognition of familiar posterior spinal landmarks and direct access to posterior element pathology including stenosis (canal, lateral recess, foramen) and synovial cysts. For fixation, the more medial bone entry point along with a caudocephalad and mediolateral screw trajectory of cortical screws allows for a more paramedial position of the segmental fixation, obviating the need for a wide lateral exposure (Fig. 10.1).

The biomechanical evaluation of cortical screws validates this novel fixation trajectory. Cortical screws are smaller than traditional pedicle screws; however, the trajectory allows the majority of the screw to pass through dense cortical bone compared with 20% cortical bone purchase of a traditional pedicle screw (Fig. 10.2). The purchase of additional cortical bone fixation despite an overall smaller screw size demonstrates equivalent pullout strength and more dense trajectory bone quality in human cadaveric lumbar spine.[5] Modifying the screw trajectory for the posterior segmental fixation from that of a traditional pedicle screw to a cortical screw trajectory establishes a durable construct using consistent anatomic landmarks even in degenerative spine pathology.

Surgical Indications

Optimal indications are one- or two-level spinal instability or deformity, including spondylolisthesis, lumbar stenosis with instability or stenosis requiring a decompression that may result in postoperative progressive deformity/iatrogenic instability, recurrent disk herniation, adjacent level degeneration to an existing fusion, and pseudoarthrosis.[6,7] In general, the surgical indications for a minimally invasive posterior lumbar interbody fusion are similar to those for an open posterior lumbar interbody fusion.

Limitations

The originally described technique uses posterior fixation with a cortical bone screw trajectory. Limitations or contraindications would include cases with no competent pedicles (e.g., fracture, neoplasm, infection) and lack of a definitive entry point at the pars and transverse process junction from a prior decompression. Biomechanical studies also identified spondylotic vertebrae as a potentially concerning pathology for placement of cortical trajectory screw fixation.[8]

Surgical Technique

The procedure steps outlined below are one example of many for how to accomplish this surgery. Each surgeon will have preferences to incorporate into the procedure including operative bed, retractor preferences, visualization aids including the microscope and/or endoscope, intraoperative imaging systems, and screw placement technique.

Minimally invasive spine surgery was born from the advancement of retractors focusing on muscle-splitting and visualization systems. Specifically, in our practice we use the MAST MIDLF retractor system; however, there are multiple other types of retractors, including tubular and expandable varieties. Often, we incorporate the use of an operative microscope into the minimally invasive lumbar fusions in place of a fiber optic lighting system. Others routinely use the endoscope.[1,9]

For intraoperative imaging we use fluoroscopy; however, increasingly computed tomography (CT) navigation systems are utilized. If used, appropriate modifications to the surgical technique, including a registration spin along with compatible hardware must be planned. The advantages to CT intraoperative guidance are surgeon comfort, real-time planning of entry point and screw trajectory, increased screw placement accuracy, and potential confirmation of screw placement.[10,11] Disadvantages are increased operative time and increased patient radiation exposure.

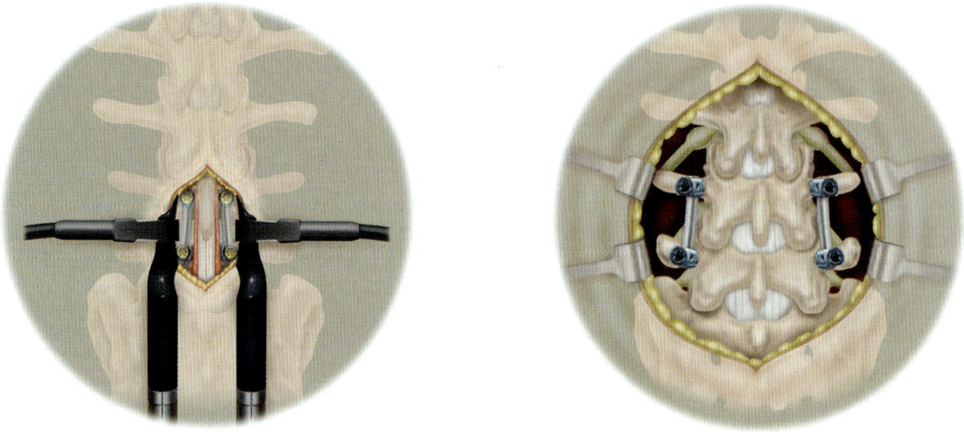

• **Fig. 10.1** Comparison of exposure windows for the minimally invasive midline lumbar fusion *(left)* and a traditional posterior segmental interbody fixation with pedicle screws *(right)*. Note the shorter length in vertical incision, approximately 4 cm, in the minimally invasive approach. Cortical screw fixation in the minimally invasive approach utilizes a more medial entry point which also reduces the necessary lateral exposure. Lateral exposure in the minimally invasive approach is sufficient once the facets are visualized as opposed to the transverse processes in traditional posterior lumbar interbody fusion approaches. (Reprinted with the permission of Medtronic, Inc., Minneapolis, MN © 2016.)

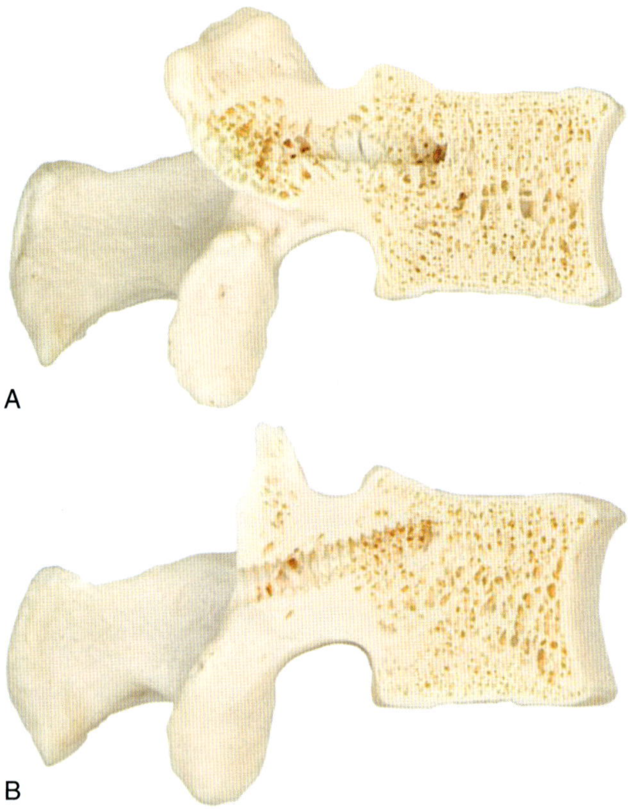

• **Fig. 10.2** The cortical screw trajectory optimizes rigid cortical bone purchase. **A.** Screw path of a traditional pedicle screw following a trajectory in line with the pedicle. Cortical bone purchase is achieved in an area amounting of approximately 20% of the screw length in the region where the pedicle is narrowest in the rostral-caudal axis. **B.** Screw path of a cortical trajectory. Cortical screws are angled caudocephalad, allowing them to navigate a longer axis of the pedicle composed of cortical bone, achieving much greater cortical bone purchase than the traditional pedicle screw trajectory. (Reprinted with the permission of Medtronic, Inc. © 2016.)

We present the cortical bone screw trajectory that uses a medial entry point compared with a traditional pedicle screw as this allows adequate visualization of the entry point without the need for further lateral muscle dissection. Percutaneous screw fixation, described in 2001,[1,2] is also another option to complement a minimally invasive approach to a posterior interbody fusion procedure.[3] Screw fixation can also be accomplished with robotic guidance systems for enhanced trajectory planning and final screw placement accuracy.[14,15]

Provided with this chapter is a detailed video demonstrating a case of a MIDLIF (Video 10.1) that follows the steps outlined below.

Step 1: Positioning. After induction of general endotracheal anesthesia and administration of preoperative antibiotics, we position the patient prone on two chest rolls on a regular table. The correct operative level is identified using fluoroscopy, and a midline incision is marked before preparing and draping in a sterile fashion.

Step 2: Incision and superficial dissection. For single level operations the incision is roughly 30 to 40 mm in length and carried down through the fascia in the midline. A speculum is then inserted on the lateral border of the spinous process to develop the subperiosteal plane between muscle and bone (Fig. 10.3A). Muscle from the spinous process and lamina of the operative levels is bluntly dissected with the speculum retractor to expose the facet (Fig. 10.3B). This process is repeated on the other side of the spinous process to accomplish a bilateral exposure. The speculum is then docked on the lamina, and a ruler on the lateral surface of the speculum blade measures out the appropriate MAST retractor blade length (Fig.10.3C). The speculum retractor is rotated 90 degrees so the blades of the speculum open parallel to the spinous process and the handle of the speculum is perpendicular to the spine (Fig. 10.4A). The blades are then opened to allow insertion of the MAST retractor blade between the blades of the speculum (Fig. 10.4B). Once the retractor blade is seated it is held in place while the speculum is withdrawn from this side of the exposure. It is then inserted

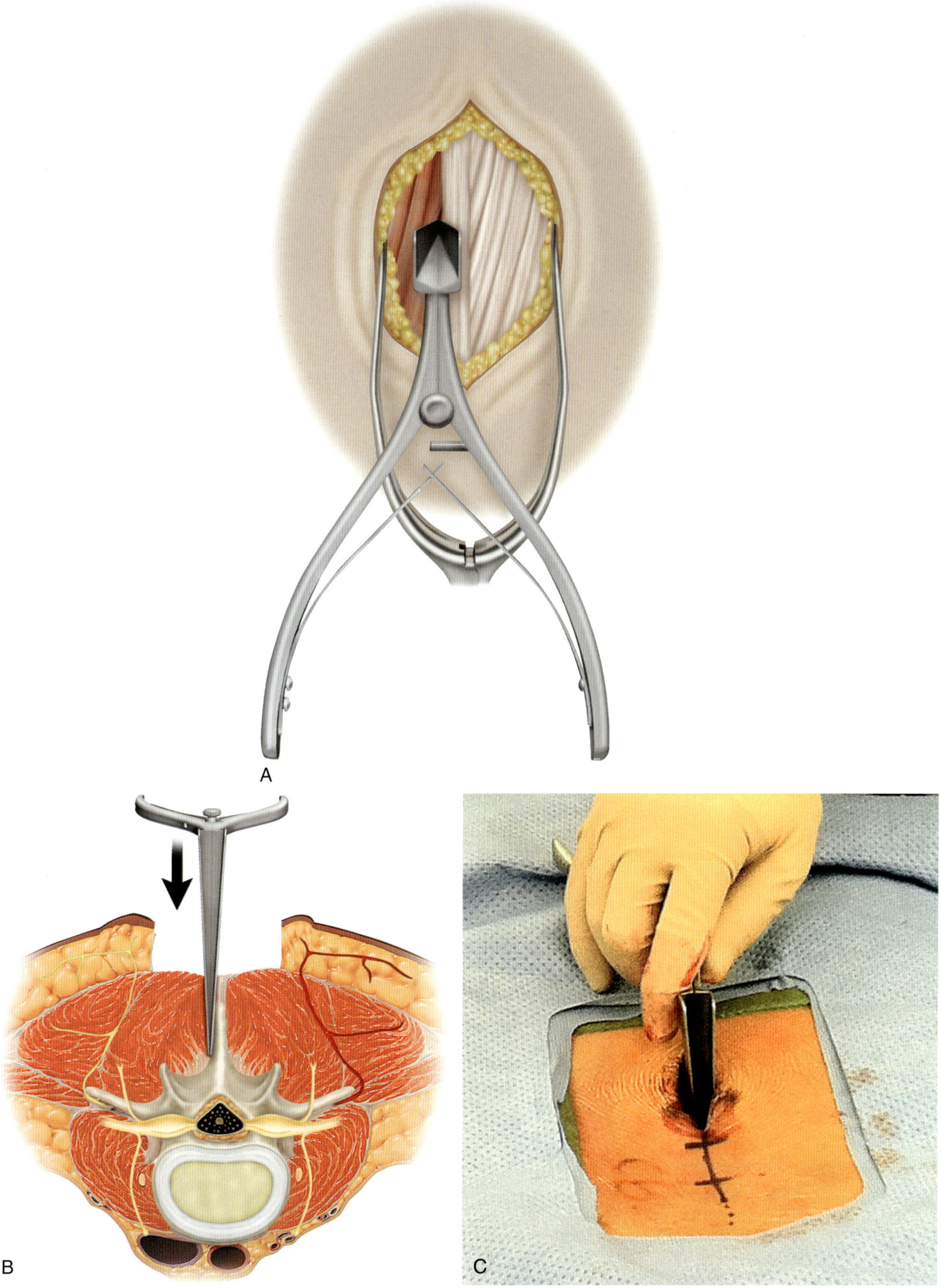

• **Fig. 10.3** Initial exposure and muscular dissection. After induction of endotracheal anesthesia, administration of preoperative antibiotics, and positioning of the patient prone on chest rolls, localization and confirmation of the correct level with fluoroscopic guidance is performed. This region is prepared and draped in the usual sterile fashion. A 4-cm midline incision is made and carried down through the fascia. **A.** A speculum is introduced on the lateral margin of the spinous process to assist in blunt subperiosteal muscle dissection, sweeping the muscle lateral over the facet joint. **B.** Axial intraoperative schematic demonstrating that once the fascia is incised a speculum is placed just lateral to the spinous process to achieve a subperiosteal dissection of the muscles laterally. The first part of this process is removing the muscle from the spinous process until the lamina is reached, requiring a predominately downward sweeping motion. Once the lamina is reached, the sweeping motion is lateral to expose the facet. **C.** Intraoperative photo demonstrating the initial dissection using the speculum. (A, B Reprinted with the permission of Medtronic, Inc. © 2016.)

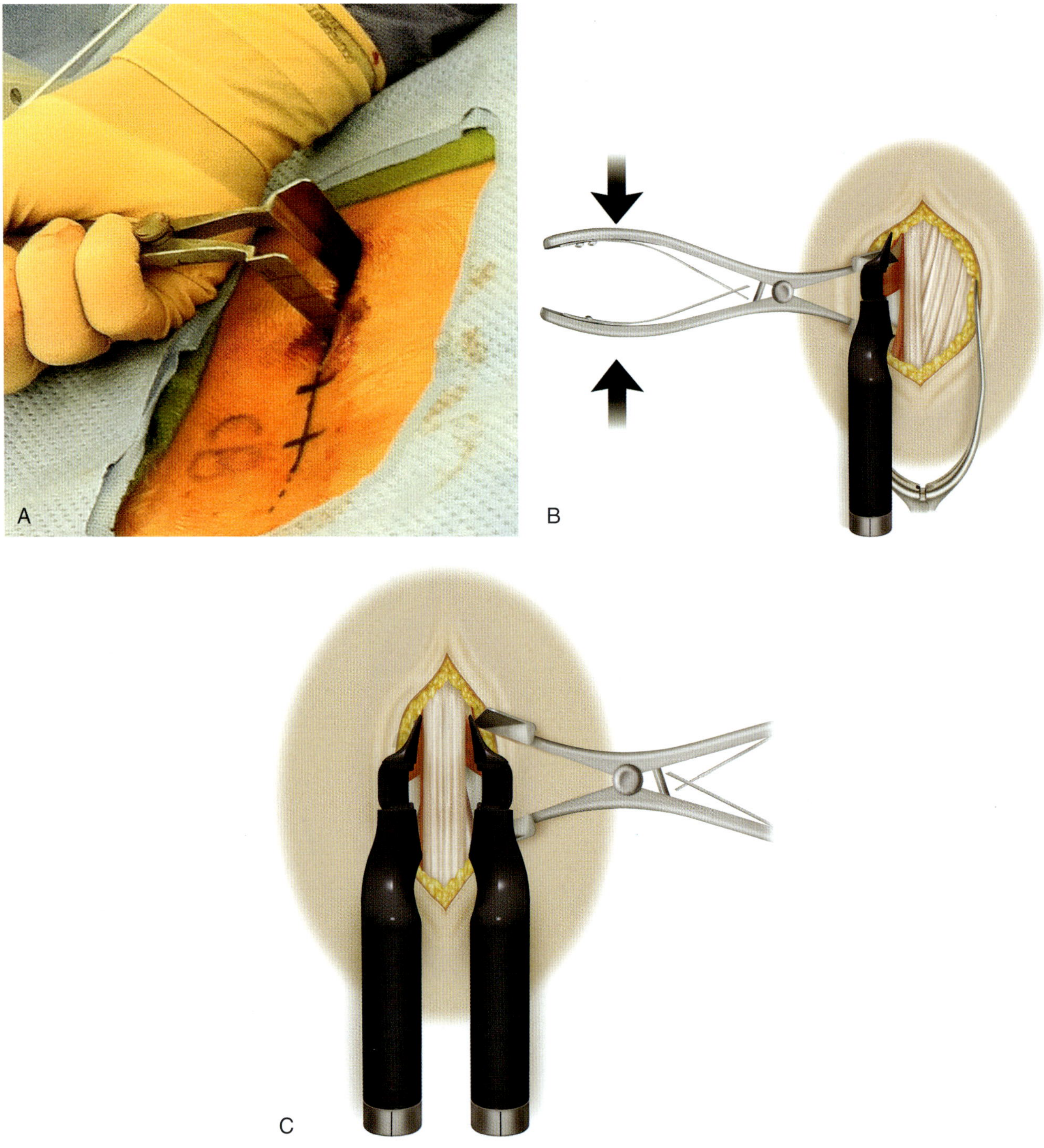

• **Fig. 10.4** Insertion of the expandable retractor. **A.** The speculum is rotated 90 degrees so the blades open parallel to the spinous process and the handles are perpendicular to the spine. **B.** The speculum is opened to allow insertion of the MAST retractor blade in the space cleared of muscle. The speculum is removed and the blade is left in place on this side. **C.** The retractor blade insertion process is repeated on the contralateral side. (B, C Reprinted with the permission of Medtronic, Inc. © 2016.)

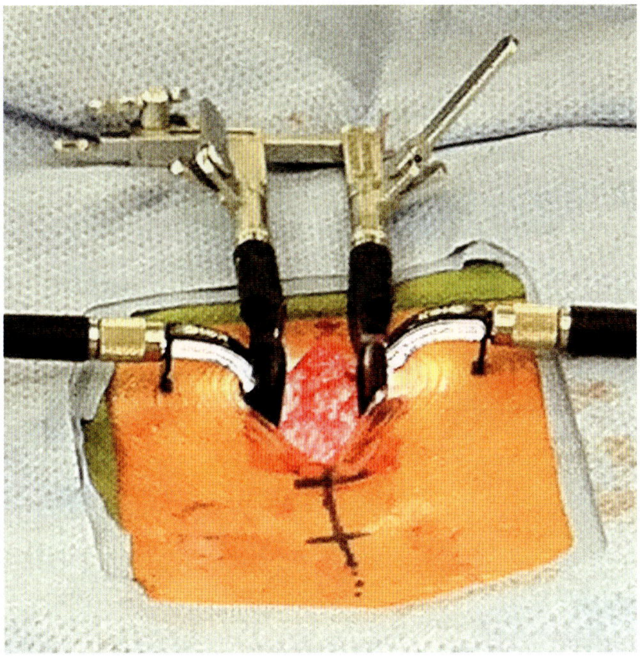

• **Fig. 10.5** Intraoperative photo demonstrating the final position of the retractor system with attachment of a fiber optic light source. Once both blades are in place they are attached to the retractor expander. The blades are rotated outward and expanded laterally to allow exposure of the operative corridor. The blades should be centered over the disk space of interest. The lateral margin of exposure should include the facets.

on the contralateral side and the retractor blade placement is repeated here (Fig. 10.4C). The final position of the MAST retractor blade should be centered over the operative disk space, which can be confirmed with fluoroscopy. The MAST blades are then attached to the retractor device, which is used to angle the blades outward laterally, maximizing the operative field visible through the incision. The retractor blades are then expanded laterally, exposing the operative corridor. The surgeon may either use the operative microscope or attach the light source to the retractor and continue the operation using loupes (Fig. 10.5).

Step 3: Facetectomy. Exposure of the interbody space begins superficially with removal of the bony facets. The inferior facets of the superior vertebral level to be fused are the most superficial bone in the field, and these are amputated using an osteotome and mallet or high-speed burr. The harvested bone is saved and ground using a bone mill to be used for autograft material in the disk space and posterior-laterally. We typically perform bilateral posterior lumbar interbody fusion (PLIF), but this can be done unilaterally if the surgeon so desires. Once the inferior facets are removed, the smooth contour of the articulating superior facet is identified. Removal of this bone begins medially, developing a space between it and the ligamentum flavum and progressing laterally into the neural foramen. The underlying superior facet of the inferior vertebrae is removed with a Kerrison rongeur. Again, harvested bone is recycled for autograft later in the case. The dura is exposed after removal of the ligamentum flavum and epidural fat (Fig. 10.6). Decompression is deemed adequate after the borders of the pedicle at the inferior level are identified with a Woodson elevator.

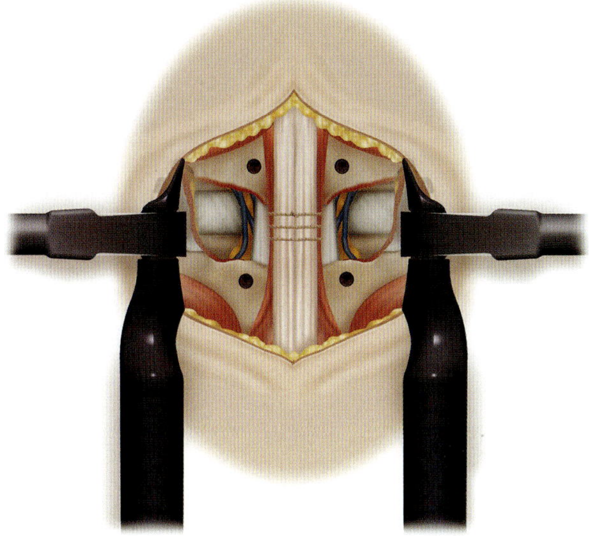

• **Fig. 10.6** Illustration of the final operative exposure after completion of bilateral facetectomies with visualization of the dura and disk space lateral and deep in the field. (Reprinted with the permission of Medtronic, Inc. © 2016.)

Step 4: Interbody fusion. The dura is gently retracted medially, if necessary. The working space is defined by the thecal sac medially, the exiting nerve root superiorly, and the pedicle inferiorly. After identification of the disk space, an annulotomy is performed. Disk material is removed with pituitary rongeurs and down pushing curettes with attention to endplate preparation. Maximal safe removal of disk material and the cartilaginous endplates optimizes the surface area for a successful fusion. Sequential dilators are used to gradually restore the disk space height, and a template is used to determine an appropriate interbody device size. With the dilator left in place for distraction, the diskectomy is repeated from the contralateral side. Once this is complete, morselized autograft, if necessary, combined with a biologic or allograft extender material, is inserted into the central disk space. Bilateral interbody devices are placed more laterally in the disk space aligned with the medial border of the pedicles to assist in restoring height, lordosis, and sagittal alignment. Caution and direct visualization are used to avoid injury to traversing or exiting nerve roots. Confirmation of interbody placement is obtained with intraoperative fluoroscopic images.

Step 5: Posterior segmental fixation. Next identify the entry points for the posterior fixation using a cortical screw trajectory. The starting point for cortical screws is just inferior to the transverse process and 4 mm medial to the lateral aspect of the pars interarticularis. Relative to the pedicle, the optimal screw insertion point can be imagined projecting from the 5 to 11 o'clock orientation in the left pedicle and 7 to 1 o'clock orientation in the right pedicle.[6] The trajectory of the screws is caudocephalad and mediolateral (Fig. 10.7). An ideal trajectory for placement of cortical screws was found to be 25 to 30 degrees cranially and 10 degrees laterally along the inferior border of the pedicle.[7]

The entry point and trajectory are confirmed using fluoroscopic imaging. Computer-assisted navigation may also be used for screw planning and placement. The entry point is made using a high-speed drill with a routing bit measuring 2 mm at the tip. During drilling we frequently pause to confirm

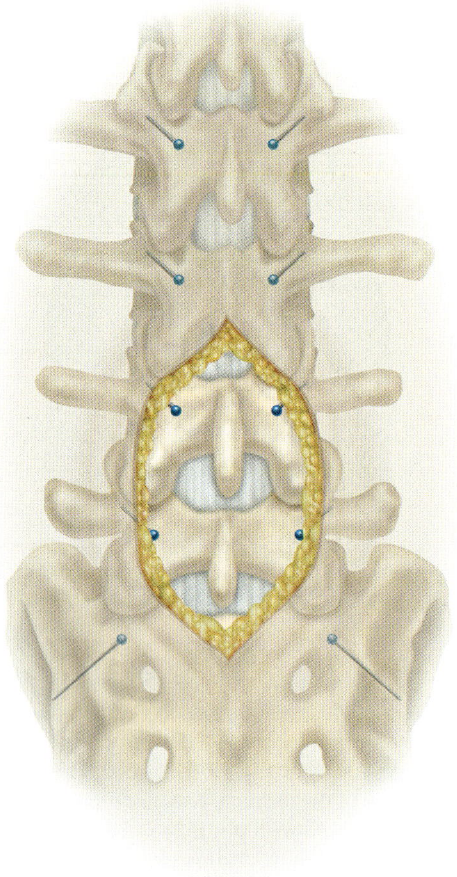

• **Fig. 10.7** **Entry points and trajectories for cortical screws in the lumbar spine.** The starting point for cortical screws is just inferior to the transverse process and 4 mm medial to the lateral aspect of the pars interarticularis. The overall direction of screw placement from this starting point can be described as "up and out." An ideal trajectory for placement of cortical screws is 25 to 30 degrees cranially and 10 degrees laterally along the inferior border of the pedicle. (Reprinted with the permission of Medtronic, Inc. © 2016.)

the tip remains in cortical bone by tapping the bit against the bottom of the hole. Anteroposterior and lateral fluoroscopy can be used to verify the correct screw trajectory (Fig. 10.8). The tip of the drill is slowly advanced to approximately 25 mm. We inspect the tract to ensure no breach has occurred before tapping with the 5.0 mm cortical thread tap (Fig. 10.9). The hole is reinspected for a breach after tapping using a ball probe and then a 5 mm by 30 or 35 mm cortical screw is then inserted. This is repeated for the remaining cortical screws to be placed (Fig. 10.10).

At S1 we identify the medial and superior borders of the S1 pedicle during the decompression. The routing drill bit is then used to drill a tract with a "straight in" trajectory into the S1 pedicle in a more conventional pedicle screw approach. We also place a larger diameter screw at this level, usually 7.5 mm.

Appropriate length rods are selected (~3 cm per level, average) and inserted into the tulip heads of the cortical screws. Set screws are placed and after final tightening of one per side, a manual compressor is placed against the screw/rod construct to optimize

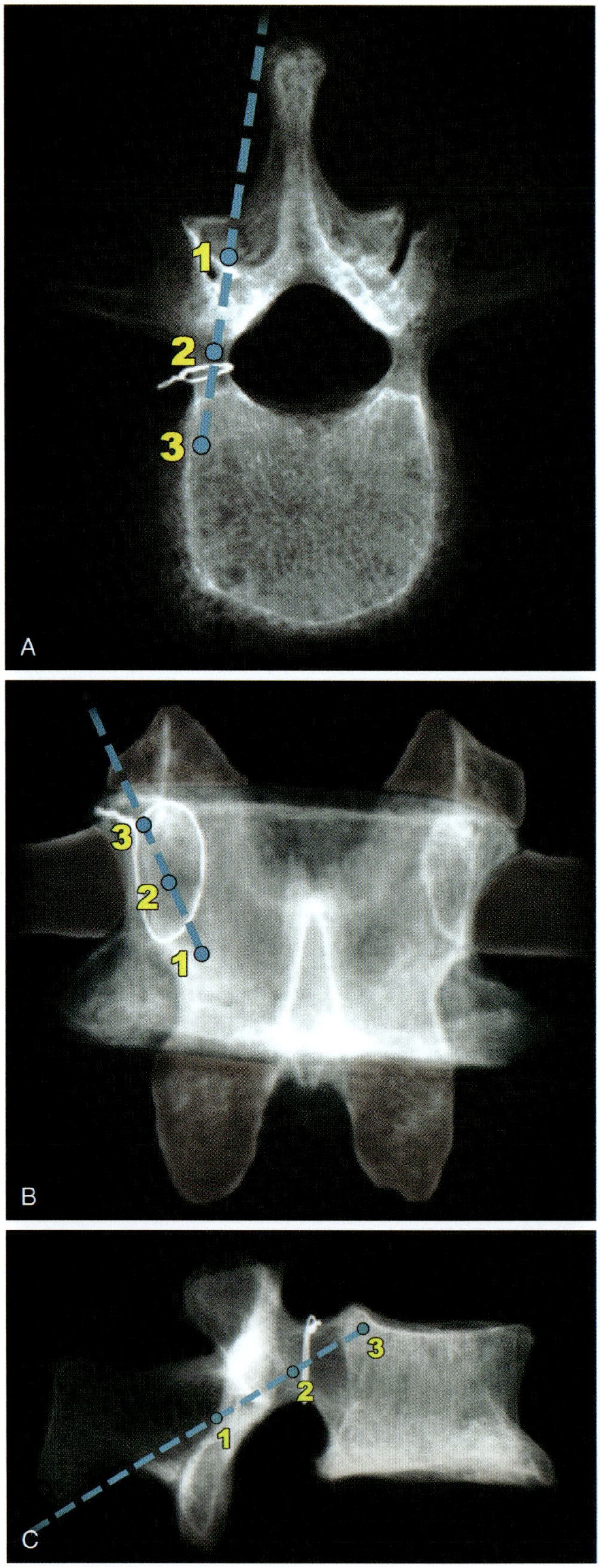

• **Fig. 10.8** Examples of fluoroscopy images for reference of the correct screw trajectory in axial (A), coronal (B), and sagittal (C) views. The x-rays are a representation of one vertebral body and corresponding drill path from starting point 1 to midpoint 2 to endpoint at around 25 mm labeled 3. (Reprinted with the permission of Medtronic, Inc. © 2016.)

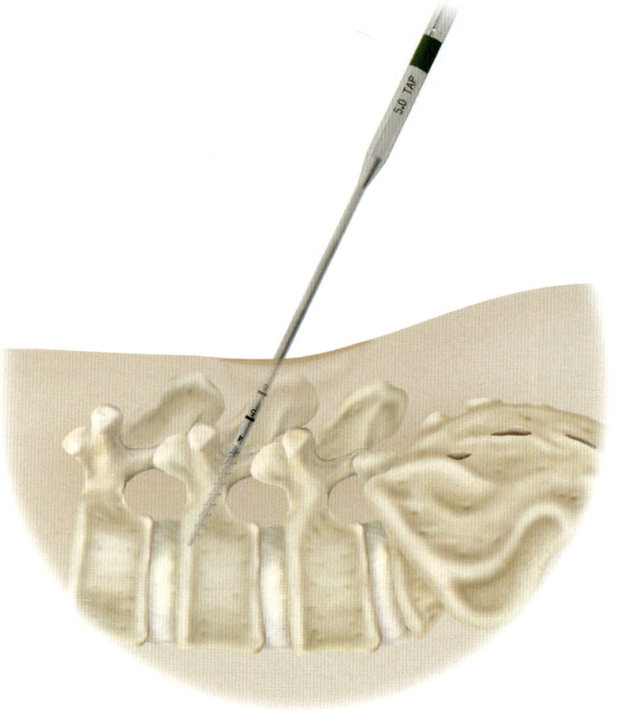

• **Fig. 10.9** Owing to density, the pilot hole is tapped its entire length and line-to-line with a sharp tap prior to final screw placement in the same trajectory as the initial drill hole. (Reprinted with the permission of Medtronic, Inc. © 2016.)

restoration of lordosis at that segment. Once this is achieved the second set screw on the same side is final tightened. This is repeated on the contralateral side of the spine. Any remaining autograft bone is placed along decorticated bone on the lateral margins of the construct.

Closure

After achieving adequate hemostasis, the wound is irrigated and lined with vancomycin powder. Closure is layered starting with the fascia followed by inverted dermal and subcuticular skin closure in a usual fashion. As a last layer, the incision is sealed with a topical skin adhesive. In our experience, surgical drains are unnecessary.

Postoperative Care

Postoperative anteroposterior and lateral x-rays are obtained in the recovery room to ensure adequate alignment and hardware placement (Fig. 10.11). Patients are admitted postoperatively to a dedicated neurosurgical floor with a fairly standardized set of routine postoperative orders. Patients receive a patient-controlled analgesia pump for the first 24 hours in addition to oral narcotic pain medication and as needed muscle relaxers. Bowel rest is observed until return of function. Mobilization and Foley catheter removal are completed on postoperative day 0 or 1, depending on the time of day the operation was completed. Retrospective review of patients undergoing the MIDLF technique as an add-on for adjacent level disease in previously instrumented thoracolumbar fusions demonstrated an average length of stay of 2.8 days,[18] which is similar to our experience.

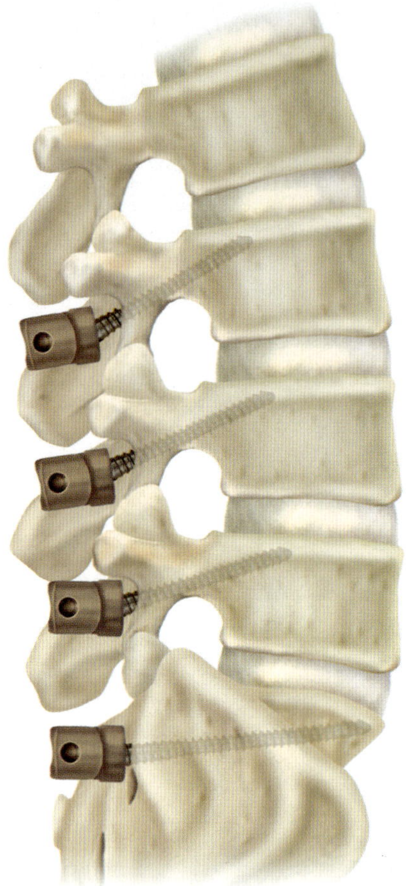

• **Fig. 10.10** Final illustration of multiple levels of cortical screw placement in lumbar spine. Notice the caudocephalad and mediolateral trajectory of the screws maximizing cortical bone purchase. Typical screw size is 5 mm by 30 or 35 mm in length. (Reprinted with the permission of Medtronic, Inc. © 2016.)

Complications/Side Effects

A meta-analysis of 856 minimally invasive lumbar interbody fusions reported an aggregate complication rate of 10.9%.[19] Potential complications can be organized into neurologic (nerve root injury, conus injury, cerebrospinal fluid leak), vascular (bleeding), infectious, and mechanical (pseudoarthrosis, instability, screw misplacement, instrumentation failure, vertebral fractures), and medical. The most common complications from this study were urinary tract infection at 4.6% and dural tear at 3.8%.

Outcomes

Large randomized analysis of the midline minimally invasive posterior interbody fusion technique are to be published, yet clinical experience is very similar to other methods of minimally invasive posterior interbody fusion approaches. Data that do exist in the literature are mainly from cohort studies.[2,19,20] After comparing minimally invasive approaches for interbody fusion with traditional approaches, these studies demonstrate that operative times were equivalent. Patients having minimally invasive procedures tended to lose less blood, were exposed to more fluoroscopy, and left the hospital sooner. Patient-reported outcomes were equivocal between the two approaches. Recent evidence suggests the rate of adjacent level disease may be lower using the MIDLIF technique[3]; however, this will need to be confirmed in future studies.

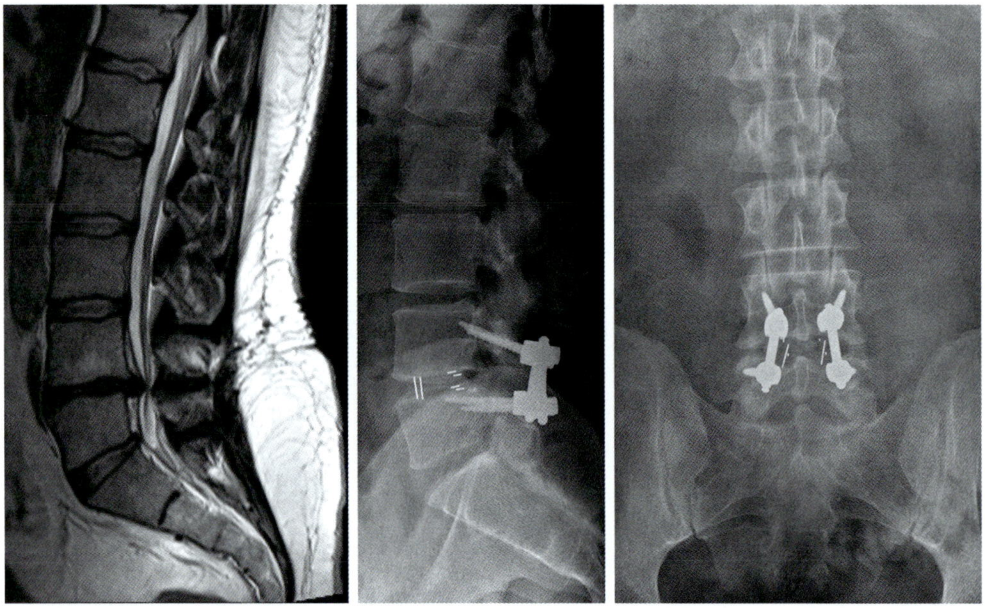

• **Fig. 10.11** Young man with multiple episodes of recurrent symptomatic disk herniation at L4-5 presented for definitive treatment with a minimally invasive midline lumbar interbody fusion. His T2 sagittal magnetic resonance image demonstrates the recurrent disk herniation followed by postoperative lateral and anteroposterior x-rays taken in the recovery room. The x-rays demonstrate the cortical screw trajectory caudocephalad through the pedicle and good placement of the interbody spacers within the disk space. Rod placement and final tightening were completed under manual compression to preserve segmental lordosis.

Conclusion

Minimally invasive techniques to the lumbar spine offers advantages including decreased muscle dissection, blood loss, length of hospital stay, and incidence of adjacent level disease. The minimally invasive midline approach allows direct visualization of familiar landmarks, and cortical bone screws utilize this exposure window to provide posterior fixation. The use of this technique should be considered in the context of an individual surgeon's experience and the pathology unique to each case. A minimally invasive decompression and fusion with cortical bone screws for segmental fixation through a small midline incision can offer the patient an efficient alternative to traditional open posterior lumbar fusion approaches.

References

1. Isaacs RE, Podichetty VK, Santiago P, et al. Minimally invasive microendoscopy-assisted transforaminal lumbar interbody fusion with instrumentation. *J Neurosurg Spine*. 2005;3:98–105. http://www.ncbi.nlm.nih.gov/pubmed/16370298. Accessed June 13, 2016.
2. Park Y, Ha JW. Comparison of one-level posterior lumbar interbody fusion performed with a minimally invasive approach or a traditional open approach. *Spine (Phila Pa 1976)*. 2007;32:537–543. http://www.ncbi.nlm.nih.gov/pubmed/17334287. Accessed June 13, 2016.
3. Li X-C, Huang C-M, Zhong C-F, et al. Minimally invasive procedure reduces adjacent segment degeneration and disease: new benefit-based global meta-analysis. *PLoS One*. 2017;12:e0171546. http://www.ncbi.nlm.nih.gov/pubmed/28207762. Accessed February 18, 2017.
4. *Medtronic introduces new procedure for minimally invasive spinal fusion [news release]*. Memphis, TN: Medtronic, Inc.; 2011.
5. Santoni BG, Hynes RA, McGilvray KC, et al. Cortical bone trajectory for lumbar pedicle screws. *Spine J*. 2009;9:366–373. http://www.ncbi.nlm.nih.gov/pubmed/18790684. Accessed June 14, 2016.
6. Satoh I, Yonenobu K, Hosono N, et al. Indication of posterior lumbar interbody fusion for lumbar disc herniation. *J Spinal Disord Tech*. 2006;19:104–108. http://www.ncbi.nlm.nih.gov/pubmed/16760783. Accessed February 18, 2017.
7. Wang JC, Mummaneni PV, Haid RW. Current treatment strategies for the painful lumbar motion segment: posterolateral fusion versus interbody fusion. *Spine (Phila Pa 1976)*. 2005;30:S33–S43. http://www.ncbi.nlm.nih.gov/pubmed/16103832. Accessed February 18, 2017.
8. Matsukawa K, Yato Y, Imabayashi H, et al. Biomechanical evaluation of lumbar pedicle screws in spondylolytic vertebrae: comparison of fixation strength between the traditional trajectory and a cortical bone trajectory. *J Neuros Spine*. 2016;24:910–915. http://www.ncbi.nlm.nih.gov/pubmed/26895531. Accessed June 13, 2016.
9. Yang Y, Liu B, Rong L-M, et al. Microendoscopy-assisted minimally invasive transforaminal lumbar interbody fusion for lumbar degenerative disease: short-term and medium-term outcomes. *Int J Clin Exp Med*. 2015;8:21319–21326. http://www.ncbi.nlm.nih.gov/pubmed/26885072. Accessed June 13, 2016.
10. Gelalis ID, Paschos NK, Pakos EE, et al. Accuracy of pedicle screw placement: a systematic review of prospective in vivo studies comparing free hand, fluoroscopy guidance and navigation techniques. *Eur Spine J*. 2012;21:247–255. http://www.ncbi.nlm.nih.gov/pubmed/21901328. Accessed February 18, 2017.
11. Innocenzi G, Bistazzoni S, D'Ercole M, et al. Does navigation improve pedicle screw placement accuracy? Comparison between navigated and non-navigated percutaneous and open fixations. *Acta Neurochir Suppl*. 2017;124:289–295. http://www.ncbi.nlm.nih.gov/pubmed/28120086. Accessed February 18, 2017.
12. Foley KT, Gupta SK, Justis JR, et al. Percutaneous pedicle screw fixation of the lumbar spine. *Neurosurg Focus*. 2001;10:E10. http://www.ncbi.nlm.nih.gov/pubmed/16732626. Accessed February 18, 2017.
13. Dickerman RD, East JW, Winters K, et al. Anterior and posterior lumbar interbody fusion with percutaneous pedicle screws. *Spine (Phila Pa 1976)*. 2009;34:E923–E925. http://www.ncbi.nlm.nih.gov/pubmed/19940722. Accessed February 18, 2017.

14. Kim H-J, Jung W-I, Chang B-S, et al. A prospective, randomized, controlled trial of robot-assisted vs freehand pedicle screw fixation in spine surgery. *Int J Med Robot*. 2017;13.
15. Kim H-J, Kang K-T, Park S-C, et al. Biomechanical advantages of robot-assisted pedicle screw fixation in posterior lumbar interbody fusion compared with freehand technique in a prospective randomized controlled trial—perspective for patient-specific finite element analysis. *Spine J*. 2017;17:671–680. http://www.ncbi.nlm.nih.gov/pubmed/27867080. Accessed February 18, 2017.
16. Matsukawa K, Yato Y, Nemoto O, et al. Morphometric measurement of cortical bone trajectory for lumbar pedicle screw insertion using computed tomography. *J Spinal Disord Tech*. 2013;26:E248–E253. http://www.ncbi.nlm.nih.gov/pubmed/23429319. Accessed June 13, 2016.
17. Matsukawa K, Taguchi E, Yato Y, et al. Evaluation of the Fixation strength of pedicle screws using cortical bone trajectory: what is the ideal trajectory for optimal fixation? *Spine (Phila Pa 1976)*. 2015;40:E873–878. http://www.ncbi.nlm.nih.gov/pubmed/26222663. Accessed June 13, 2016.
18. Rodriguez A, Neal MT, Liu A, et al. Novel placement of cortical bone trajectory screws in previously instrumented pedicles for adjacent-segment lumbar disease using CT image-guided navigation. *Neurosurg Focus*. 2014;36:E9. http://www.ncbi.nlm.nih.gov/pubmed/24580010. Accessed June 8, 2016.
19. Goldstein CL, Macwan K, Sundararajan K, et al. Comparative outcomes of minimally invasive surgery for posterior lumbar fusion: a systematic review. *Clin Orthop Relat Res*. 2014;472:1727–1737. http://www.ncbi.nlm.nih.gov/pubmed/24464507. Accessed June 13, 2016.
20. Sidhu GS, Henkelman E, Vaccaro AR, et al. Minimally invasive versus open posterior lumbar interbody fusion: a systematic review. *Clin Orthop Relat Res*. 2014;472:1792–1799. http://www.ncbi.nlm.nih.gov/pubmed/24748069. Accessed June 13, 2016.

11

Lateral Transpsoas Approach to Interbody Fusion

ZACHARY J. TEMPEL, DAVID J. SALVETTI, AND ADAM S. KANTER

Introduction

The transpsoas lateral lumbar interbody fusion (LLIF) technique was first introduced by Pimenta and Taylor in 2006 as an alternative to traditional anterior lumbar interbody fusion.[1] Over the past decade, LLIF has established itself as an effective means and adjunct when treating an array of spinal pathologies.[2–6] The technique enables access to the spine laterally via the retroperitoneal corridor by splitting the fibers of the psoas muscle longitudinally. Lateral tissue planes and the adjacent anatomic structures are often less familiar to traditional spine surgeons; thus it remains essential to develop an understanding of the numerous complexities of the LLIF procedure prior to performing this technique. This chapter discusses the unique anatomy, surgical technique, surgical indications, and postoperative care relevant to the LLIF technique. Patient outcomes are also briefly described.

To understand the LLIF and its potential uses and limitations, the surgeon must have a thorough understanding of the relevant anatomy to this approach. The psoas muscle originates from the transverse processes and the anterolateral aspect of the lumbar vertebral bodies. It descends deep to the inguinal ligament until it meets the iliacus muscle and inserts into the lesser trochanter of the femur. The psoas muscle becomes more robust as it descends caudal from its L1 origin owing to additional contributions from each lumbar segment. It is innervated by the L2-4 nerve roots and functions as the primary hip flexor muscle.

The LLIF corridor runs in proximity to the complex anatomy of the lumbar plexus, which is enveloped by the psoas muscle adjacent to the lateral vertebral bodies and disk spaces (Fig. 11.1).[7–10] In general, the plexus migrates anteriorly as it descends caudally along the psoas (Fig. 11.2). The iliohypogastric and ilioinguinal nerves arise at L1 and remain posterior until the L4-5 level, where they take a sharp turn anteriorly. The genitofemoral nerve arises from the L1 and L2 nerve roots and descends within the psoas muscle parallel to the spine until it emerges from the muscle and runs along the superficial surface around L3. The largest nerve within the lumbar plexus is the femoral nerve, originating from the L2, L3, and L4 nerve roots. It lies deep within the psoas and courses anteriorly as it descends along the spine, often crossing the L4-5 disk space. Here, the nerve has two branches as the descending nerve accepts its final contribution from the L4 root. Of note, the L4-5 disk space is the most challenging lumbar level to access via the LLIF approach owing to the close proximity of the femoral nerve, and the risk of nerve injury is highest at this level.[7–10]

Surgical Indications

The LLIF can successfully be utilized to treat an array of spinal conditions, including (1) degenerative disk disease, (2) recurrent disk herniations (without fragment extrusion), (3) mild to moderate lumbar stenosis, (4) grades I and II spondylolisthesis, (5) adjacent level degeneration after previous arthrodesis, (6) far lateral disk herniations, (7) diskitis, (8) pseudarthrosis, and (9) degenerative scoliosis. In general, much of the same pathology traditionally treated with posterior arthrodesis and decompressive techniques can be addressed with LLIF. The primary difference from open surgical procedures is that LLIF relies on indirect decompression and ligamentotaxis to decompress neural elements as compared with direct visualization and bony decompression.

Limitations

Selection of the appropriate surgical candidate for an LLIF procedure relies heavily on understanding the structural and anatomic limitations that may compromise the success and safety of the procedure. First, despite being a very useful decompressive technique, LLIF has limitations in the extent that neural elements may be decompressed. Patients with severe central canal stenosis are not ideal LLIF candidates because indirect decompression may prove inadequate. Furthermore, if neural compression is primarily caused by posterior pathology, such as hypertrophied ligamentum flavum, LLIF may not be suitable for decompression. Other examples would include extruded disk fragments, facet cysts, osteophytic disease, or severely hypertrophied facets. Similarly, grade II or higher spondylolisthesis is better approached through a posterior corridor as the disk center may be difficult to access without injuring the adjacent neural structures, or the anterior longitudinal ligament.

Another anatomic consideration unique to the LLIF approach involves the position of the iliac crest relative to the lower levels of the spine, particularly L4-5. Plain anteroposterior (AP) radiographs are most helpful to assess the iliac crest and determine if lateral access is possible (Fig. 11.3). As previously noted, as the femoral nerve travels distal, it courses anteriorly, limiting the safe working space within the psoas at L4-5 and the subsequent risk of femoral nerve traction/injury is higher.[9] The position of the psoas muscle relative to the vertebral body should be examined; it should rest immediately lateral to the vertebral body just anterior to the transverse

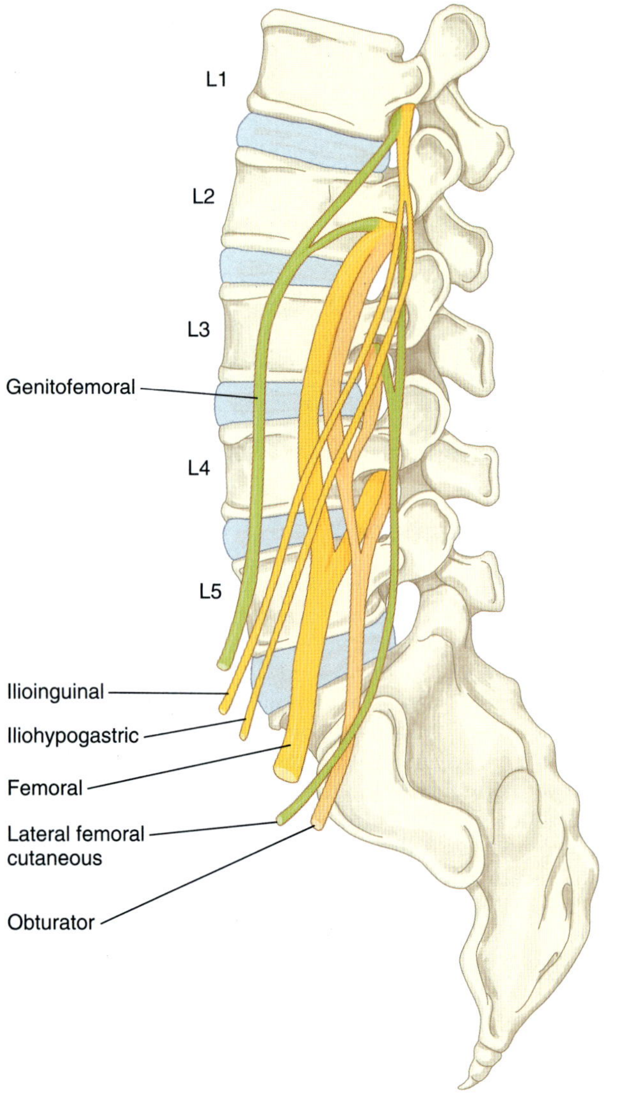

• **Fig. 11.1** Figure depicting complex relationship of neural elements in the lumbar plexus with ilioinguinal, iliohypogastric, and genitofemoral nerves coursing at various points potentially directly through the surgical corridor. Proper use of neuromonitoring and surgical technique is paramount to protecting these structures. (From Miller MD, Chhabra AB, Shen FH, et al. *Orthopaedic Surgical Approaches*, 2nd ed. Philadelphia: Elsevier; 2015: Fig. 5.61.)

process. Occasionally, the psoas can be found anterolateral to its typical position, thus displacing the neural elements with it. Failure to recognize, anticipate, and adjust for this anatomic variant will increase the risk of vascular and/or neural injury. The position of the great vessels must be evaluated, particularly in the setting of deformity as their anatomic position can be severely disturbed. The ribs can limit lateral access superiorly, necessitating either traversal of the intercostal space or resection of a portion of the rib. Importantly, these anatomic structures can be visualized with magnetic resonance imaging and/or computed tomography (CT) myelography. Also notable, prior retroperitoneal surgery predisposes the patient to internal adhesions and fibrosis, further increasing the complexity and risk of the LLIF approach. Lastly, consideration of supplemental hardware (lateral plating, pedicle screw, or spinous process fixation) is influenced by the patient's intrinsic bone quality as

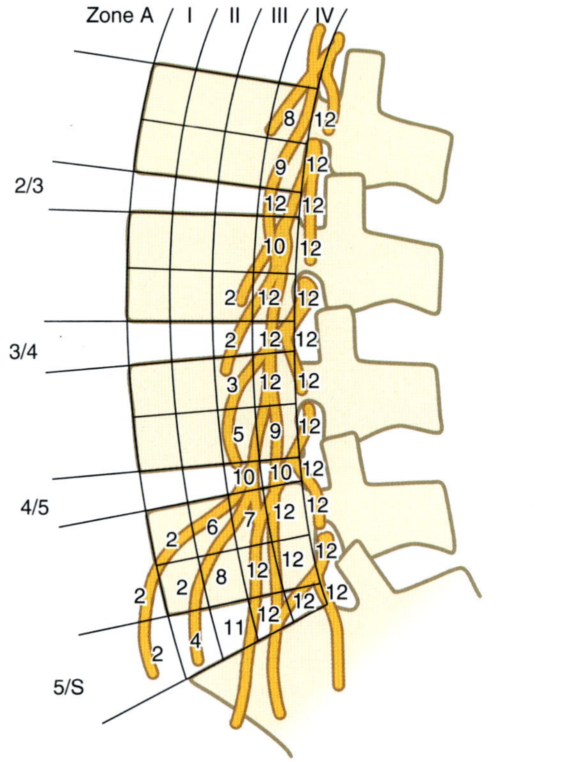

• **Fig. 11.2** Figure depicting summary of cadaveric study depicting the anterior progression of the lumbar plexus as it descends caudally. The safe working corridor for a transpsoas approach thus narrows caudally. In general, the anterior half of the vertebral body is considered safe. (Images provided by Medtronic.) (From Quinones-Hinojoas A, ed. *Schmidek and Sweet Operative Neurosurgical Techniques*, vol 6. Philadelphia: Elsevier; 2012: Fig. 172-3.)

well as intraoperative disruption of the anterior longitudinal ligament (ALL), and endplate violation.[11,12]

Surgical Technique

Step 1: Required Equipment

To perform LLIF, the required equipment consists of a series of dilators, a table-mounted lateral access retractor with light source, a neuromonitoring system, and specially designed instruments for disk resection. Neuromonitoring is critically important to ensure the safety of the LLIF procedure. An appropriate neuromonitoring platform consists of electromyography (EMG) and allows for direct stimulation of the instruments through all steps of the procedure beginning with serial dilation through the psoas to disk space until the retractor is firmly anchored in place. Once the retractor is docked and prior to incising the disk space, a stimulation probe permits direct stimulation of any tissue overlying the disk space and excludes the presence of a motor nerve. Successful use of EMG and neuromonitoring during the LLIF procedure requires the avoidance of neuromuscular blockade during anesthesia.

Other equipment needed includes an operative table with the capability to articulate between the greater trochanter and the iliac crest. Like many minimally invasive techniques, direct visualization is limited, and a significant portion of the procedure is carried out with fluoroscopic guidance. Accurate fluoroscopic imaging during LLIF is technically challenging and paramount to successfully performing the procedure. Therefore, it is recommended that the fluoroscope is managed by an experienced fluoroscopy technician.

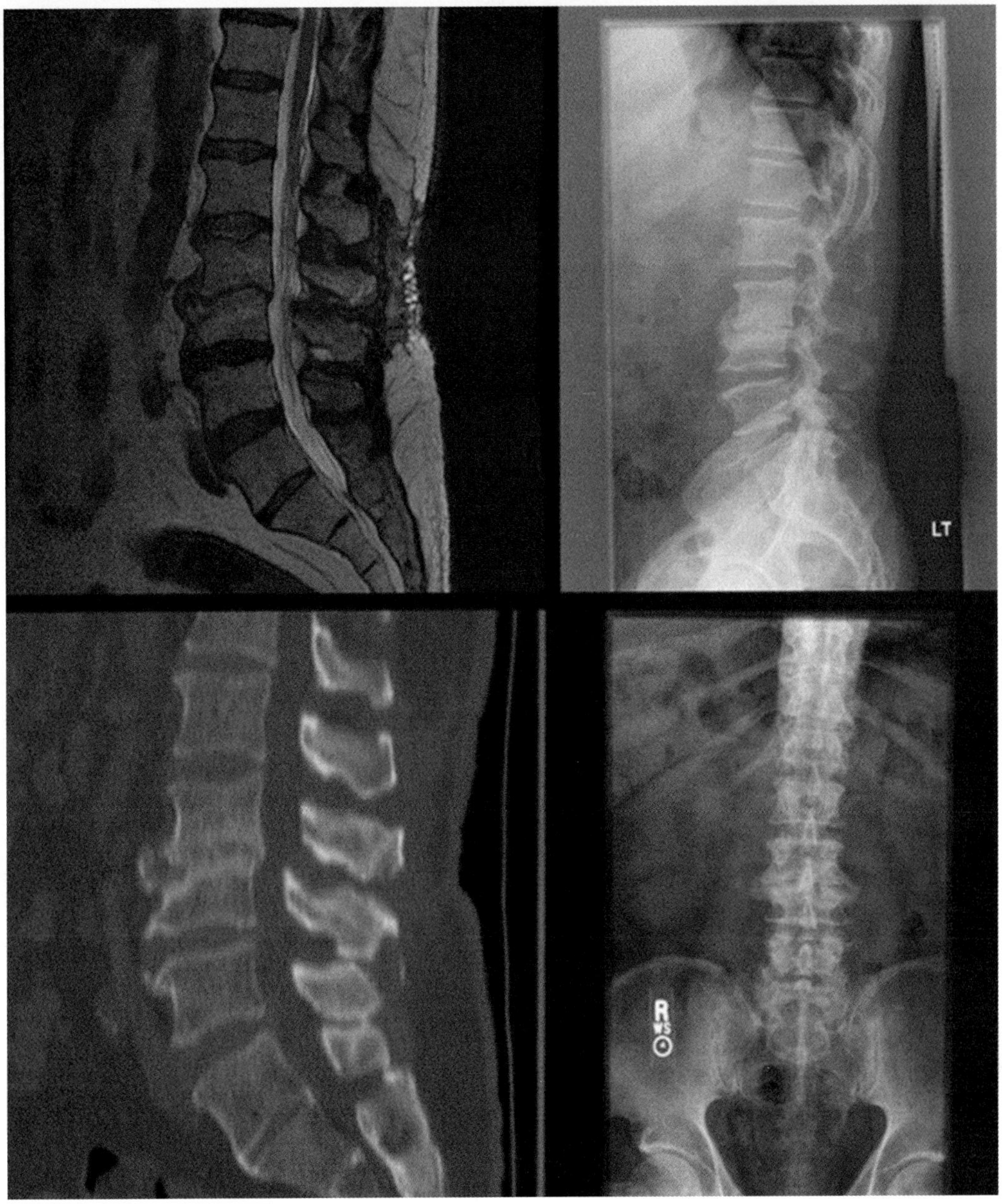

• **Fig. 11.3** A patient suited for the lateral lumbar interbody fusion (LLIF) technique. Note the lack of severe central canal stenosis; the operative level is also well above the iliac crest as noted on the lateral radiographs. (From Ozgur BM, Aryan HE, Pimenta L, Taylor WR. Extreme lateral interbody fusion (XLIF): a novel surgical technique for anterior lumbar interbody fusion. *Spine J* 2006;6:435–443, Fig. 1.)

Step 2: Positioning

The patient should be positioned in the operating room in the lateral decubitus position with the knees slightly flexed to approximately 30 degrees to relax the psoas muscle, and the articulation point of the table should be equidistant between the greater trochanter and the top of the iliac crest. The back and shoulders should be parallel just medial to the edge of the bed with an axillary roll placed under the dependent axillae. Padding of dependent and exposed bony prominences is ensured. If the patient is positioned too close to the edge, the bed frame may obstruct the fluoroscopic images. A pillow is typically placed between the knees. Finally, a pillow is placed folded in half between the arms with the dependent arm supported by an arm board (Fig. 11.4). It is important to position the arms of the patient in 90 degrees of forward flexion to create a clear path for the fluoroscope. Once the patient is positioned satisfactorily, three-inch cloth tape is used to fix the patient to the table at the upper torso superiorly and around the iliac crest inferiorly. When applying tape inferiorly, it is important run the tape inferior to the articulation point of the table. Another point of fixation is accomplished by running tape from the iliac crest to the anterior inferior corner of the table, thus maximizing the costopelvic angle, and enabling a secure lateral jack-knife position (Fig. 11.5). Securing the patient in this manner allows for rotation of the operative table in order to obtain the correct orientation of the spine. The table is then brought into reverse Trendelenberg position and the back of the table is brought down to create the lateral jackknife position. Care must be taken to avoid excessive breaking of the table as neural stretch can occur from positioning with resultant neurapraxia.[13,14]

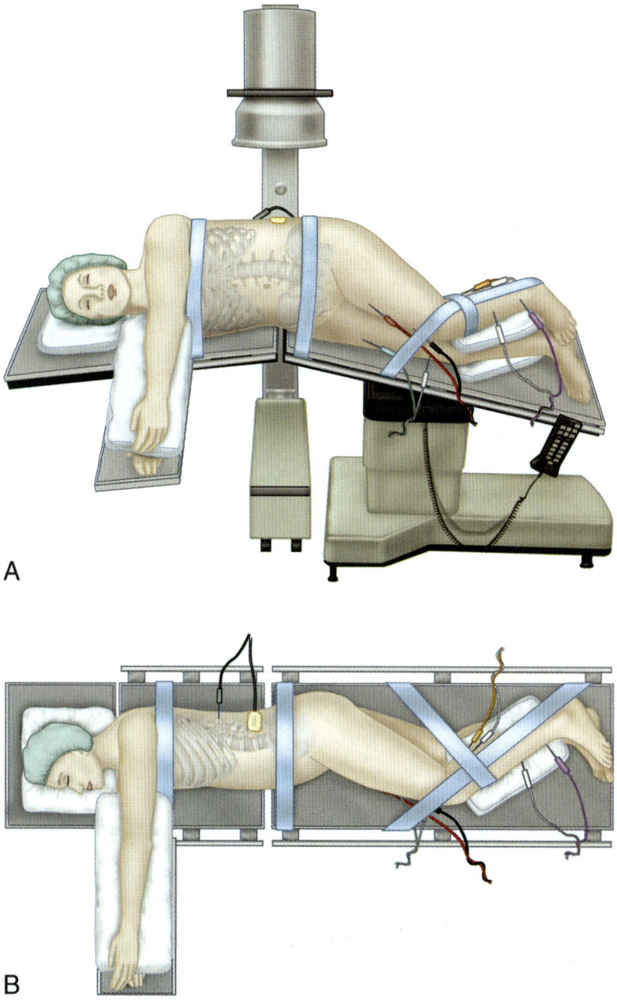

• **Fig. 11.4** Frontal (A) and top-down (B) views of proper patient positioning. Note the patient is positioned on the table such that the break is between the greater trochanter and iliac crest to allow for side bending for easier access to the disk space. The goal is to have the operative level directly perpendicular to the floor. (Images provided by Medtronic.) (From Quinones-Hinojoas A, ed. *Schmidek and Sweet Operative Neurosurgical Techniques*, vol 6. Philadelphia: Elsevier; 2012: Fig. 172-4.)

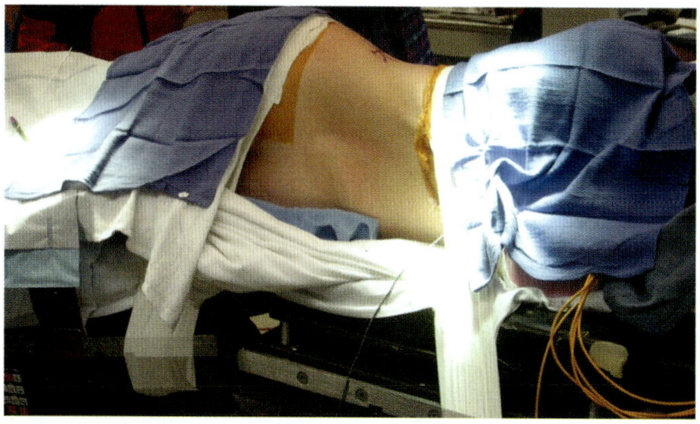

• **Fig. 11.5** Implementation of patient positioning in the operating room (OR). Note the axillary roll, padding of bony prominences, break in bed, and tape to secure patient. (From author's collection.)

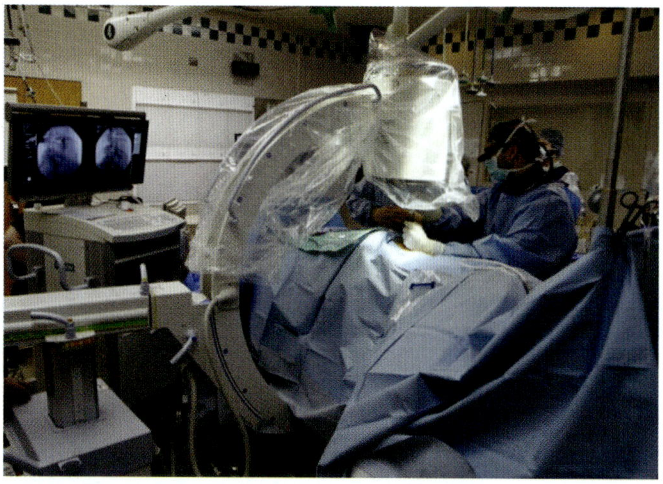

• **Fig. 11.6** Typical operating room setup with fluoroscope brought into field from the opposite side of the patient from the surgeon. The surgeon stands at the patient's back with the head toward anesthesia. The fluoroscope screen is best placed toward the feet. (From author's collection.)

Step 3: Flouroscopy Setup and Incision Planning

Fig. 11.6 demonstrates the typical operating room (OR) setup for the LLIF approach (Fig. 11.6). The OR tables is positioned with the head toward anesthesia. The surgeon and surgical technician are located posterior to the patient, and the C-arm is brought in from the abdominal side of the patient with the fluoroscopy monitor at the feet. The two most common incision techniques used to access the retroperitoneal space are the single and double incision method. The nuances of these two incisions are compared below. Regardless of which technique is chosen, the first step in incision planning is to obtain a true AP radiograph with a C-arm in a cross table orientation (Fig. 11.7). To accomplish this, the C-arm is brought into the field such that the long axis of the machine matches the lordotic angle of the targeted disk space. The operative table is then rotated left or right with the C-arm remaining at 0 degree to obtain a true AP view by lining up the spinous processes symmetrically between the pedicles. If a multilevel surgery is planned, the C-arm and the patient may require repositioning for each level, depending on the anatomy, to ensure proper positioning and approach trajectory. This is critically important in patients with scoliosis with a significant rotatory component.

To mark the incision, the C-arm is rotated into the lateral position, and a true lateral radiograph is obtained by lining up the endplates and pedicles of the targeted level such that the disk space and neural foramen are sharply defined. To mark the disk space, a K-wire is then placed on the patient's flank (Fig. 11.8) and positioned until it is radiographically parallel with the disk space with the tip of the K-wire located at the anterior border of the disk space (Fig. 11.9). After marking the skin, it is common to define and mark the posterior aspect of the disk space with the K-wire. Some surgeons find it advantageous to mark the different quartiles of the disk space as well in order to define their planned docking location. The incision line should then be drawn approximately one-third of the distance from the posterior to anterior spinal line at the same angle. For multiple levels, especially in scoliotic cases, a true lateral must be obtained and the disk space marked at each level. This is accomplished by adjusting the operative table using the Trendelenburg and reverse Trendelenburg positions and maintaining the C-arm at 90 degrees. For surgery involving multiple levels, it is often beneficial to draw the anterior and posterior spinal lines on the flank of the patient with

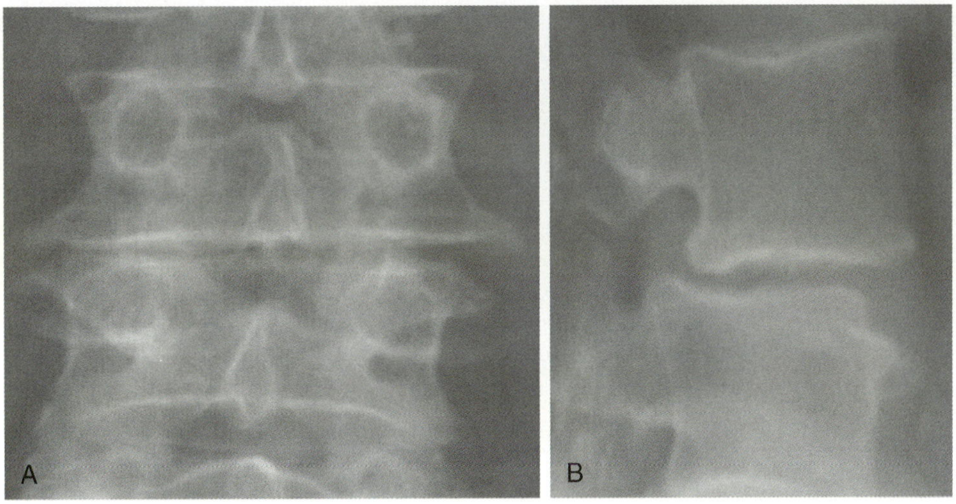

• **Fig. 11.7** Anteroposterior (A) and lateral (B) radiographs depicting well aligned endplates and pedicles with the spinous process in between indicating appropriate patient positioning for a lateral lumbar interbody fusion (LLIF). (From Quinones-Hinojoas A, ed. *Schmidek and Sweet Operative Neurosurgical Techniques*, vol 6. Philadelphia: Elsevier; 2012: Fig. 172-7.)

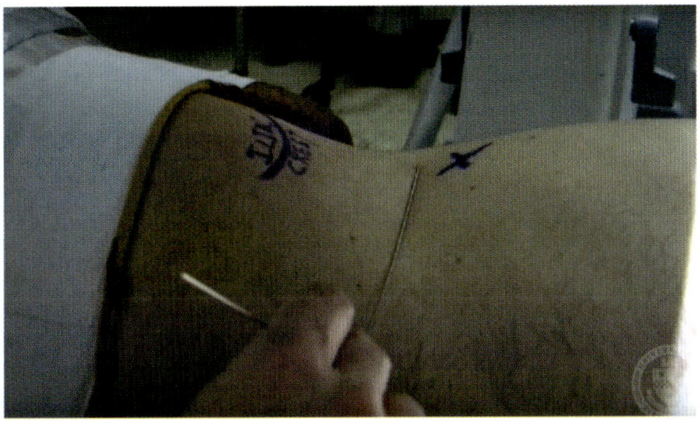

• **Fig. 11.8** A k-wire placed on patient's flank during incision planning. The goal is to have the k-wire parallel to the endplates of the operative level with the tip of the k-wire at the anterior margin of the disk space. (From author's collection.)

disk spaces marked (Fig. 11.10). Often, multiple levels can be accessed through a single incision by creating an incision the takes a more diagonal course from posterior/superior to anterior/inferior (simulating the course of the lumbar plexus) between the targeted disk spaces.

Step 4: Retroperitoneal Access

There are two primary techniques to access the retroperitoneal space, a single and double incision method. For a single incision technique, the skin is incised on the center line as described above. Using a blunt dissection technique, a plane is created through the layers of the external oblique, internal oblique, transversalis muscle, and fascia (Fig. 11.11). This can be accomplished by utilizing either a hemostat, blunt scissors, or by manual digital dissection. When in the retroperitoneal space, the viscera overlying the psoas muscle is gently swept anteriorly above and below the exposure. With the finger in contact with the psoas muscle, the first dilator is gently guided onto the surface of the psoas muscle. Neurostimulation is utilized during each pass of the dilators to minimize nerve contact and injury.

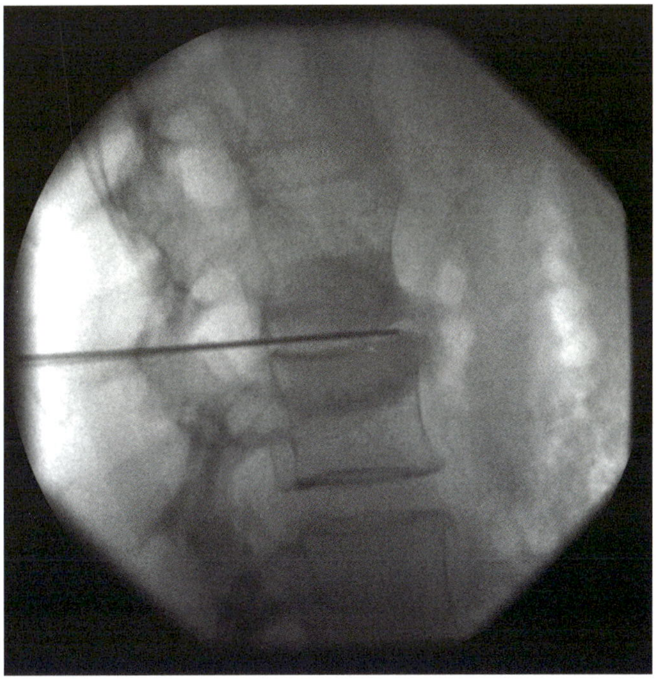

• **Fig. 11.9** Flouroscopic image depicting k-wire parallel to the endplates of the operative level with the tip of the k-wire at the anterior margin of the disk space during incision planning. (From author's collection.)

For the two incision technique, in addition to the true lateral incision overlying the disk, a short posterolateral incision is made along the edge of the paraspinal musculature (Fig. 11.12). Utilizing blunt dissection at an angle of approximately 45 degrees toward the floor, the abdominal wall is dissected in a similar fashion as above. Periodically checking with blunt finger dissection, when a clear pathway has been created into the retroperitoneal space, resistance to digital palpation should cease and viscera should be palpable. Correct location can be confirmed by palpation of the tip of the transverse process. The hand is then turned palm up with index finger sliding along the inner abdominal wall until the tip of the finger is underneath

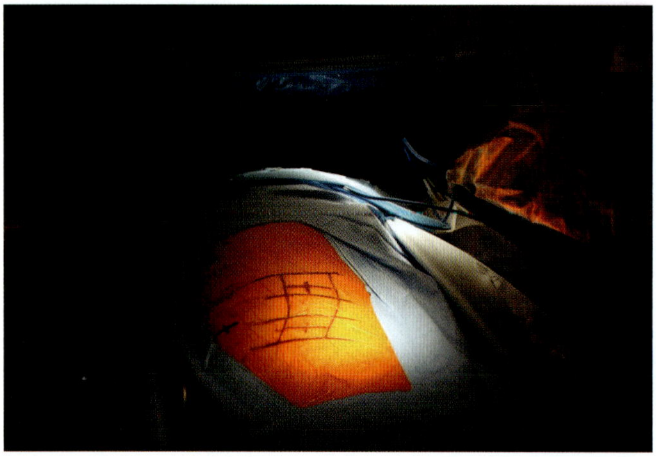

• **Fig. 11.10** Incision planning for multiple levels involves drawing out the anterior and posterior spinal lines with disk spaces clearly marked. The incision can then be made in an oblique fashion mimicking the course of the lumbar plexus; frequently multiple levels can be accessed through a single incision. (From author's collection.)

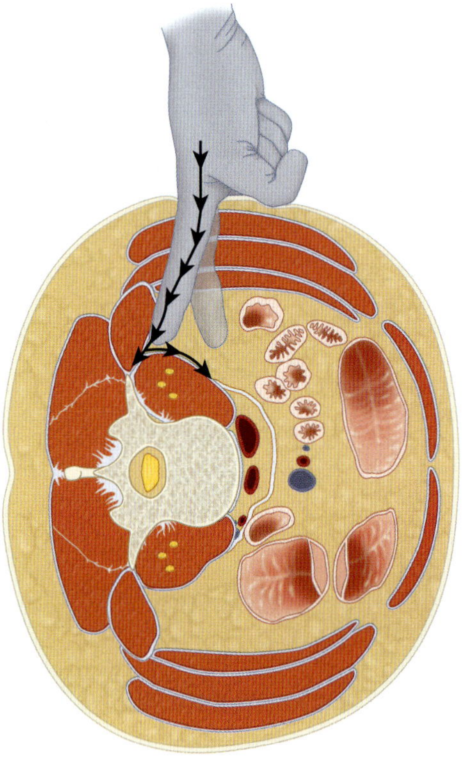

• **Fig. 11.11** Figure depicting layers of the abdominal wall that must be traversed including external and internal obliques, transverse abdominus, deep fascia, and retroperitoneal fat. In the single incision technique, blunt dissection with a finger is utilized to mobilize retroperitoneal contents forward and out of the operative corridor. (Images provided by Medtronic.) (From Quinones-Hinojoas A, ed. *Schmidek and Sweet Operative Neurosurgical Techniques*, vol 6. Philadelphia: Elsevier; 2012: Fig. 172-5.)

the planned flank incision. The viscera should be swept forward using this technique. The flank incision is then performed and the dilator passed onto the tip of the finger and guided to the border of the psoas muscle. A cosmetic variation of this technique involved a larger single skin incision that extends posteriorly and creating two distinct fascial openings as an alternative to making two separate skin incisions.

Step 5: Transpsoas Dilation and Retractor Placement

Neuromonitoring is performed via sequential dilation through the psoas muscle as each is passed to the disk space. The dilators have localizable EMG electrodes to provide directional stimulation to determine the proximity and direction of the motor nerves relative to the dilators (Fig. 11.13). The C-arm is used to confirm the position of the initial dilator in the lateral position, following which a K-wire is passed into the disk space to secure its position (Fig. 11.14). The aim is to land anterior to the motor nerves of the lumbar plexus at the approximate midpoint of the disk space. An AP image is then obtained, and the sequential dilators and retractor are passed to rest flush with the disk space (Fig. 11.15). As each item is passed, it is tested with directional EMG to ensure the safety of the nerve of the lumbar plexus. The retractor is secured to the articulating arm and locked; the aperture is opened slightly in the AP and craniocaudal directions and the dilators removed. Fiberoptic lighting is used to illuminate the surgical corridor.

Direct visualization and blunt probe EMG stimulation is performed to verify a safe trajectory through the working corridor to the disk space. A shim is then inserted down the posterior blade and tapped into the disk space under fluoroscopic and visual guidance; this serves as the posterior margin of the discectomy (Fig. 11.16). A thin retractor is then inserted between the craniocaudal blades to retract residual muscle tissue anteriorly and visually identify the ALL; it is then gently advanced approximately 1 cm deep along the anterior border of the ALL as confirmed by fluoroscopic imaging. This tool is secured to the index retractor and serves as the anterior border of the safe operative field and protects the ALL as well as the anterior visceral and vascular structures. Caution is taken to avoid excessive retractor distraction and toeing of the blades as this increases the risk of injury to the psoas muscle and neural structures, as well as the segmental arteries, which are direct branches off the aorta and can result in significant hemorrhage if lacerated (Fig. 11.17).

Step 6: Discectomy

An ipsilateral annulotomy is performed with a bayonetted knife beginning 1 cm behind the ALL and extending to the posterior shim along each endplate. A cobb elevator is then inserted along the endplates into the disk space down to the contralateral annulus to separate the cartilaginous disk material under fluoroscopic guidance; careful palpatory feedback and fluoroscopic confirmation are used to prevent endplate breach (Fig. 11.18). Once resistance is met at the contralateral annulus, the cobb elevator is carefully advanced with a mallet to breach it. The diskectomy is then performed utilizing various pituitary rongeurs and curettes, being sure to respect the ALL and endplates above and below. If disk access proves challenging, a disk space dilator can be gently tapped between the vertebrae to assist in creating a working corridor (Fig. 11.19). In cases of sagittal imbalance where lordosis restoration is necessary, the ALL retractor can be advanced across the disk space, and the ALL can be carefully sectioned with a guillotine blade, thus enabling anterior distraction at the level of the disk space and hyperlordotic graft placement when necessary. Fig. 11.20 is a view of the disk space during lateral diskectomy.

Step 7: Interbody Graft Placement

The next step involves placing various sized trials into the disk space to determine proper graft size (Fig. 11.21). It is imperative that all nuclear disk material is meticulously removed, as failure to do so

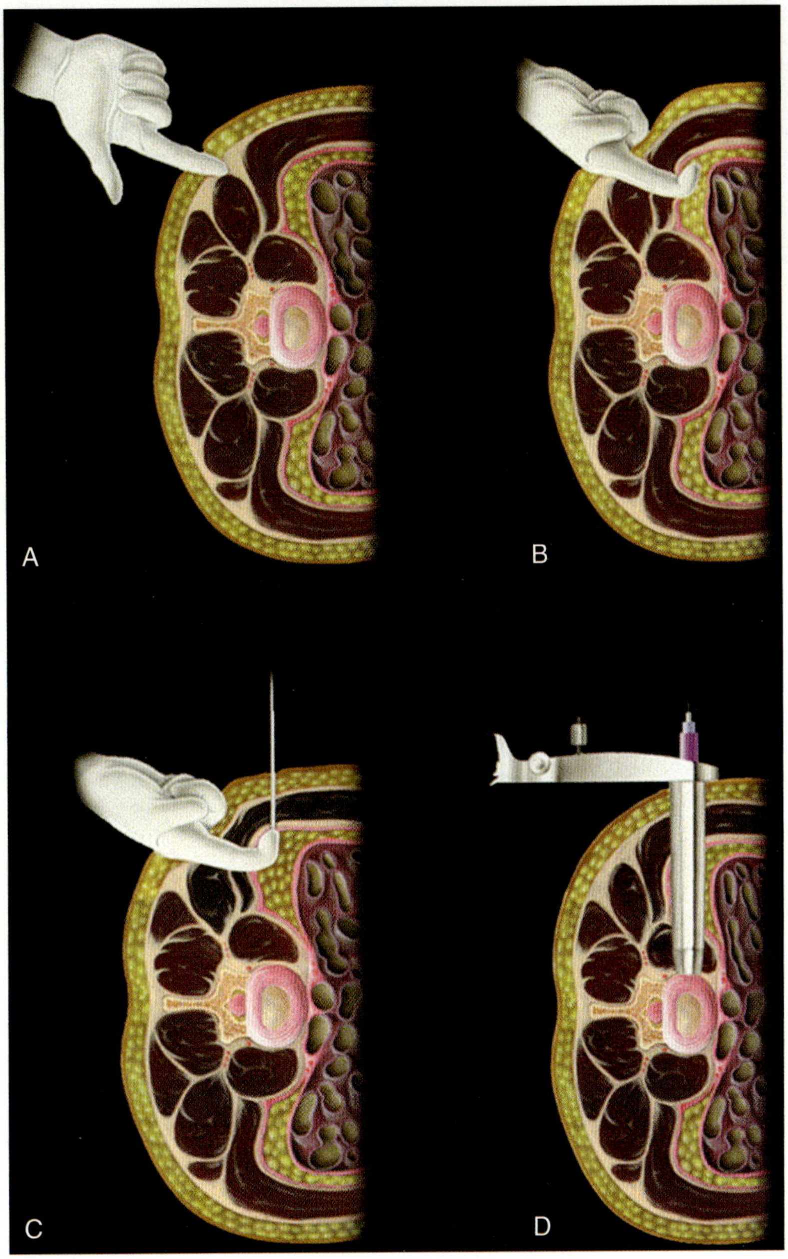

• **Fig. 11.12** The two-incision technique as another means of ensuring the safety of retroperitoneal contents. (A) A posterolateral incision is utilized to traverse the abdominal wall lateral to the paraspinal muscles. (B) Blunt finger dissection is utilized to sweep retroperitoneal contents forward creating space for dilator. (C) Finger guides k-wire into place avoiding visceral injury. (D) Retractor is positioned. (From Ozgur BM, Aryan HE, Pimenta L, Taylor WR. Extreme lateral interbody fusion (XLIF): a novel surgical technique for anterior lumbar interbody fusion. *Spine J* 2006;6:435–443, Fig. 4.)

prior to graft trialing may cause its extrusion through the annulus resulting in contralateral nerve root impingement. The length of the trial should span the entire width of the disk space in the AP dimension and occupy the anterior and central disk space on lateral imaging mimicking the final graft. Selection of the ideal interbody graft placement requires consideration of several general principles and patient-specific factors. In general, the graft should be sufficiently large, anatomically contoured to the disk space, and span the lateral borders of the entire apophyseal ring. Greater surface contact between the graft and the robust apophyseal ring dramatically improves the load-sharing properties of the construct to resist graft subsidence.[12] The height of the graft should permit restoration of the neural foramina and disk space while avoiding over distraction.[15] Appropriate graft height may be predicted by measuring the height of a nonpathologic adjacent segment. Next, the specific goal of the operation for an individual patient may further refine graft selection. For instance, if neurofaminal decompression and ligamentotaxis is the primary goal for a patient with symptoms of claudication or radiculopathy, the surgeon may choose to be slightly more aggressive in placing a larger graft to aid in this goal. In contrast, in a patient with a low-grade spondylolisthesis and primarily back pain, graft height can be tailored for an appropriate mechanical fit without focusing on aggressive distraction of the disk space. Moreover, lordotic grafts (10 degrees) and hyperlordotic grafts (20 and 30 degrees) can be utilized as an adjunct means of improving sagittal balance and spinopelvic realignment. These are commonly utilized in patients with scoliosis who are undergoing

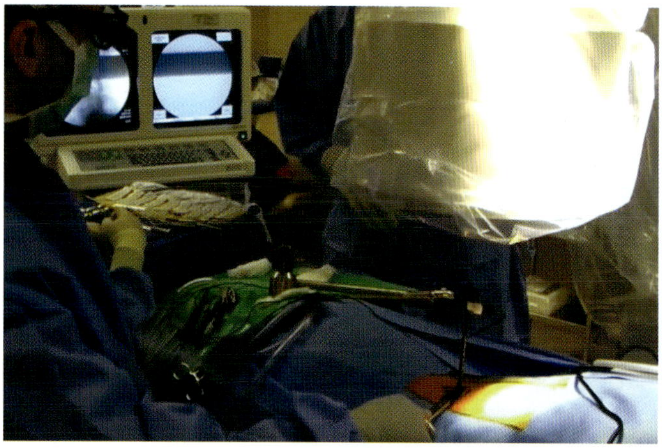

• **Fig. 11.13** Initial dilator with localizable electromyography (EMG) attached as it is being passed and docked on the disk space. Flouroscopic images are taken during this process to ensure proper positioning. (From author's collection.)

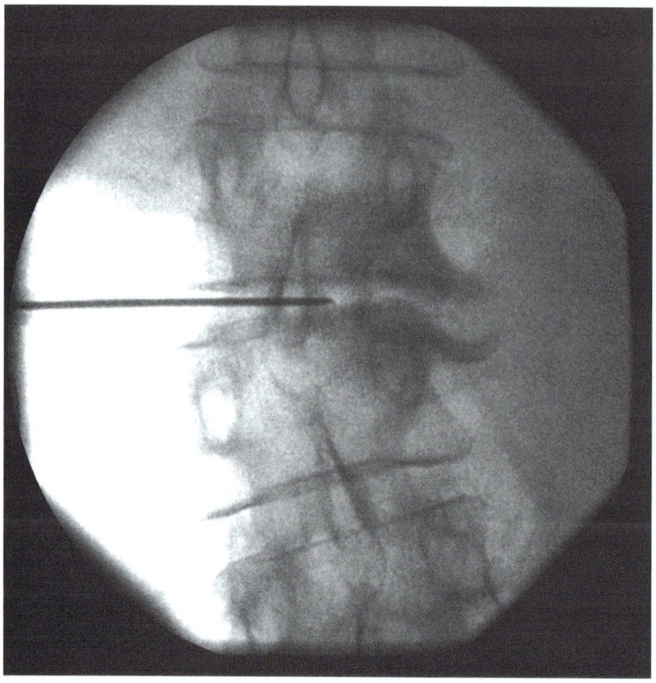

• **Fig. 11.14** After the initial dilator is confirmed to be in an appropriate position, a k-wire is inserted into the disk space to hold the position of the dilators. (From author's collection.)

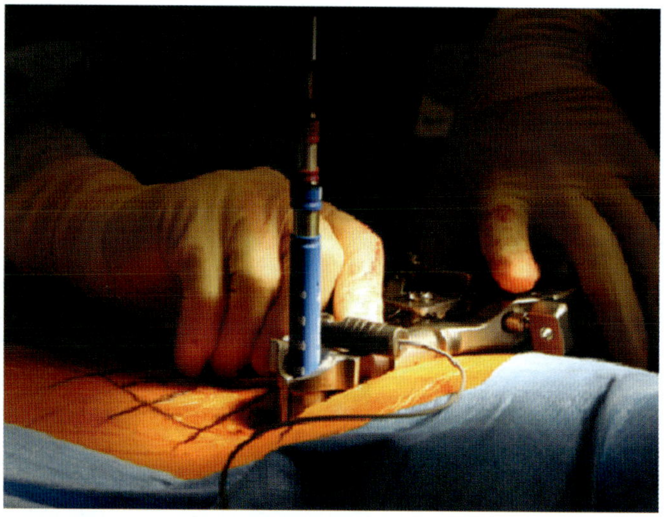

• **Fig. 11.15** Sequential dilators and retractor placed over the dilators. Each dilator is stimulated while being passed through the psoas to assess for proximity of neural structures. (From author's collection.)

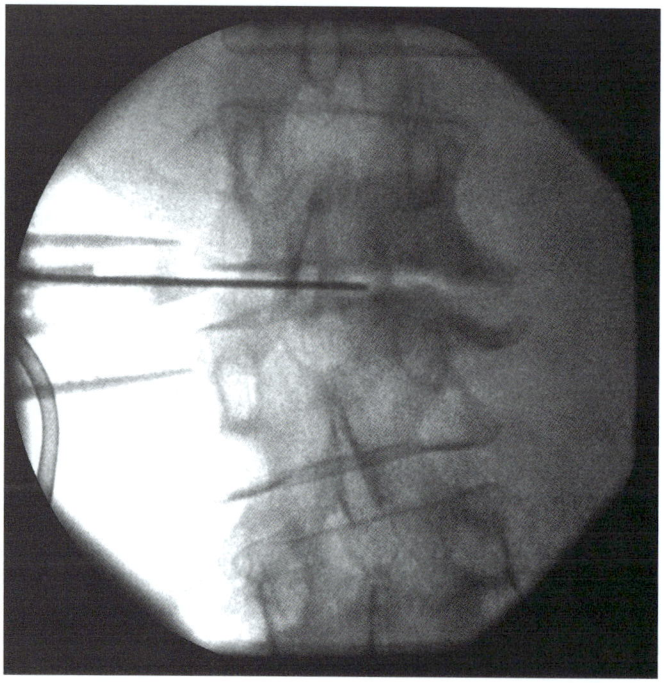

• **Fig. 11.16** Radiograph depicting retractor dilated and shim inserted just into the disk space marking the posterior border of working corridor. (From author's collection.)

staged procedures, but even for single-level operations, modern spine surgeons are focusing more attention on spinopelvic parameter restoration and maintenance.

After final selection, the interbody graft is filled with a bone growth extender; a variety of allograft and synthetic options are available from demineralized bone matrix in chip, gel, or putty form, to ceramics and calcium phosphates, to bone morphogenic protein.. The filled graft is then inserted to its final position similar to the trial (Fig. 11.22). There are subtle nuances to selecting the final position of the graft that can be advantageous depending on surgical goals. For instance, a more posterior graft position can be advantageous if correcting neuroforaminal narrowing is the primary goal (e.g., far lateral disk herniation). Fluoroscopic imaging is obtained to confirm placement of the trials and final implant prior to closure.

Consideration of supplemental hardware (lateral plating, pedicle screw, or spinous process fixation) is influenced by the patient's intrinsic bone quality as well as intraoperative disruption of the ALL and endplate violation.[11,12] At the surgeon's discretion, lateral plating can be performed to enhance stability and minimize motion in the lateral bending plane through the same incision. This is performed by utilizing self-tapping screws and traversing the lateral vertebral body, being sure to maintain a parallel screw trajectory to minimize bicortical breach and injury to the contralateral neural and vascular structures. Alternatively, some surgeons will place minimally invasive pedicle screws, which can be done either in the same lateral position as the LLIF, or the patient can be moved to a more traditional prone position.

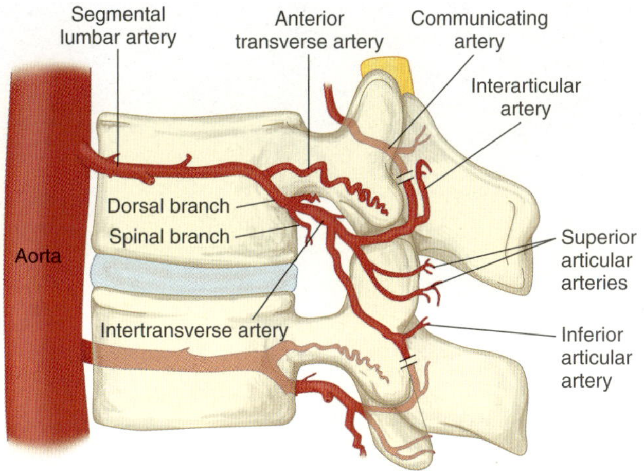

• **Fig. 11.17** The segmental branches of the aorta can result in significant hemorrhage if lacerated and care must be taken to avoid doing so in the transpsoas approach. (From Benzel EC, ed. Spine Surgery: Techniques, Complication Avoidance, and Management, vol 1. Philadelphia: Elsevier; 2012: Fig. 57.3a.)

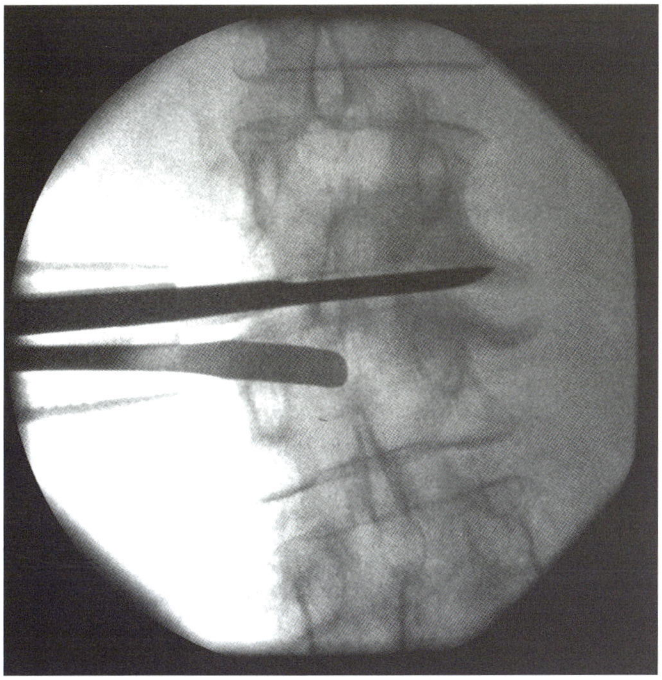

• **Fig. 11.18** Flouroscopic image of cobb elevator malleted across disk space during the diskectomy. (From author's collection.)

Closure

After copious irrigation of the surgical corridor and removal of any residual graft packing material, the blades of the retractor may be undilated. The shim is then removed from the posterior blade and the articulating locking arm released. The retractor is slowly elevated under direct visualization and hemostasis performed as necessary, being careful not to cauterize the neural structures as they return to their native position. After removal of the retractor, the superficial tissues are inspected for additional bleeding. The transversalis fascia can be closed at the surgeon's discretion; however, doing so may require sewing in close proximity to peritoneal structures. The superficial fascia and subcutaneous tissue are closed in layers with interrupted absorbable sutures, and the skin reapproximated in subcuticular fashion using thin absorbable monofilament sutures (Fig. 11.23).

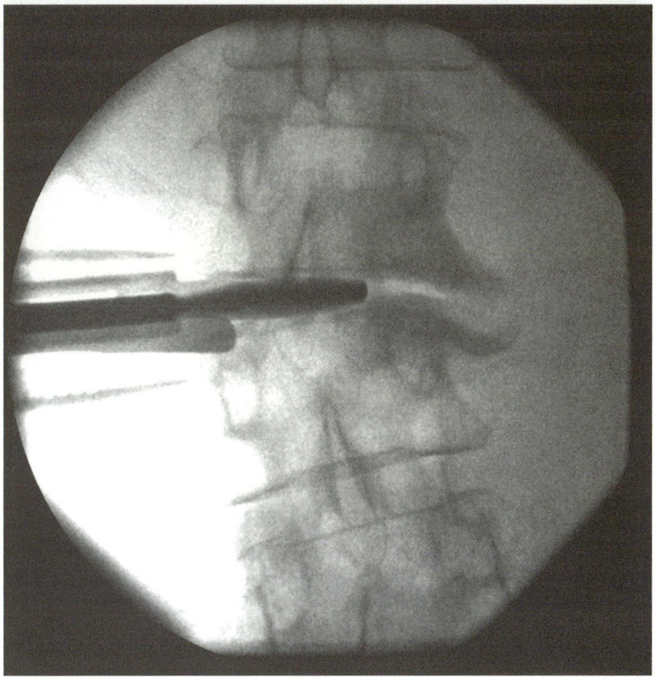

• **Fig. 11.19** Flouroscopic image of disk space dilator inserted to assist in creating a working corridor for discectomy. (From author's collection.)

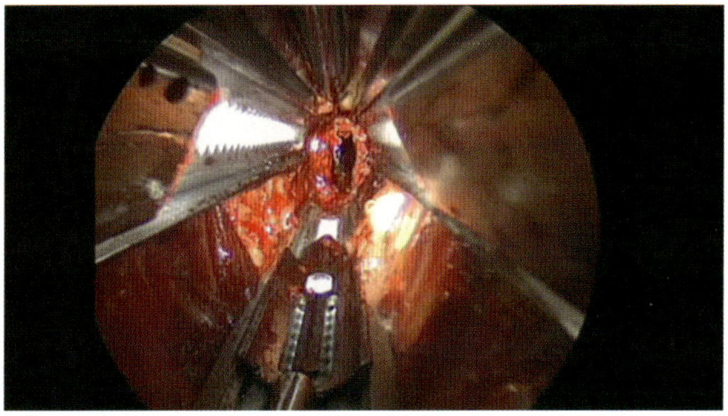

• **Fig. 11.20** Disk space seen through retractor after diskectomy is complete. (From author's collection.)

Postoperative Care

No firm guidelines exist regarding appropriate postoperative imaging following LLIF, and some physicians are satisfied with intraoperative fluoroscopic images if they are of good quality. However, it is common practice to obtain AP and lateral radiographs and/or a noncontrasted lumbar CT scan postoperatively. In the author's practice, a postoperative CT scan is obtained to evaluate for endplate violation, as evidence of graft translation (ALL violation), and to provide a baseline to compare with future imaging. In complex cases or in patients with a concern for bowel injury (e.g., thin patients with scoliosis), a postoperative abdominal CT scan with oral dye load can be obtained. In patients undergoing a staged correction for scoliosis or adult deformity, it is our practice to obtain standing 36-inch radiographs postoperatively prior to the second stage to assess the degree of correction.

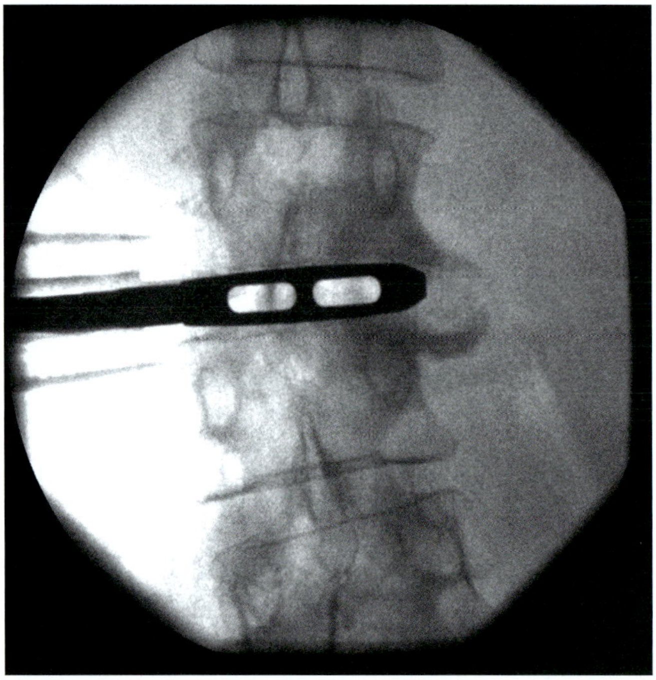

• **Fig. 11.21** Flouroscopic image of appropriately sized interbody trial. Note that the trial spans the width of the apophyseal ring mimicking an appropriately sized graft. (From author's collection.)

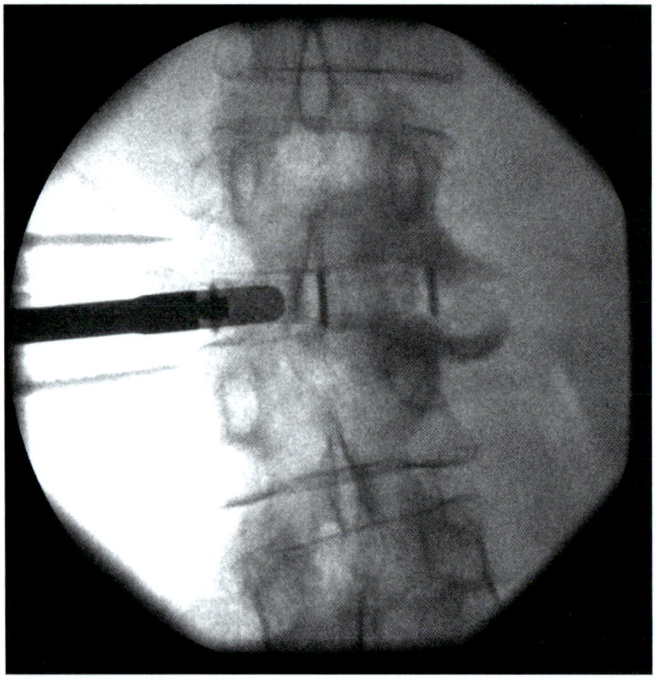

• **Fig. 11.22** Anteroposterior flouroscopic radiograph of appropriately sized graft being inserted. The disk height is restored but not over distracted. (From author's collection.)

The postoperative course of patients undergoing this approach varies widely, depending on the number of levels performed and the indication for the procedure. For instance, a single-level LLIF portends a vastly easier recovery then a multilevel fusion performed to correct a spinal deformity. Patients who undergo single-level procedures are mobilized the same day as surgery and discharged the subsequent morning with only oral pain control.

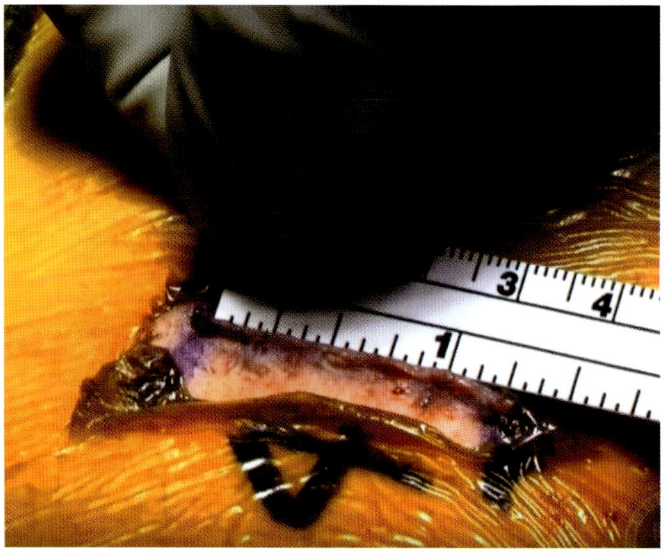

• **Fig. 11.23** A closed 3-cm incision through which a single-level lateral lumbar interbody fusion (LLIF) was performed. (From author's collection.)

For multilevel deformity corrections, early mobilization is still the goal, however variable, as the patient's status may be more dependent on the alteration in spinal alignment than the procedure itself. Activity restriction is consistent with other types of spinal arthrodesis, with limitation in bending, twisting, or lifting more than 10 pounds for a period of approximately 6 weeks.

Complications

Two commonly reported complications from the LLIF approach potentially should better be called side-effects owing to their commonality and resultant likely resolution. Patients can report anterior thigh or groin numbness and paresthesias secondary to genitofemoral nerve stretch. Additionally, hip flexor weakness can result from psoas muscle dilation. The incidence can range from 15% to 40%, and the vast majority resolve within 4 to 12 weeks.[16–20] The best defense to mitigating these confounds is to minimize surgical time in the psoas. Understandably, the risk is higher when performing LLIF at multiple levels with repeated psoas dilations, particularly at the lower lumbar spine levels. Both of these issues tend to be present immediately postoperatively if they are going to occur.

Another relatively unique complication to this approach can be the development of a pseudohernia in the abdominal wall. This results from injury to the motor nerves innervating the abdominal wall causing loss of muscle tone and an outpouching of the abdomen. It is not a true hernia because no abdominal contents protrude through the defect, but can appear clinically similar. The ilioinguinal, subcostal, and iliohypogastric nerves all contribute to innervation of the three muscle layers of the abdomen. Utilizing blunt dissection and preserving any traversing nerves while dissecting through the abdominal musculature helps avoid this complication. A CT scan of the abdomen can rule out a true hernia.

Graft subsidence is a complication that can result in the need for revision surgery and there are both technical and intrinsic contributions to its development. Avoiding a technical error during surgery resulting in endplate breach is the primary defense in avoiding subsidence. Fig. 11.24 demonstrates immediate postoperative imaging and delayed 6-month follow-up imaging of a patient with

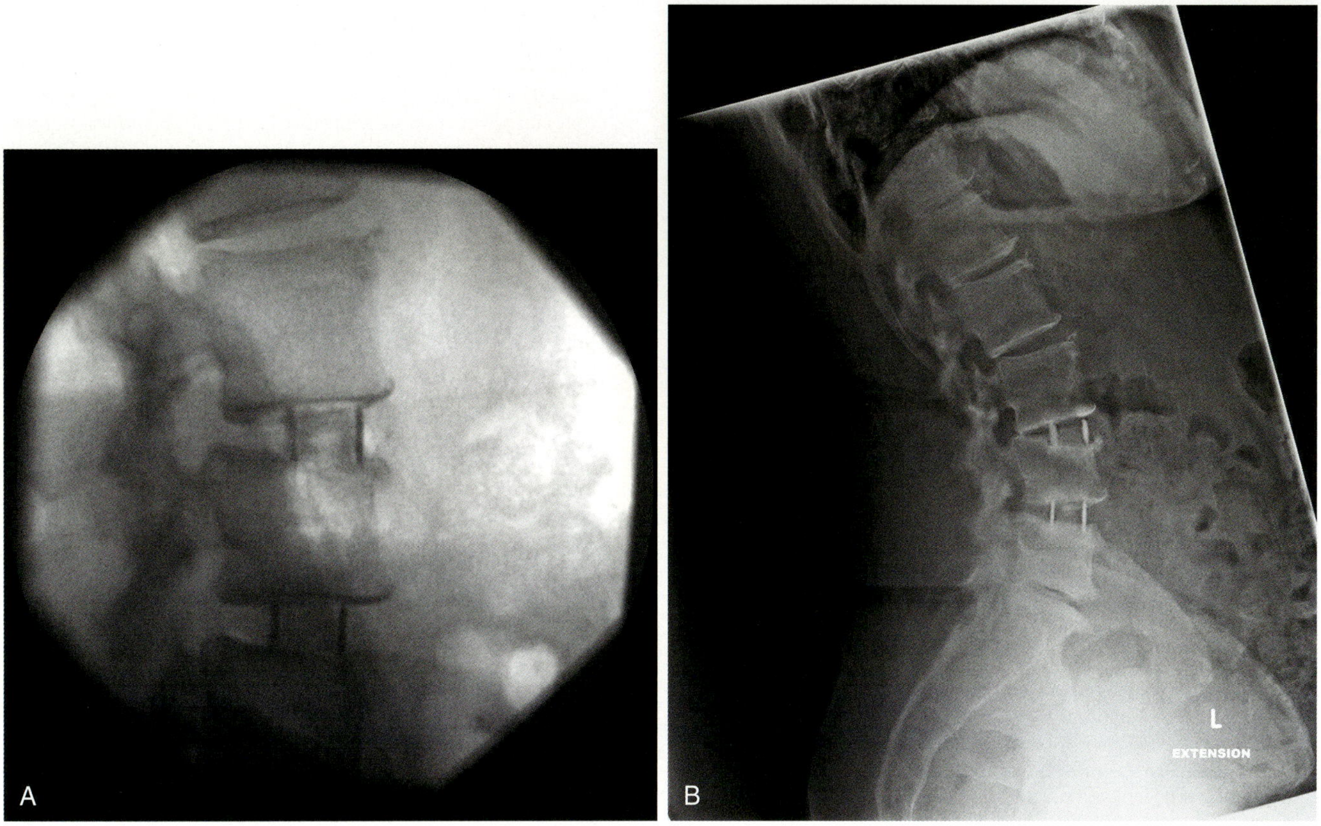

• **Fig. 11.24** (A) Intraoperative image of a patient with a subtle endplate breach placing the patient at risk for subsidence. (B) The same patient's delayed 6-month follow-up film demonstrating graft subsidence with a decrease in the neuroforaminal height restoration that was achieved initially. (From author's collection.)

an intraoperative endplate breach that resulted in graft subsidence (Fig. 11.24). Whether detected intraoperatively or on postoperative imaging, supplemental instrumentation should be considered to help avoid subsidence. However, subsidence can still occur in a delayed fashion with a technically flawless LLIF, particularly in patients with impaired bone quality. If indirect decompression is compromised owing to failed ligamentotaxy and disk height loss, direct decompression and supplemental instrumentation may be necessary.[11,12]

Infection, although rare, tends to manifest as a psoas abscess. These can typically be seen on spinal imaging but sometimes better visualized with a CT abdomen scan with contrast. In our experience, these infections may be successfully treated with a course of antibiotics; removal of the graft is extremely uncommon.

Lastly, the most notorious and serious of complications from the LLIF approach are vascular injury and bowel injury. Careful and judicious study of preoperative imaging is the best method to avoid vascular injury. It is imperative to consider this anatomy in determining laterality in the approach, and it is often a compromise in choosing between the easier side to access the disk space and the safest. Of note, even smaller aortic branches typically that cannot be seen on preoperative imaging can result in significant hemorrhage if lacerated. If vascular injury occurs, control of the bleeding should be attempted and, if unachievable, appropriate specialty care should be sought immediately. Similarly, if a bowel injury is suspected intraoperatively, appropriate surgical specialty assistance should be promptly engaged.

Outcomes

The LLIF approach was designed as a minimally invasive alternative to traditional anterior (ALIF) and posterior/transforminal (PLIF/TLIF) approaches to the thoracolumbar spine. Several large single- and multicenter studies have demonstrated that LLIF is associated with favorable complication rates as well as less blood loss, OR time, and length of stay when compared with open anterior and posterior approaches.[2–6,16–20] In patients with significant comorbid conditions or advanced age, LLIF is further associated with fewer perioperative complications and reduced mortality rates.[16,17]

The LLIF technique has steadily proved to be an effective treatment option for a variety of spinal pathologies, producing significant improvements in health-related quality of life (HRQOL) metrics. A recent multicenter study by Sembrano et al.[3] demonstrated statistically significant, but equivalent improvements in visual analog scale (VAS) for back/leg pain, Oswestry disability index (ODI), and Short Form 36 (SF-36) outcome measures (MCS), as well as reduced narcotic use in patients with low-grade degenerative spondylolisthesis treated with LLIF.[3] At 1- and 2-year follow-up, minimum clinically important difference and substantial clinical benefit (SCB) were similar between the minimally invasive LIF (MITLIF) and LLIF cases.[3] In 2015, Lehmen and Gerber[6] conducted a systematic literature review of 237 articles discussing the LLIF approach and identified 47 articles that specifically discussed outcomes. In their review, the authors found improvement in VAS, ODI, and overall patient satisfaction rates up to 90%, 89%, and 100%, respectively, with successful arthrodesis occurring in greater than 90% of patients. They concluded that the complication profile and clinical outcomes of LLIF are well characterized in the literature and at least comparable to clinical outcomes of traditional approaches.[3]

Conclusions

Lateral interbody fusion techniques are increasingly being utilized as a minimally invasive approach to treat an array of spinal pathology. The approach requires consideration of factors not typically considered in traditional spine surgery, utilizing specialized equipment and neuromonitoring techniques to maximize the safety and reproducibility of the approach. When carefully performed in properly selected patients, surgical outcomes are consistent with other interbody fusion techniques with minimal morbidity, and a quick return to daily life activities.

References

1. Ozgur BM, Aryan HE, Pimenta L, et al. Extreme lateral interbody fusion (XLIF): a novel surgical technique for anterior lumbar interbody fusion. *Spine J.* 2006;6:435–443.
2. Ahmadian A, Bach K, Bolinger B, et al. Stand-alone minimally invasive lateral lumbar interbody fusion: multicenter clinical outcomes. *J Clin Neurosci.* 2015;22(4):740–746.
3. Sembrano JN, Tohmeh A, Isaacs R, et al. Two-year comparative outcomes of MIS lateral and MIS transforaminal interbody fusion in the treatment of degenerative spondylolisthesis. Part I: clinical findings. *Spine (Phila Pa 1976).* 2016;41(suppl 8):S123–S132.
4. Youssef JA, McAfee PC, Patty CA, et al. Minimally invasive surgery: lateral approach interbody fusion. Results and review. *Spine (Phila Pa 1976).* 2010;35(suppl 26):S302–S311.
5. Ozgur BM, Agarwal V, Nail E, et al. Two-year clinical and radiographic success of minimally invasive lateral transpsoas approach for the treatment of degenerative lumbar conditions. *SAS J.* 2010;4(2):41–46.
6. Lehmen JA, Gerber EJ. MIS lateral spine surgery: a systematic literature review of complications, outcomes, and economics. *Eur Spine J.* 2015;24(suppl 3):287–313.
7. Dakwar E, Vale FL, Uribe JS. Trajectory of the main sensory and motor branches of the lumbar plexus outside the psoas muscle related to the lateral retroperitoneal transpsoas approach. *J Neurosurg Spine.* 2011;2:290–295.
8. Guerin P, Obeid I, Gille O, et al. Safe working zones using the minimally invasive lateral retroperitoneal transpsoas approach: a morphometric study. *Surg Radiol Anat.* 2011;8:665–671.
9. Uribe JS, Arredondo N, Dakwar E, et al. Defining the safe working zones using the minimally invasive lateral retroperitoneal transpsoas approach: an anatomical study. *J Neurosurg Spine.* 2010;2:260–266.
10. Kepler CK, Bogner EA, Herzog RJ, et al. Anatomy of the psoas muscle and lumbar plexus with respect to the surgical approach for lateral transpsoas interbody fusion. *Eur Spine J.* 2011;4:550–556.
11. Marchi L, Abdala N, Oliveira L, et al. Radiographic and clinical evaluation of cage subsidence after stand-alone lateral interbody fusion. *J Neurosurg Spine.* 2013;19(1):110–118.
12. Pimenta L, Turner AW, Dooley ZA, et al. Biomechanics of lateral interbody spacers: going wider for going stiffer. *Scientific World Journal.* 2012;2012:381814.
13. Berjano P, Lamartina C. Minimally invasive lateral transpsoas approach with advanced neurophysiologic monitoring for lumbar interbody fusion. *Eur Spine J.* 2011;9:1584–1586.
14. O'Brien J, Haines C, Dooley ZA, et al. Femoral nerve strain at L4-L5 is minimized by hip flexion and increased by table break when performing lateral interbody fusion. *Spine (Phila Pa 1976).* 2014;39:33–38.
15. Kepler CK, Sharma AK, Huang RC, et al. Indirect foraminal decompression after lateral transpsoas interbody fusion. *J Neurosurg Spine.* 2012;16(4):323–329.
16. Rodgers WB, Gerber EJ, Patterson J. Intraoperative and early postoperative complications in extreme lateral interbody fusion: an analysis of 600 cases. *Spine (Phila Pa 1976).* 2011;14:31–37.
17. Karikari IO, Grossi PM, Nimjee SM, et al. Minimally invasive lumbar interbody fusion in patients older than 70 years of age: analysis of peri- and postoperative complications. *Neurosurgery.* 2011;68:897–902.
18. Le TV, Burkett CJ, Deukmedjian AR, et al. Postoperative lumbar plexus injury after lumbar retroperitoneal transpsoas minimally invasive lateral interbody fusion. *Spine (Phila Pa 1976).* 2013;1:E13–E20.
19. Moller DJ, Slimack NP, Acosta FL Jr, et al. Minimally invasive lateral lumbar interbody fusion and transpsoas approach-related morbidity. *Neurosurg Focus.* 2011;31:E4.
20. Barbagallo GM, Albanese V, Raich AL. Lumbar lateral interbody fusion (LLIF): comparative effectiveness and safety versus PLIF/TLIF and predictive factors affecting LLIF outcome. *Evid Based Spine Care J.* 2014;5(1):28–37.

12 Pre-psoas (Oblique) Lateral Interbody Fusion

NEEL ANAND, JASON COHEN, AND RYAN COHEN

Introduction

Lumbar interbody fusion (LIF) is a well-accepted treatment for spinal pathologies. Traditionally, LIF is performed using posterior approaches. These open strategies require broad dissection of the paraspinal musculature and nerve root retraction to access the disk space for interbody fusion. A more refined minimally invasive method, transforaminal lumbar interbody fusion (TLIF), approaches the disk space through a tube via a more posterior oblique trajectory. Access to the disk space is gained through the Kambin's triangle. This posterior variant approach preserves the contralateral musculoligamentous elements and avoids excessive manipulation of the dural sac. Therefore, many of the complications associated with traditional open posterior approaches are mitigated. TLIF remains an important interbody fusion strategy. Nonetheless, the technique relies on a small surgical window—a particularly limiting factor when attempting more extensive diskectomy, graft placement, and fusion.

Anterior lumbar interbody fusion (ALIF) affords the most impressive fusion area of any surgical technique. The improvements in arthrodesis can be attributed to superb visualization of the disk space. This allows for robust removal of the disk and placement of the graft with maximal biological footprint. Other theoretic benefits of ALIF include avoidance of the spinal canal and the potential for more impressive degrees of correction via sectioning of the anterior longitudinal ligament (ALL). Nonetheless, ALIF is not without significant risks. ALIF requires entry in the abdominal cavity, which may be intraperitoneal or retroperitoneal, and careful dissection of important vascular structures. This puts the patient at risk for potentially devastating hollow-viscous and large-vessel injuries (including the iliac and great vessels). Other important considerations include ureteral injury, sexual dysfunction, and the need for a secondary access surgeon.

Various strategies have been proposed to improve on ALIF. These include laparoscopic, endoscopic, and mini-open approaches. Although strong proponents of these respective methods remain, many now consider laparoscopic strategies as historical stepping-stones. Laparoscopic methods, however, have laid the foundation for the more modern lateral lumbar interbody fusion strategies (LLIF). These include a number of synonyms, namely the direct lateral (DLIF) and extreme lateral (XLIF) approaches.

The LLIF technique allows for lateral exposure of the disk space through a retroperitoneal route. The traditional approach is a transpsoas approach, which allows for clearance of the disk tissue in the anterior column. This approach affords access to the disk space, avoiding the spinal canal posteriorly, and abdominal cavity and large vessels anteriorly. Other benefits of LLIF include no need for a secondary access surgeon, reduced incidence of ileus, preservation of the ALL, lack of bony resections, reduced operative time, reduced hospital stay, and reduced analgesic requirements. These features have slowly made the LLIF an acceptable method for lumbar interbody fusion. Nonetheless, certain issues remain if the transpsoas LLIF is to be embraced as a gold-standard interbody fusion strategy. Chief among them include injury to the lumbar plexus with neurologic injury and access to the lumbosacral junction. In a broader sense, it remains to be seen whether minimally invasive (MIS) techniques such as this can, as a whole, accomplish comparable metrics in global coronal and sagittal alignment.

In this chapter, we discuss an alternative lateral interbody approach, the pre-psoas (oblique) lateral interbody fusion (OLIF) technique. We review anatomic considerations of the approach including the rationale for the shift from a transpsoas to a pre-psoas trajectory and limitations of accessing the L5-S1 disk space via the lateral approach. Our discussion offers a step-by-step description of the technique including patient positioning, preoperative planning, operative procedure, and closure. We discuss common complications and management strategies. In our discussion, we review the available literature for preliminary outcome data and discuss future endeavors moving forward. Finally, we introduce relatively new techniques, such as lordotic cages, used to improve global alignment—a primary limiting factor in MIS correction.

Limitations and Anatomic Considerations

A thorough anatomic understanding is a vital tool in the spinal surgeon's armamentarium. This is particularly important given the shift toward minimally invasive methods. Surgeons once trained in posterior approaches must now familiarize themselves with the novel anatomic landscape of OLIF.

Landmarks

A comprehensive review must not overlook key anatomic landmarks. The intercrestal line is the theoretic plane between respective superior iliac crests. The landmark classically represents the L4-5 interspace. Surgeons must be weary of variations based on abdominal circumference, body mass index, age, gender, and degree of flexion.[1,2] Furthermore,

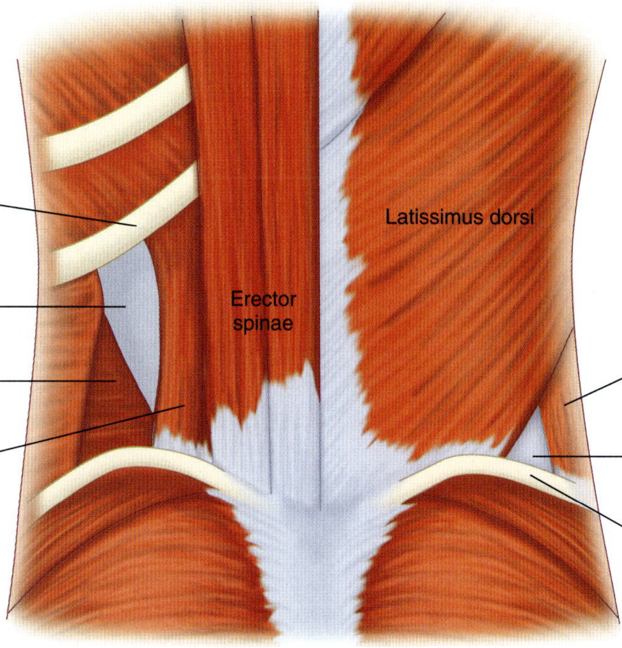

• **Fig. 12.1** Diagram of superior and inferior lumbar triangle (Petit's triangle). (From Lillie GR, Deppert E. Inferior lumbar triangle hernia as a rarely reported cause of low back pain: a report of 4 cases. *J Chiropr Med.* 2010:9(2);73–76, Fig. 1.)

the intercrestal line denotes the lower limit of the minimally invasive transpsoas lateral approach as the iliac crest hinders lateral L5-S1 disk space entry. An oblique anterior pre-psoas approach (OLIF) allows surgeons access to the lumbosacral junction avoiding the iliac crest and this could be a distinct advantage of OLIF over LLIF.

Superficial Musculature

The abdominal musculature consists of the external oblique, internal oblique, and transverse abdominis from superficial to deep. It is important to note the direction of the respective muscle fibers. In particular, the external oblique travels diagonally from the superior-lateral to the inferior-medial direction. This plane is followed during superficial dissection in order to improve cosmesis with closure. Another important consideration is the inferior lumbar triangle, also known as Petit's triangle (Fig. 12.1). This anatomic space is bordered by the iliac crest inferiorly, latissimus dorsi posteriorly, and external abdominal oblique anteriorly. The area could be targeted during the initial dissection in order to gain access to the retroperitoneal space.

Deep Musculature

The psoas muscle lies posterior to the retroperitoneal space. It traverses on the lateral surface of vertebral bodies and intervertebral spaces and originates from the anterior surface of the transverse processes from T12 to L5 and eventually inserts inferiorly on the lesser trochanter of the femur. Embedded within the muscle fibers of the psoas run key components of the lumbosacral plexus. Careful attention must be given in order to avoid damage to these neuronal structures. Another important deep muscle is the quadratus lumborum. This spinal stabilizer attaches to the transverse processes, 12th rib, and iliac crest. Fig. 12.2 illustrates the musculature of the lumbar spine.

Lumbosacral Plexus

The lumbosacral plexus arises from the ventral rami of T12-S3. The major terminal branches of the lumbar plexus include the iliohypogastric (L1), ilioinguinal (L1), genitofemoral (L1-2), lateral femoral cutaneous (L2-3), femoral (L2-4), and oburator (L2-4) nerves (Fig. 12.3). These branches have mixed motor and sensory innervation with the exception of the lateral femoral cutaneous nerve, a purely sensory nerve. The plexus originates posterior and medial to the psoas muscle and descends in an anterior and lateral direction, traversing through the fibers of the psoas muscle.

Benglis et al.[3] measured the ratio of the plexus location relative to the disk length on three cadavers. The plexus migrated in a progressively ventral direction with a ratio of 0 at L1-2 and 0.28 at L4-5. Moro et al.[4] detailed the distribution of the lumbar plexus based on six cadaveric specimens. From L1-5, vertebral bodies were divided into four zones from anterior to posterior. All parts of the lumbar plexus were found in zone IV and dorsally at levels L2-3 and above. Excluding the genitofemoral nerve, the plexus was found posterior to zone II from L4-5 and above (Fig. 12.4). Uribe et al.[5] dissected 20 lumbar segments and divided vertebral bodies into 4 similar zones to identify anatomic "safe zones" during the lateral retroperitoneal transpsoas approach. These safe zones were found at the midpoint of zone III and posterior from L1-4 and at the midpoint of the vertebral body at the L4-5 disk space.

Positioning

The patient is placed in the lateral decubitus position (LDP). A right LDP (with left side facing up) is preferred as it avoids the inferior vena cava and right common iliac vein that lies slightly right and anterior to the vertebral body, especially at L4-5. We prefer to access the left side always with the OLIF approach. The

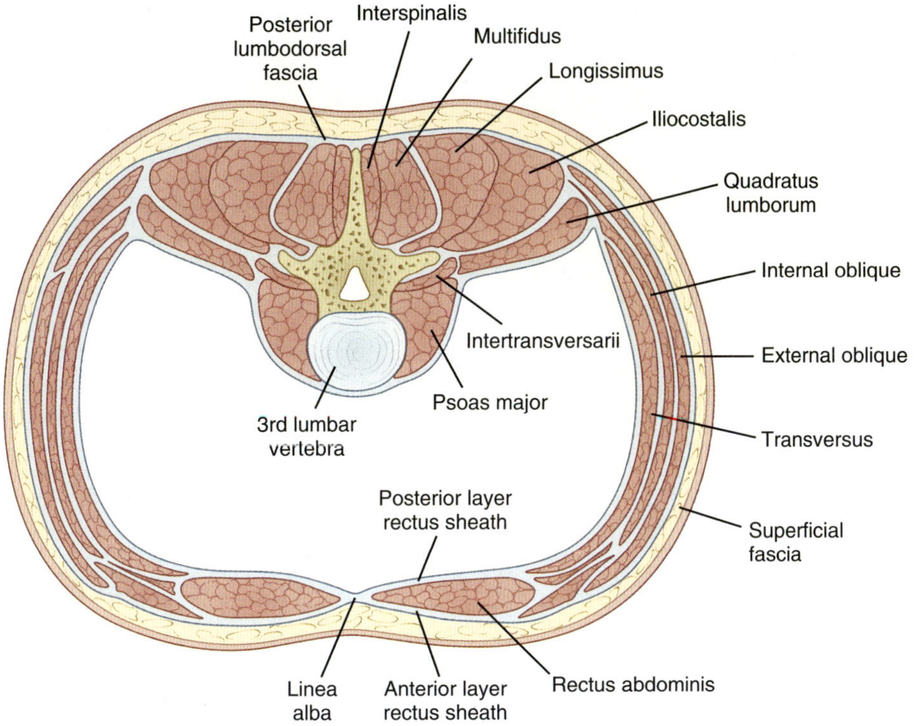

• **Fig. 12.2** Coronal section of lumbar musculature. (From Mayer TG, Mayer EAK, Reese D. Lumbar musculature: anatomy and function. In: Herkowtiz HN, Garfin SR, Eismont FJ, et al, eds. *Rothman-Simeone The Spine*. Philadelphia: Elsevier; 2012:85, Fig. 5.4.)

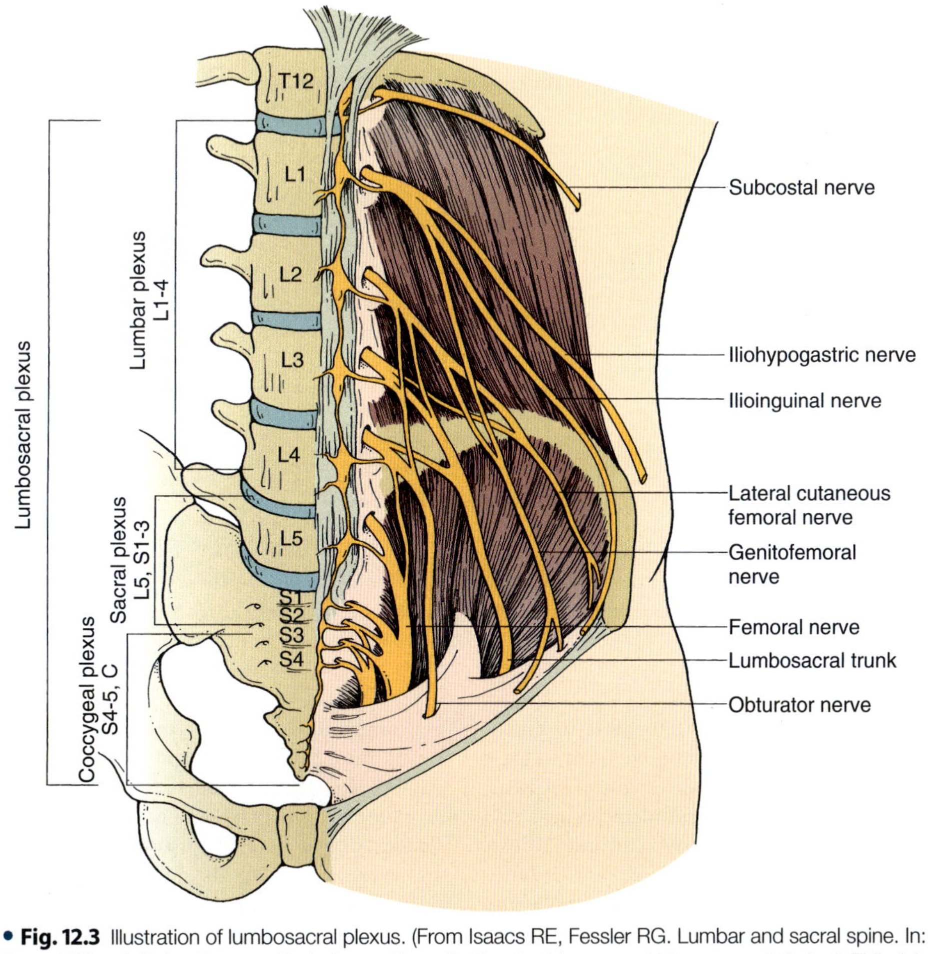

• **Fig. 12.3** Illustration of lumbosacral plexus. (From Isaacs RE, Fessler RG. Lumbar and sacral spine. In: Benzel EC, ed. *Spine Surgery: Techniques, Complication Avoidance, and Management*. 3rd ed. Philadelphia: Elsevier; 2012:359, Fig. 36.8.)

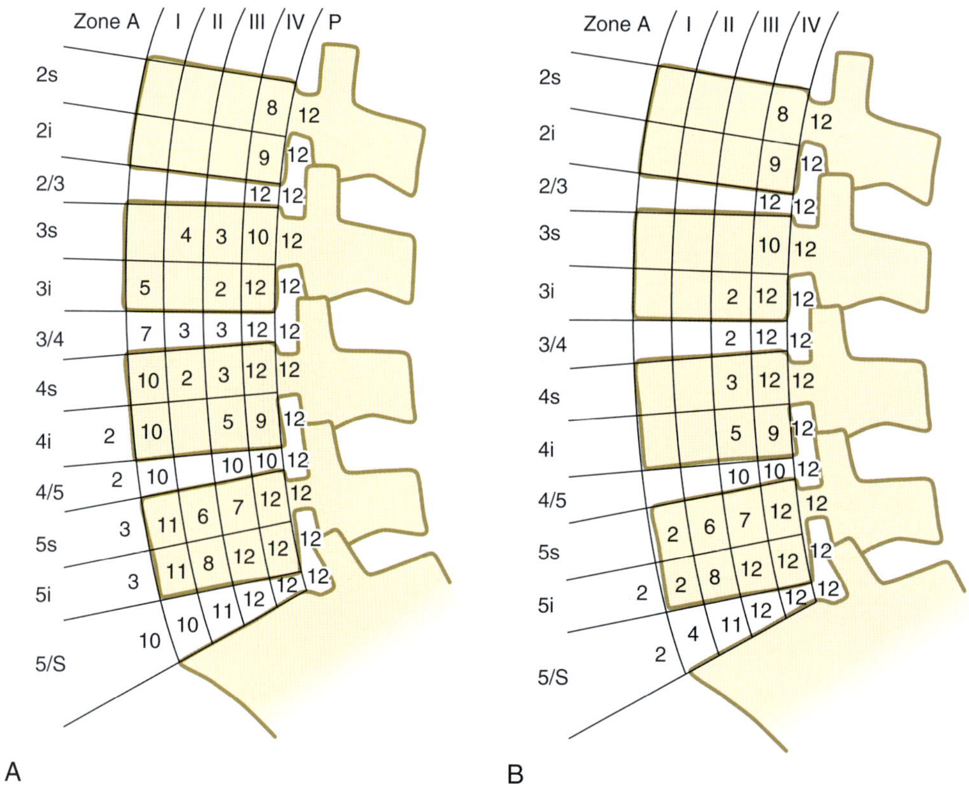

• **Fig. 12.4** Distribution of lumbar plexus and exiting nerve roots (A) in its entirety and (B) excluding the genitofemoral nerve. (From Moro T, Kikuchi SI, Konno SI, et al. An anatomic study of the lumbar plexus with respect to retroperitoneal endoscopic surgery. *Spine* 2003:28(5);423–427, Fig. 3.)

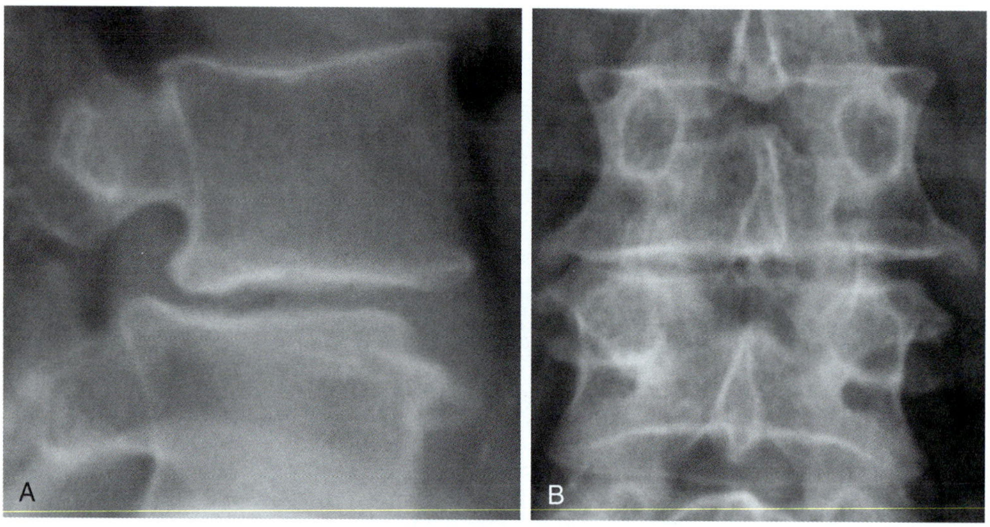

• **Fig. 12.5** True lateral *(left)* and anteroposterior *(right)* radiographs of the lumbar spine. (From Sugrue PA and Liu, JC. Lateral Lumbar Interbody Fusion. In Kim DH, Vaccaro AR, Dickman CA, et al. eds., *Surgical Anatomy and Techniques to the Spine*. 2nd ed. Philadelphia, PA: Elsevier/Saunders. 2013: 459-469. Fig. 47.8.)

iliac crest is placed slightly below the kidney rest table to maximize the opening between the ribs and iliac crest when the kidney rest is elevated. With the OLIF procedure, unlike the transpsoas procedure, the iliac crest is not as much of a problem because the incision is anterior and avoids the iliac crest. We continue to use short-latency somatosensory evoked potentials (SSEP) with both real time and triggered electromyography (EMG), although again with the pre-psoas approach it may not be needed as the lumbar plexus is not transgressed. Generous padding, axillary rolls, and tape are used to maintain the patient's position, prevent stretching or compression injuries, and minimize skin abrasion. Neutral positioning of the head is particularly important in avoiding brachial plexus disturbances.

Fluoroscopic images are next obtained with the C-arm perpendicular to the floor. Adjustments to obtain a true-lateral image are made by tilting the table rather than rotating the C-arm. This ensures that the surgical intervention remains perpendicular relative to the floor and maintains the surgeon's sense of the spinal anatomy. A true-lateral image must clearly delineate superimposed pedicles and a "flat" superior endplate (Fig. 12.5). It is

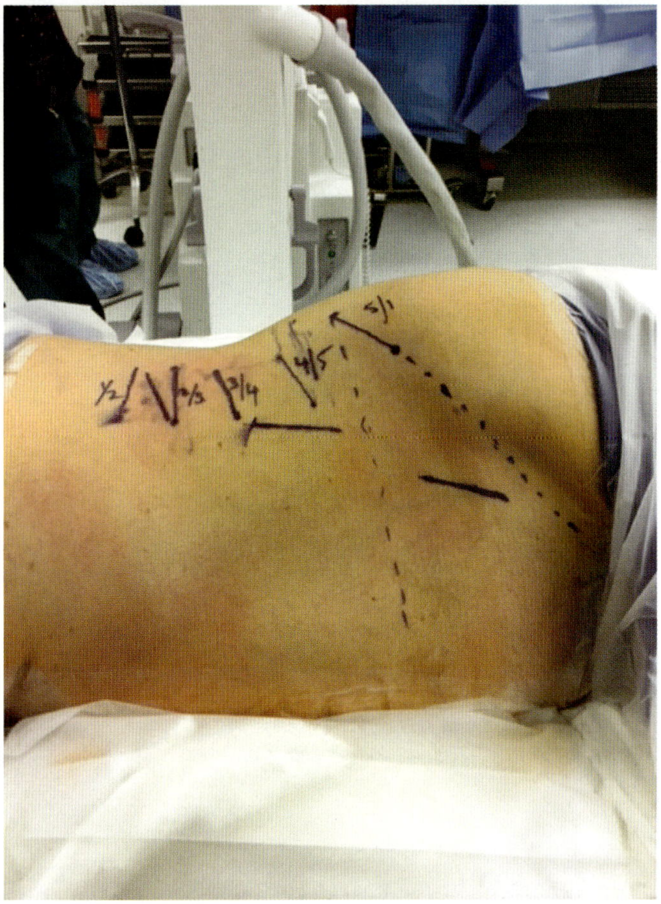

• **Fig. 12.6** Positioning of the patient in the right lateral decubitus position with left side up and incisions marked for oblique lateral interbody fusion from L1-2 to L5-S1.

also possible to perform the procedure with intraoperative 3D image acquisition and navigation. Some systems allow one to navigate all instruments and implants, thus no need for intraoperative fluoroscopy.

Procedure

The true lateral image is obtained to confirm the relative anatomy and identify the appropriate disk space. Anatomic landmarks, including the iliac crest, help pinpoint the lumbar triangle (Petit's triangle). The disk spaces are marked and an incision is marked two finger breadths anterior to the anterior margin of the disk. We tend to access the L4-5 and L3-4 with one incision, L2-3 and L1-2 through another, and the L5-S1 is accessed separately (Fig. 12.6). The patient is prepared and draped in the usual manner. The incision is made splitting the fibers of the external and internal oblique muscle along their orientation. The surgeon then uses a single finger to push through the transversalis fascia toward the iliac crest and sweep the peritoneum off the inside of the iliac crest and over the psoas to gain entry to the retroperitoneal space.

The anatomy of retroperitoneal space is explored using tactile stimuli. Upon entering the retroperitoneal space, the quadratus lumborum can be palpated posterolaterally. Following the muscle medially, the transverse process of the respective vertebrae and overlying psoas can be recognized. The under surface of the rib and inner surface of the iliac crest can also be palpated to confirm entry into the retroperitoneal space. Fig. 12.7 is an illustration of the retroperitoneal space along with the relative anatomy.

A retractor is brought in to reflect the anterior contents of the abdomen and expose the anterior border of the psoas muscle (Fig. 12.8). A sponge stick or peanut dissector may be used to dissect the soft tissue over the psoas to expose the anterior border of the psoas. Once the relevant anatomy is appreciated, a blunt dilator is guided down to the disk just anterior to the psoas muscle (Fig. 12.9A). A lateral fluoroscopic image is obtained to confirm the appropriate position of the first dilator anterior to the psoas (Fig. 12.9B). The ideal position for the dilator is the anterior third of the disk space just behind the ALL.[6] A more anterior approach reduces potential injury to the lumbosacral plexus and its branches housed within the psoas muscle. Once a satisfactory position is confirmed, triggered-EMG (t-EMG) is used to stimulate the dilator and confirm safe distance from neural elements. The guidewire is then advanced through the initial dilator and into the disk space. Fluoroscopic images are obtained to confirm the final location of the guidewire. Dilators are placed with sequentially larger diameters to retract the surrounding soft tissue (Fig. 12.10A,B).

t-EMG is repeated with placement of each successive dilator to ensure safe dissection of the psoas. Readings in excess of 10 mA are considered acceptable. Once the final dilator is placed, a corresponding marking is used to determine the optimal length of the retractor blades. The retractors are positioned and attached to the EMG monitoring system. The retractor blades are locked into place by anchoring the retractor-articulating arm to the bed, establishing a window to the disk space. Additionally, a threaded pin may be used to fix the retractor system to the vertebral body. Anteroposterior (AP) fluoroscopy is used to confirm the position of the retractor blades.

Once the retractors are firmly in place, the field is inspected for any neuronal structures. This is especially important in lower lumbar segments where more anterior elements of the lumbosacral plexus can be encountered. Although a more anterior oblique trajectory should largely mitigate the risk of facing such a structure, surgeons must be wary of anatomic variants. If a nerve is encountered, a Penfield dissector can be used to gently sweep the nerve behind the retractor. Rarely, the approach may have to be aborted altogether.

In the absence of any obstructing structures, the disk space should be clearly visualized. It is important to identify the anterior border of the disk space as well as the ALL. Preserving the ALL minimizes the risk for injury to vascular structures positioned directly anterior and facilitates proper graft placement and fixation. In patients with severe preoperative sagittal imbalance, some surgeons may opt to resect the ALL in order to gain extra degrees of lordosis. In our experience we have not felt the need to perform an ALL release in patients with degenerative or adult idiopathic scoliosis when they have not had a prior fusion. We reserve ALL release for patients who have had an L4 to sacrum fusion and there is proximal junctional failure (PJF) with kyphosis at L3-4 or similarly PJF at L2-3 following a fusion at L3 to Sacrum.[6]

The disk is incised using a no. 15 blade. Diskectomy is performed using pituitary rongeurs targeted to the anterior two-thirds of the disk space, making sure not to dissect the ALL. Under fluoroscopic guidance, a cobb elevator is advanced across the disk space using a mallet. The contralateral annulus is released and the cobb elevator rotated 90 degrees to further stretch and release the annulus. This is a vital step in accomplishing robust coronal correction in patients with scoliosis (Fig. 12.10C).

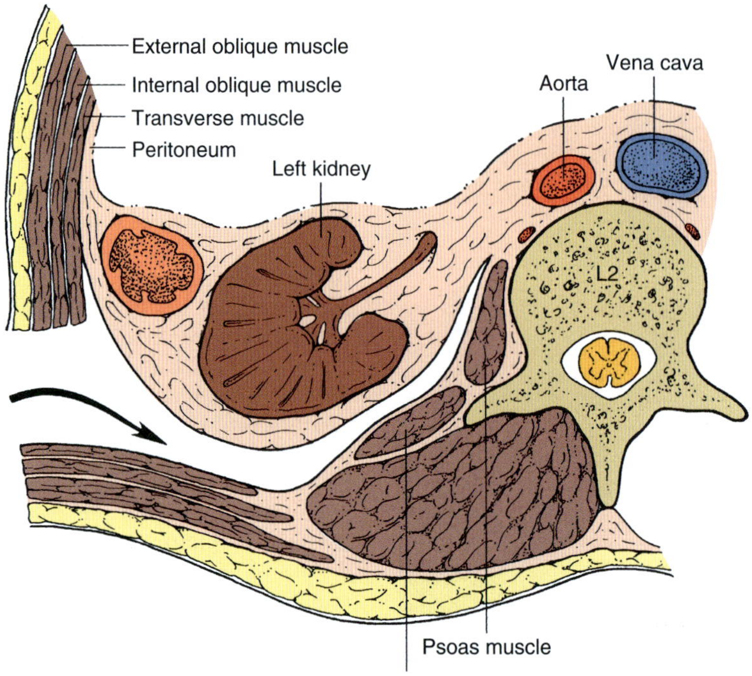

• **Fig. 12.7** Coronal representation of retroperitoneal approach to the lumbar spine. (From Isaacs RE, Fessler RG. Lumbar and sacral spine. In: Benzel, EC, ed. *Spine Surgery: Techniques, Complication Avoidance, and Management. 3rd ed.* Philadelphia: Elsevier; 2012:368)

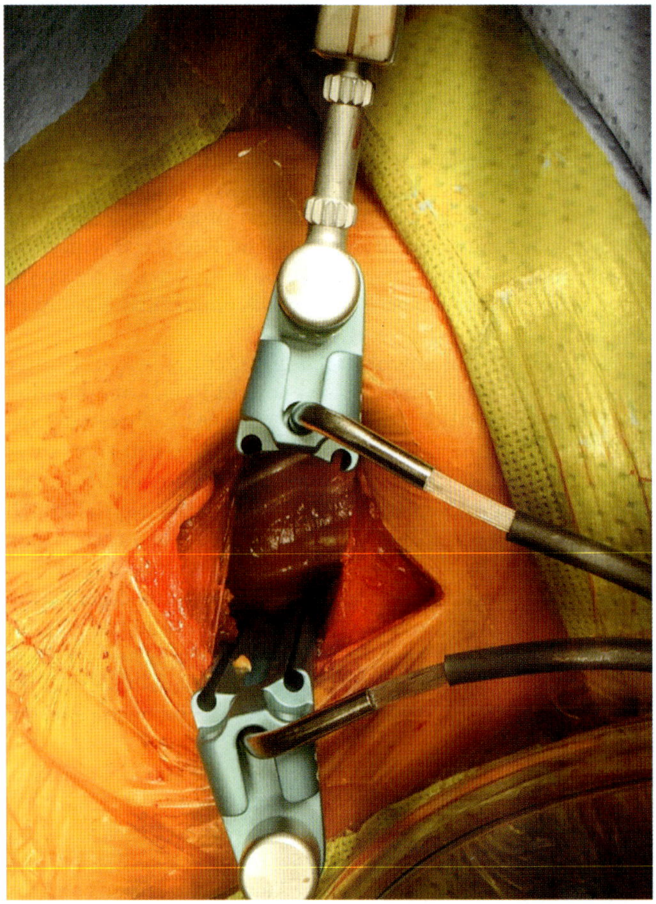

• **Fig. 12.8** Intra-operative picture showing the anterior border of the psoas following an oblique lateral interbody fusion approach.

The disk spaces and endplates are prepared for implant placement using a series of curettes, rasps, box cutting curettes, and shavers as needed. Prior to placing the implant, serial trial spacers are placed and removed using a slap hammer. Based on the preoperative imaging, some surgeons may opt for a hyperlordotic cage in order to gain additional degrees of lordosis. Usually, we tend to use a 12 mm by 12 degree cage most of the time. The cage is next filled with bone graft or other biologic material and inserted into a graft-retaining device. We prefer to use 3 to 4 mg of recombinant bone morphogenic protein-2 (rhBMP-2 [Infuse] combined with Grafton putty demineralized bone matrix (DBM) and local bone to fill the cage. The cage is impacted into place using fluoroscopic guidance. In order to maximize correction in the sagittal plane, the device should be placed as anteriorly as possible within the disk space. This maximizes the gains in segmental lordosis achieved with each interbody device.[6] However, surgeons must be careful not to violate the ALL. A lateral and anteroposterior image is obtained prior to removing the graft inserter to ensure proper positioning of the graft (Fig. 12.11).

Closure

The surgical field is irrigated vigorously with saline solution. Prior to removing the dilator, the area is examined for any bleeding and hemostasis is achieved with bipolar cautery. Once all instrumentation has been removed from the field, final anteroposterior and lateral images are obtained to confirm proper graft placement. Moreover, the imaging allows the surgeon to assess the overall sagittal and coronal alignment. The fascia is closed using buried Vicryl sutures. Finally, the skin is closed using subdermal stiches and Steri-Strips.

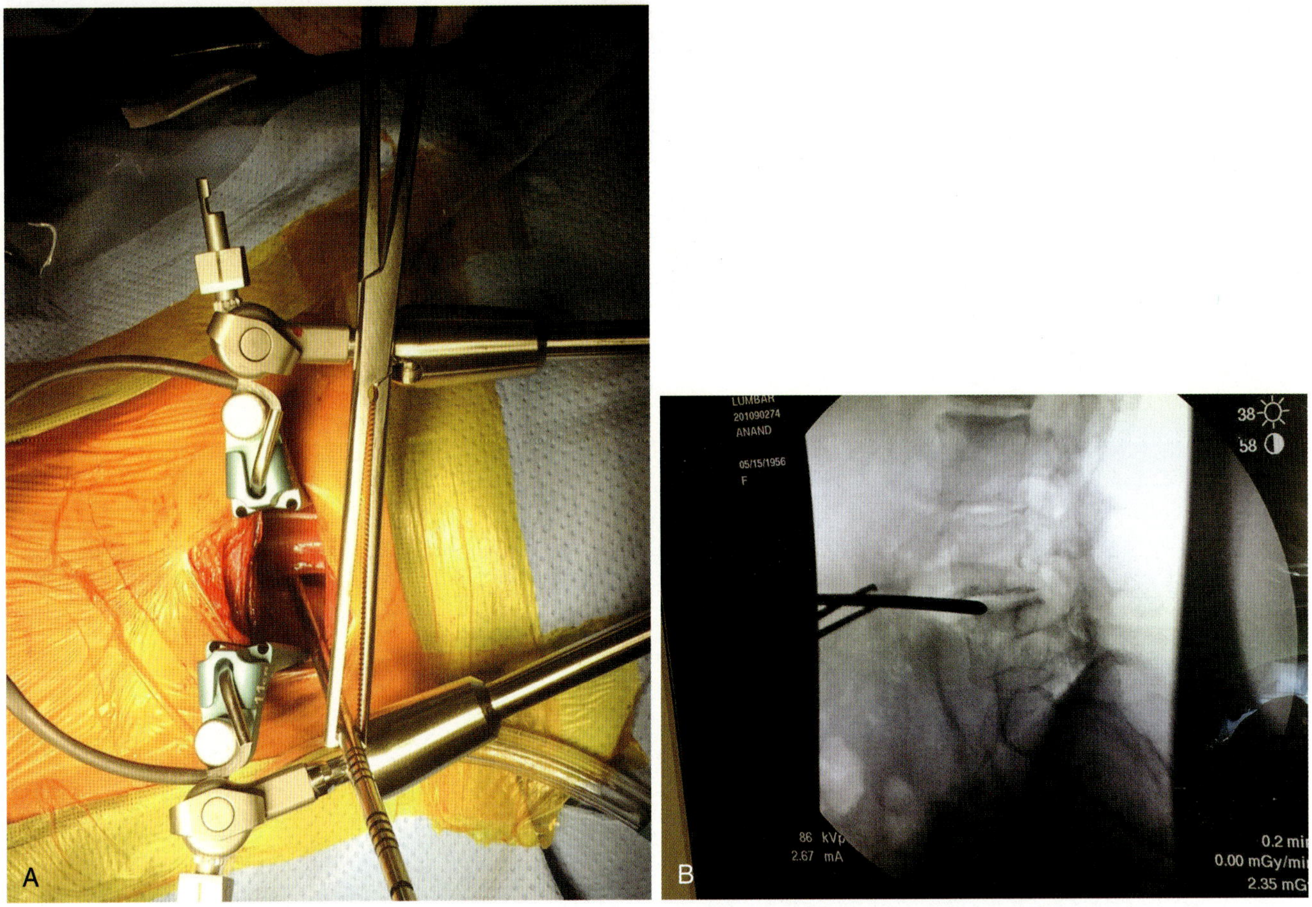

• **Fig. 12.9** Intraoperative picture (A) showing placement of first dilator on the disk anterior to the psoas and (B) fluoroscopic picture confirming placement of first dilator in anterior third of disk space.

Complications

Despite its relative safety compared with alternative approaches, LLIF or OLIF is not without a considerable risk of complications. The reduced surgical footprint of minimally invasive techniques still poses a risk for damage of neuronal, muscular, and vascular structures. Moreover, as with any instrumentation-based operation, the device may be suboptimal or fail all together. It is important to identify the potential causes of morbidity and understand management strategies that can optimize the minimally invasive approach. Neuromuscular injuries, lumbar plexopathies, vascular insults, and graft subsidence are some of the important complications to consider.

Neuromuscular Injuries and Lumbar Plexopathies

Both LLIF and OLIF pose a unique risk to the lumbosacral plexus housed within the psoas muscle. Injuries of this sort are referred to as lumbar plexopathies. The LLIF because of its approach that is essentially transpsoas is more at risk than OLIF which is a pre-psoas approach.[7] Postoperatively, it is imperative to perform a detailed clinical examination of the patient's sensory and motor function. Careful attention should be paid to the dermatomal distribution of the patient's symptomatology. Muscle weakness should be localized to a particular muscle or group of muscles. Combining these neurologic findings helps pinpoint the specific injured element of the lumbar plexus.

The genitofemoral branch is particularly susceptible to injury during LLIF, with a reported incidence ranging from 0 to 75%.[8] A deficit secondary to a genitofemoral nerve insult classically manifests as anterior groin pain or numbness. Its potential for injury, as expected, has much to do with its anatomy. The nerve originates from the L1-2 roots, traverses through the substance of the psoas, and emerges on the anterior surface of the muscle at the L3-4 level. It then splits into two distinct branches—the femoral and genital branches. The former supplies the skin anterior to the upper part of the femoral triangle and the latter supplies the cremasteric muscle in male patients and the skin of the mons pubis and labia major in female patients. These nerve fibers may be encountered adjacent to the anterior quarter of the vertebral body from L3-5 and the anterior half of the vertebral body at L2-3.[5] This anatomic location makes the nerve fibers susceptible to injury both through a direct insult or indirect trauma secondary to retraction. Some have also theorized that genitofemoral nerve disturbances may be attributed to neuropraxia or a psoas muscle's inflammatory response.

The ilioinguinal, iliohypogastric, and lateral femoral cutaneous branches are also at risk for injury during dissection in the retroperitoneal space.[5] The lateral femoral cutaneous branch, which is made up of dorsal branches of the ventral rami, poses a special risk when accessing the L4-5 disk space. The nerve often sits posterior to the retractor and can be pressed against the anterior iliac crest or lateral anterior sacrum. Clinical manifestations of a lateral femoral cutaneous nerve insult include numbness or pain of the outer thigh.

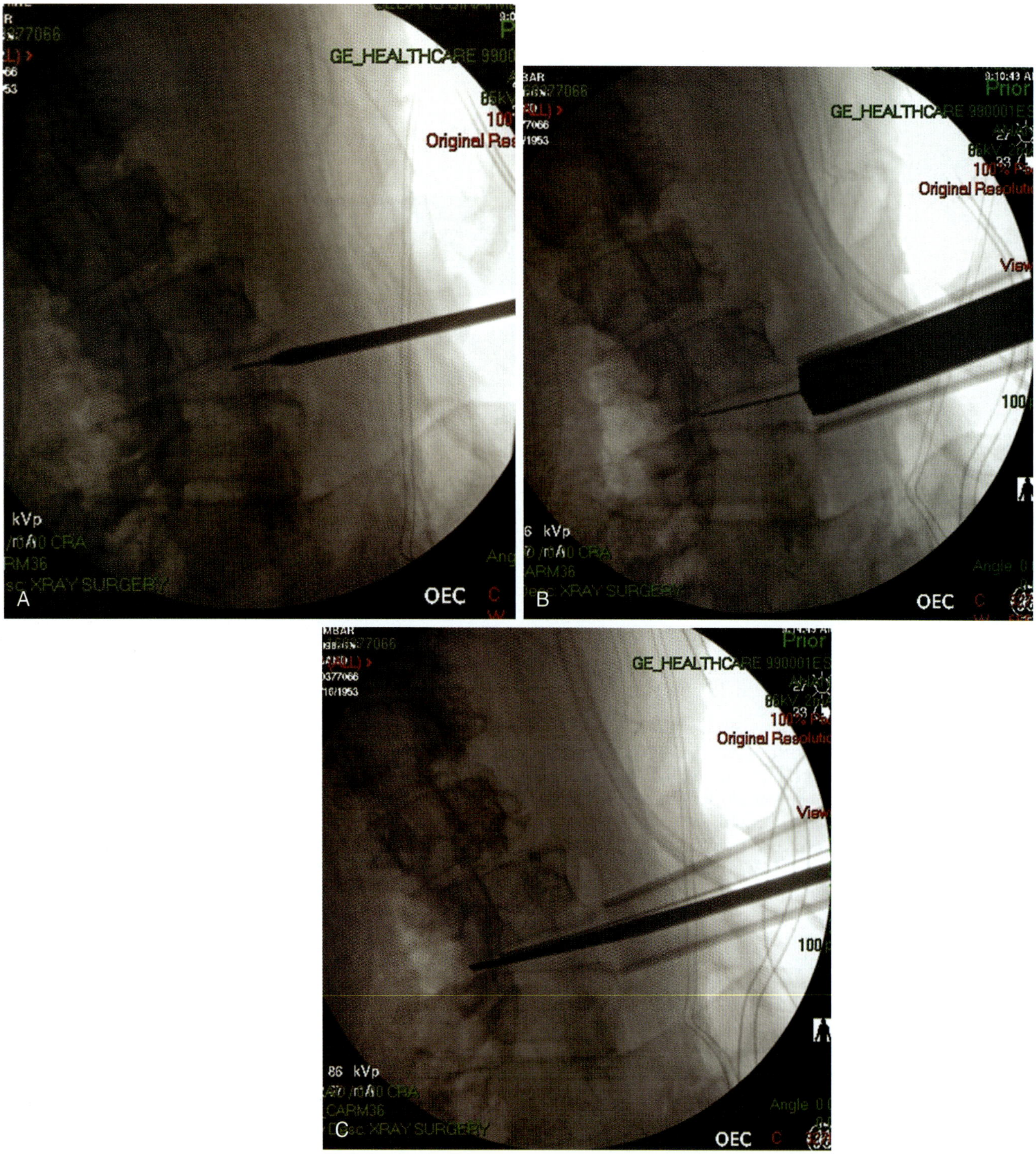

• **Fig. 12.10** **A.** Fluoroscopic image of first dilator with guidewire to level of disk space. **B.** Placement of serial dilators with retractor. **C.** Fluoroscopic image with cobb elevator passed to the opposite annulus.

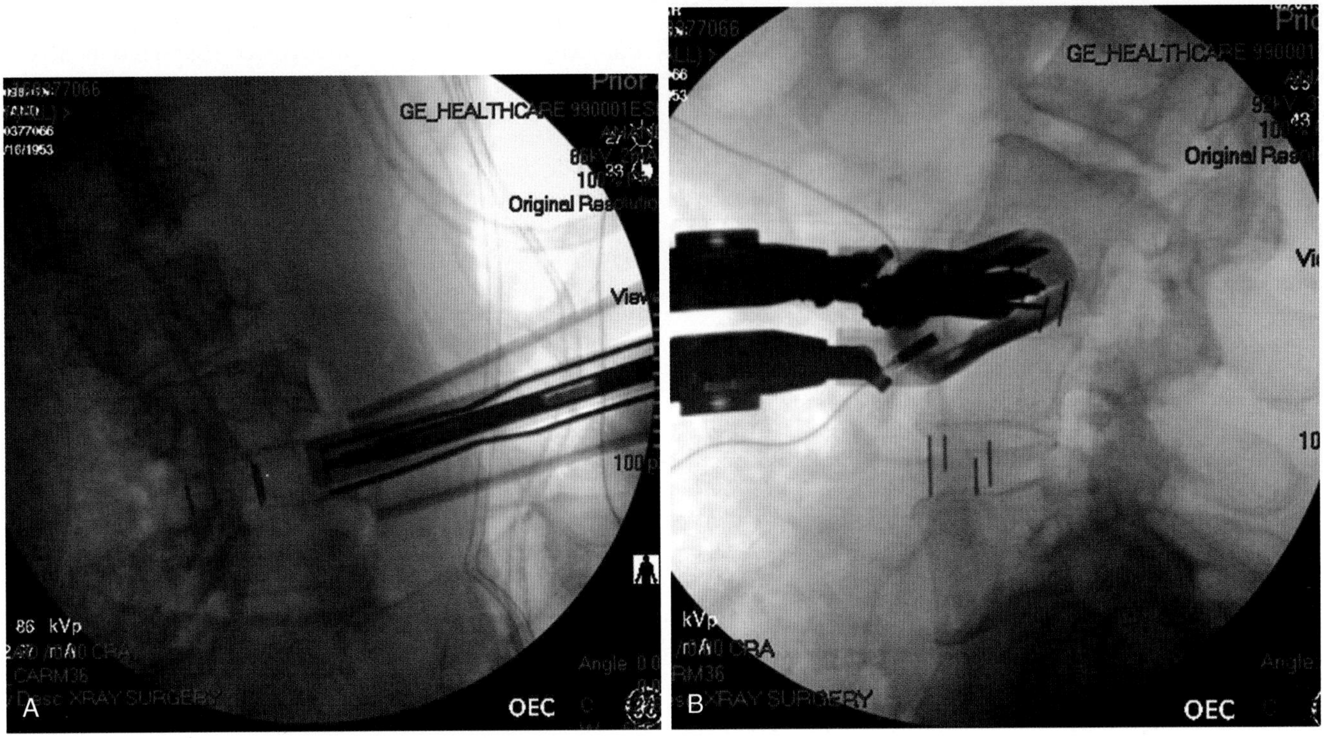

• **Fig. 12.11 A.** Anteroposterior fluoroscopic view of placement of interbody polyetheretherketone prostheses in disk space. **B.** Lateral fluoroscopic view of Interbody prosthesis in disk space.

Along with sensory deficits, it is important to note the motor effects of nerve damage. Damage to the femoral nerve, the largest branch of the lumbar plexus, may result in significant quadriceps weakness or palsy. The femoral nerve arises from the dorsal branches along the posterior division of the lumbar plexus, eventually, branching to include the femoral cutaneous nerve branch. Its relatively posterior anatomic position provides the nerve with some added protection from direct traumatic injury. Nonetheless, there is potential for indirect insults or inflammatory changes to the nerve. If persistent, injury can progress to significant muscle atrophy. A study of 118 patients by Cahill et al.[9] found a 4.8% rate of femoral nerve injuries, all of which occurred after surgery of the L4-5 disk space. Anand et al.[10] reported 2 cases of quadriceps palsy in 28 patients that underwent LLIF. Of note, all patients recovered within 6 months.

Dissection of the psoas muscle itself may also result in motor weakness. Damaging the integrity of muscular fibers along with the added damage of nerve insults to the psoas can, at the very least, cause transient clinical consequences. Lee et al.[11] evaluated the degree of psoas muscle injury in LLIF using a digital dynamometer on 33 patients.[11] The study found a statistically significant reduction of hip flexor strength on the operated side. However, after 2 weeks' follow-up, the values returned to baseline.

Although neuromuscular elements are at risk during LLIF, fortunately most deficits appear to resolve within 6 months. There appears to be a learning curve and, with increasing experience, authors have reported a reduction in the incidence of neural injuries.[12] Spinal surgeons have taken measures to mitigate these risks. Spontaneous EMG and triggered EMG have been used to monitor nerve firings during psoas dissection. To optimize intraoperative neuromonitoring, others have added transcranial electrical stimulation with motor evoked potential (TESMEP) to previously described monitoring using spontaneous EMG (s-EMG) and peripheral stimulation (triggered EMG: tEMG). Berends et al.[13] reported that TESMEP has additional value to s-EMG and t-EMG during XLIF procedure: (1) it informed about otherwise unnoticed events, and (2) it confirmed and added information to events measured using s-EMG.[13]

Uribe et al.[14] also reported that retraction time was significantly longer in those patients with symptomatic neuropraxia vs. those without ($P = .031$). Stepwise logistic regression showed a significant positive relationship between the presence of new postoperative symptomatic neuropraxia and total retraction time ($P < .001$), as well as change in t-EMG thresholds over time ($P < .001$)[14]

Furthermore, when traversing the psoas muscle, an anterior trajectory to the disk space may prove the safest route, reducing the risk of direct injury of those nerves traversing or lying posterior to the muscle. The "oblique" approach (OLIF) preserves more of the psoas muscular fibers as the access is anterior to the psoas and avoids traversing the substance of the psoas. It appears that early reports are showing a reduced incidence of lumbar plexopathies with the OLIF pre-psoas approach as opposed to the transpsoas LLIF approach.[7] Careful attention must be paid to visually inspect the surgical field and appreciate any exposed nerves. A visualized nerve combined with EMG analysis is ample justification to abort lateral fusion at that spinal level in favor of an alternative approach. Importantly, surgeons must keep in mind that many anatomic variants of the lumbar plexus may exist. Additionally, it should be noted that certain nerves are outside the capabilities of our EMG monitoring systems.

Vascular Injuries[15–18]

Both LLIF and OLIF avoid direct manipulation of the great vessels, a major advantage compared with more invasive anterior approaches. Nonetheless, injury to the aorta can occur with either. During instrumentation, if the ALL is violated, anterior displacement of the interbody cage can insult the adjacent aorta. However, this phenomenon is very rare. Vascular injuries include injury to the common iliac vein, ascending iliolumbar vein, and segmental arteries. Bleeding from these vessels can be managed intraoperatively with clipping or cautery. Formal vascular repair and, in rare instances, stenting of the vessel may be needed to control the bleeding. Retroperitoneal hematoma may develop postoperatively, especially if a bleed is overlooked or insufficiently controlled. Generally, retroperitoneal hematomas should be observed, with evacuation by a vascular surgeon reserved only for more severe cases. Fortunately, these events usually resolve spontaneously.

Graft Subsidence

Graft subsidence is defined as an interbody device "sinking" into either the adjacent superior or inferior vertebral body. In radiographic terms, this can be measured by a reduction in disk space relative to a postoperative reduction of greater than 2 to 3 mm. The phenomenon can be attributed to a myriad of factors including age, gender, body mass index (BMI), bone quality, cage design and positioning, use of biologics, and surgical approach.[19,20] Graft subsidence is particularly troubling for minimally invasive fusion techniques that rely on indirect decompression of the disk space.

Le et al.[21] evaluated subsidence in 140 patients who underwent minimally invasive LIF from L1 to L5. Polyetheretherketone (PEEK) cages filled with either allograft (1.05–2.10 mg rhBMP-2 [Infuse, Medtronic, Minneapolis, MN]) mixed with bone extender hydroxyapatite and tricalcium phosphate per level (Formagraft, NuVasive) or 5 mL of cadaveric cancellous bone mixed with mesenchymal stem cells (Osteocel, NuVasive). There were 102 patients in the former group and 38 patients in the latter group. Subsidence was defined as any violation of the vertebral endplate. Based on these criteria, radiographic subsidence occurred in 14.3% and clinical subsidence in 2.1%. The rate of subsidence was significantly higher using cages 18-mm wide compared with cages 22-mm wide.

Malham et al.[19] assessed rates of subsidence after minimally invasive LIF using computed tomography (CT) imaging in 128 patients (178 treated levels). The cage was filled with either of the following: (1) AttraX (NuVasive, Inc., San Diego, CA), which is an osteoinductive synthetic bone putty composed of 95% β-TCP (tricalcium phosphate) and 5% hydroxyapatite, or (2) a combination of rhBMP-2 (Infuse, Medtronic, Inc.) and Mastergraft β-TCP granules (Medtronic, Inc.). Infuse had a fixed concentration of 1.5 mg/mL, and the dose used per level was volume dependent (i.e., the internal volume of the cage equaled the Infuse volume in milliliters). They used a small Infuse kit (2.8 mL, providing a 4.2-mg dose). No Infuse was placed outside the cage. Subsidence was defined as any compromise of either endplate. The study found a subsidence rate of 10% in patients (8% in treated levels), 3% of whom exhibited clinical subsidence. In patients who developed subsidence, there was a statistically significant increase in the rate of pseudoarthrosis at 6 months; however, the findings did not persist by 12 months.

Marchi et al.[20] compared the rate of subsidence in two groups undergoing XLIF—46 patients (61 lumbar levels) with a cage 18 mm wide and 28 patients (37 lumbar levels) with a cage 22 mm wide. They reported bone graft materials included calcium phosphate bone graft material and no mention of use of rhBMP-2. Subsidence was confirmed using standing lateral radiograph and classified based on loss of disk height as follows: Grade 0: 0 to 24% loss, grade I: 25% to 49% loss, grade II: 50% to 74% loss, and grade III: 75% to 100% loss. The study found a significant difference in subsidence between the cohorts at 6 weeks, 3 months, and 12 months. Furthermore, when stratifying patients based on subsidence grade, female sex and age were risk factors for developing high-grade subsidence.

Mitigating the risk of subsidence is an important goal for minimally invasive interventions because it may contribute to inadequate decompression, global misalignment, and pseudoarthrosis. To prevent subsidence during LLIF, careful attention of certain measures must be met. Spinal surgeons should take heed of preoperative factors including age, gender, BMI, and bone quality. Proper patient selection based on these criteria can rule out poor surgical candidates. Further, careful attention must be paid to evacuate the disk space thoroughly. Endplate preparation and preservation comprise a vital step in maintaining the structural integrity of the construct and providing an optimal surface for fusion. With the use of rhBMP-2, it is important to preserve the endplate as it has been postulated that endplate violation may result in aggressive osteoclastic response by the rhBMP-2, resulting in weakening of the bone further subsidence. Surgeons should consider supplementing graft placement with internal fixation, especially in patients with risk factors. Furthermore, the biomechanical properties and design of the graft must not be overlooked—in particular, the preventative effect of wider grafts on subsidence.[20,21]

Outcomes

Early studies reporting on the efficacy and clinical outcomes of LLIF have been reassuring. Isaacs et al.[22] prospectively evaluated 107 patients who underwent transpsoas XLIF with or without posterior fusion for treatment of degenerative scoliosis. Although an XLIF was required in the treatment of these cases, the addition of supplemental instrumentation (anterior, lateral, or posterior), the use of direct decompression, the addition of a posterior approach (using either open or minimally invasive techniques), and the inclusion of L5–S1 was left to the choice of the surgeon. The cohort had a mean age of 68 years and mean levels treated of 4.4. Mean operative time was 178 minutes, blood loss was 50 to 100 mL and mean hospital stay was 2.9 days (unstaged) and 8.1 days (staged). The rate of major complications was 12.1%, including 1.9% medical and 11.2% surgical.

Anand et al.[23] assessed 2- to 5-year outcomes of 71 patients who underwent minimally invasive correction for adult spinal deformity. All patients underwent direct lateral interbody fusion as part of the treatment. The cohort had a mean age of 64 years and mean follow up of 39 months. Average blood loss was 412 mL (1-stage) and 314 mL (2-stage). Surgical time was 291 minutes (1-stage) and 183 minutes (2-stage). Mean hospital stay was 7.6 days. The study reported a mean preoperative cobb angle of 24.7 degrees corrected to 9.5 degrees, coronal balance of 25.5 mm corrected to 11 mm, and sagittal balance of 31.7 mm corrected to 10.7 mm. Within the cohort, 14 patients reported adverse events requiring intervention as follows: 4 pseudoarthrosis, 4 persistent stenosis, 1 osteomyelitis, 1 adjacent segment discitis, 1 late wound infection, 1 proximal junctional kyphosis, 1 screw prominence, 1 idiopathic cerebellar hemorrhage, and 2 wound dehiscence.

Kotwal et al.[24] assessed 118 patients who underwent minimally invasive LLIF with at least a 2-year follow up. In terms of clinical outcomes, visual analog scale (VAS), Oswestry disability index (ODI), and mental component of the Short Form-12 (SF-12) improved significantly. Radiographic measures, including disk height and coronal angulation at each levels as well as the cobb angle, were restored in a significant manner. Fusion was successful in 88% of levels. The most frequent complication was transient thigh pain occurring in 36% of patients.

Silvestre et al.[25] reported on 179 patients who underwent OLIF at one institution. Patients were age 54.1 ± 10.6 with a BMI of 24.8 ± 4.1 kg/m. The procedure was performed in the lumbar spine at L1-2 in 4, L2-3 in 54, L3-4 in 120, L4-5 in 134, and L5-S1 in 6 patients. It was done at 1 level in 56, 2 levels in 107, and 3 levels in 16 patients. Surgery time and blood loss were, respectively, 32.5 ± 13.2 minutes and 57 ± 131 mL per level fused. There were 19 patients with a single complication and 1 with two complications, including 2 patients with postoperative radiculopathy after L3-5 OLIF. There was no abdominal weakness or herniation.

Kim et al.[26] reported 29 patients having had an OLIF procedure. All patients also underwent percutaneous pedicle screw fixation in the prone position, with additional posterior laminectomy in 3 patients. The average VAS score for back/leg improved from 6.3/6.5 to 3.1/2.1 at the last follow up (both, $P < .001$). The average ODI score improved from 50.4 preoperatively to 27.2 at the last follow up ($P < .001$). Radiologic evidence of fusion on CT scans was noted in 57.0% of the patients in 6 months and 92.9% in 12 months. Subsidence during the follow up periods occurred in 8 (21.6%) of 37 OLIF levels in 29 patients. Lumbar plexopathy was noted in 4 (13.5%) patients: it consisted of transient motor weakness in 3 (10.3%) patients and numbness in 3 (10.3%) patients (Sensory Dermal Zone III in 2, II in 1). All lumbar plexopathy symptoms resolved within 4 weeks postoperatively. Evidence of sympathetic injury on physical examination and digital infrared thermal imaging was noted in 4 (13.5%) patients.

Woods et al.[27] reported a total of 137 patients who underwent fusion at 340 levels. An overall complication rate of 11.7% was seen. The most common complications were subsidence (4.4%), postoperative ileus (2.9%), and vascular injury (2.9%). Ileus and vascular injuries were seen only in cases including OLIF at L5-S1. No patient suffered neurologic injury. No cases of ureteral injury, sympathectomy affecting the lower extremities, or visceral injury were seen. Successful fusion was seen at 97.9% of surgical levels.

Anand et al.[7] in another publication compared their old protocol with the TLLIF approach with their new protocol using the pre-psoas approach (OLIF). They reported a significant drop in both major and minor complications and no instance of quadriceps palsy with the pre-psoas OLIF approach as compared with a 5% incidence with the transpsoas LLIF approach.[7]

The overall consensus of prior studies demonstrates improvements in radiographic correction and clinical outcomes, as well as a moderate rate of morbidity. Higher level-of-evidence prospective studies are needed to make more definite conclusions about the efficacy of minimally invasive approaches. Nonetheless, early results are promising, which is fueling further innovation and advancement in the field.

Conclusion

As a whole, minimally invasive spinal surgery is a field in its relative infancy. Recent studies have begun comparing these approaches, such as LLIF, with more invasive open and hybrid procedures. Haque et al.[28] compared 184 patients who underwent either a minimally invasive (42 patients), hybrid (33 patients), or open (109 patients) correction for adult spinal deformity. The study found the minimally invasive group had a significantly smaller mean lumbar cobb-angle, SVA correction, and postoperative thoracic kyphosis compared with the open group. Compared with the hybrid group, the minimally invasive group had a smaller curve correction and mean change in pelivic incidence minus lumbar lordosis (PI-LL) mismatch. Of note, no significant difference was noted in clinical outcome measures between the groups and major complications were lower in the minimally invasive group compared with the open group.

These findings underline the potential benefits and possible shortcomings of LLIF and OLIF moving forward. Clinical results appear, at the very least, to be comparable to more invasive strategies. Moreover, there are inherent advantages to the minimally invasive philosophy, including less blood loss and improved cosmesis. However, achieving sagittal balance remains a challenge using minimally invasive techniques; more importantly, sagittal alignment has been shown to be an important radiographic indicator of patient outcome.[29]

As a consequence of this radiographic shortcoming, many surgeons restrict minimally invasive techniques to mild or moderate deformity cases. In recent years, efforts have been made to improve the standard of attainable correction. One such novelty is the use of interbody cages with additional degrees of lordosis, known as "hyperlordotic cages." These implants can presumably achieve excess gains in segmental lordosis while maintaining the benefits of an MIS approach.[30]

Modifications in surgical technique appear to be improving as well. TLIF studies have shown that by using cantilever effects and placing the interbody in the anterior portion of the disk space, there is a greater ability to create and maintain lumbar lordosis.[31] By meticulously placing interbody cages anteriorly at multiple levels, OLIF may be able to provide robust sagittal correction, and harmonious global alignment.[6] Anand et al.[7] have shown significant improvement in sagittal balance with their strategically staged protocol for circumferential minimally invasive treatment of adult spinal deformity.

More nuanced innovations are being explored as well. Advancements in cage design, biologics, and nanotechnologies are on the horizon. Technical innovations, including staged protocols and rod contouring, also show promise. With advances in the field, coupled with increasing strides forward in the learning curve, we may greatly broaden the scope and merit of minimally invasive fusion. On the heels of these improvements, minimally invasive approaches, such as LLIF and OLIF, may one day become the gold standard for deformity correction.

References

1. Lin N, Li Y, Bebawy JF, et al. Abdominal circumference but not the degree of lumbar flexion affects the accuracy of lumbar interspace identification by Tuffier's line palpation method: an observational study. *BMC Anesthesiol.* 2015;15:9.
2. Kim JT, Jung CW, Lee JR, et al. Influence of lumbar flexion on the position of the intercrestal line. *Reg Anesth Pain Med.* 2003;28: 509–511.
3. Benglis Jr DM, Vanni S, Levi AD. An anatomical study of the lumbosacral plexus as related to the minimally invasive transpsoas approach to the lumbar spine: laboratory investigation. *J Neurosurg Spine.* 2009;10:139–144.
4. Moro T, Kikuchi S, Konno S, et al. An anatomic study of the lumbar plexus with respect to retroperitoneal endoscopic surgery. *Spine (Phila Pa 1976).* 2003;28:423–428; discussion 427–428.
5. Uribe JS, Arredondo N, Dakwar E, et al. Defining the safe working zones using the minimally invasive lateral retroperitoneal transpsoas approach: an anatomical study: laboratory investigation. *J Neurosurg Spine.* 2010;13:260–266.
6. Anand N, Khandehroo B, Cohen J, et al. The influence of lordotic cages on creating sagittal balance in the CMIS treatment of adult spinal deformity. *Int J Spine Surg.* 2017;11:23.

7. Anand N, Cohen JE, Cohen RB, et al. Comparison of a newer versus older protocol for circumferential minimally invasive surgical (CMIS) correction of adult spinal deformity (ASD)—evolution over a 10-year experience. *Spine Deform*. 2017;5:213–223.
8. Pumberger M, Hughes AP, Huang RR, et al. Neurologic deficit following lateral lumbar interbody fusion. *Eur Spine J*. 2012;21: 1192–1199.
9. Cahill KS, Martinez JL, Wang MY, et al. Motor nerve injuries following the minimally invasive lateral transpsoas approach. *J Neurosurg Spine*. 2012;17:227–231.
10. Anand N, Rosemann R, Khalsa B, et al. Mid-term to long-term clinical and functional outcomes of minimally invasive correction and fusion for adults with scoliosis. *Neurosurg Focus*. 2010;28:E6.
11. Lee YP, Regev GJ, Chan J, et al. Evaluation of hip flexion strength following lateral lumbar interbody fusion. *Spine J*. 2013;13:1259–1262.
12. Le TV, Burkett CJ, Deukmedjian AR, et al. Postoperative lumbar plexus injury after lumbar retroperitoneal transpsoas minimally invasive lateral interbody fusion. *Spine (Phila Pa 1976)*. 2013;38: E13–E20.
13. Berends HI, Journee HL, Racz I, et al. Multimodality intraoperative neuromonitoring in extreme lateral interbody fusion. Transcranial electrical stimulation as indispensable rearview. *Eur Spine J*. 2016;25:1581–1586.
14. Uribe JS, Isaacs RE, Youssef JA, et al. Can triggered electromyography monitoring throughout retraction predict postoperative symptomatic neuropraxia after XLIF? Results from a prospective multicenter trial. *Eur Spine J*. 2015;24(suppl 3):378–385.
15. Aichmair A, Fantini GA, Garvin S, et al. Aortic perforation during lateral lumbar interbody fusion. *J Spinal Disord Tech*. 2015;28:71–75.
16. Assina R, Majmundar NJ, Herschman Y, et al. First report of major vascular injury due to lateral transpsoas approach leading to fatality. *J Neurosurg Spine*. 2014;21:794–798.
17. Kueper J, Fantini GA, Walker BR, et al. Incidence of vascular complications during lateral lumbar interbody fusion: an examination of the mini-open access technique. *Eur Spine J*. 2015;24:800–8009.
18. Uribe JS, Deukmedjian AR. Visceral, vascular, and wound complications following over 13,000 lateral interbody fusions: a survey study and literature review. *Eur Spine J*. 2015;24(suppl 3):386–396.
19. Malham GM, Parker RM, Blecher CM, et al. Assessment and classification of subsidence after lateral interbody fusion using serial computed tomography. *J Neurosurg Spine*. 2015:1–9.
20. Marchi L, Abdala N, Oliveira L, et al. Radiographic and clinical evaluation of cage subsidence after stand-alone lateral interbody fusion. *J Neurosurg Spine*. 2013;19:110–118.
21. Le TV, Baaj AA, Dakwar E, et al. Subsidence of polyetheretherketone intervertebral cages in minimally invasive lateral retroperitoneal transpsoas lumbar interbody fusion. *Spine (Phila Pa 1976)*. 2012;37:1268–1273.
22. Isaacs RE, Hyde J, Goodrich JA, et al. A prospective, nonrandomized, multicenter evaluation of extreme lateral interbody fusion for the treatment of adult degenerative scoliosis: perioperative outcomes and complications. *Spine (Phila Pa 1976)*. 2010;35: S322–S330.
23. Anand N, Baron EM, Khandehroo B, et al. Long-term 2- to 5-year clinical and functional outcomes of minimally invasive surgery for adult scoliosis. *Spine (Phila Pa 1976)*. 2013;38:1566–1575.
24. Kotwal S, Kawaguchi S, Lebl D, et al. Minimally invasive lateral lumbar interbody fusion: clinical and radiographic outcome at a minimum 2-year follow-up. *J Spinal Disord Tech*. 2015;28: 119–125.
25. Silvestre C, Mac-Thiong JM, Hilmi R, et al. Complications and morbidities of mini-open anterior retroperitoneal lumbar interbody fusion: oblique lumbar interbody fusion in 179 patients. *Asian Spine J*. 2012;6:89–97.
26. Kim JS, Choi WS, Sung JH. 314 Minimally invasive oblique lateral interbody fusion for L4-5: clinical outcomes and perioperative complications. *Neurosurgery*. 2016;63(suppl 1):190–191.
27. Woods KR, Billys JB, Hynes RA. Technical description of oblique lateral interbody fusion at L1-L5 (OLIF25) and at L5-S1 (OLIF51) and evaluation of complication and fusion rates. *Spine J*. 2017;17:545–553.
28. Haque RM, Mundis Jr GM, Ahmed Y, et al. Comparison of radiographic results after minimally invasive, hybrid, and open surgery for adult spinal deformity: a multicenter study of 184 patients. *Neurosurg Focus*. 2014;36:E13.
29. Schwab F, Patel A, Ungar B, et al. Adult spinal deformity-postoperative standing imbalance: how much can you tolerate? An overview of key parameters in assessing alignment and planning corrective surgery. *Spine (Phila Pa 1976)*. 2010;35:2224–2231.
30. Uribe JS, Smith DA, Dakwar E, et al. Lordosis restoration after anterior longitudinal ligament release and placement of lateral hyperlordotic interbody cages during the minimally invasive lateral transpsoas approach: a radiographic study in cadavers. *J Neurosurg Spine*. 2012;17:476–485.
31. Anand N, Hamilton JF, Perri B, et al. Cantilever TLIF with structural allograft and RhBMP2 for correction and maintenance of segmental sagittal lordosis: long-term clinical, radiographic, and functional outcome. *Spine (Phila Pa 1976)*. 2006;31:E748–E753.

13

Pre-psoas (Oblique) Lateral Interbody Fusion at L5-S1

MARK B. FRENKEL AND DAVID J. HART

Introduction

The pre-psoas oblique lateral approach to the lumbar spine was first described by Mayer et al. in 1997.[1] At that time, the approach was described only for the L2-5 disk spaces and the authors recommended an anterior transabdominal approach to the L5-S1 disk space owing to the anatomic considerations surrounding its access. The aortic bifurcation and iliocaval junction typically occur at or just below the L4 vertebral body[2] and, as the iliac vessels course inferolaterally from their origin, they commonly overlie the anterolateral aspect of the L5-S1 disk space (Fig. 13.1).

After the initial description of oblique lateral interbody fusion (OLIF) by Mayer, there were only scattered reports of OLIF in the literature while alternative interbody fusion techniques (transforaminal lumbar interbody fusion [TLIF], anterior lumbar interbody fusion [ALIF], posterior lumbar interbody fusion [PLIF]) were predominantly used to access the L5-S1 interspace. This was true until 2012, when a retrospective study of 179 patients who underwent OLIF was published.[3] This study included six patients who had two-level interbody fusions from L4-S1. The authors also introduced a "sliding window" mini-open technique to access multiple disk levels through one small incision. To our knowledge, this is the first reported L5-S1 OLIF procedure in the literature, although the specific technique has since been modified by other authors to facilitate easier access to the L5-S1 level.[3]

In 2014, another group[4] performed a cadaveric study attempting to access L2-S1 disks from a lateral decubitus position. They found that in all of their 20 specimens they were able to access the L5-S1 disk space medial to the iliac vessels, elucidating the surgical corridor used for modern L5-S1 OLIF. The authors noted that an advantage of this technique is in being able to access all levels from L2-S1 while keeping the patient in a lateral decubitus position without a break in the table. It has only been since the publication of this study and the discovery of this corridor that reports of isolated L5-S1 OLIFs have begun to appear in the literature. In addition, at least one company (Medtronic Inc., Memphis, TN) has begun producing and marketing a retractor and instrumentation system designed specifically for this procedure.

One case report described two OLIFs performed at L5-S1 accompanied by posterior fixation and reported good results without complications. In their discussion, the authors supported the concept of being able to access disks at multiple levels and perform fusion from L1-S1 with the patient in the lateral decubitus position.[5] Another case report presented OLIFs performed at L2-3, 3-4, 4-5, and 5-1 in a single procedure with good results. The authors also commented on the benefit of being able to perform the L5-S1 interbody work through the same incision as the other levels.[6]

From an anatomic standpoint, a recent retrospective magnetic resonance imaging study[2] explored the oblique access to L5-S1, which the authors defined transversely from the midsagittal line of the inferior endplate of L5 to the medial border of

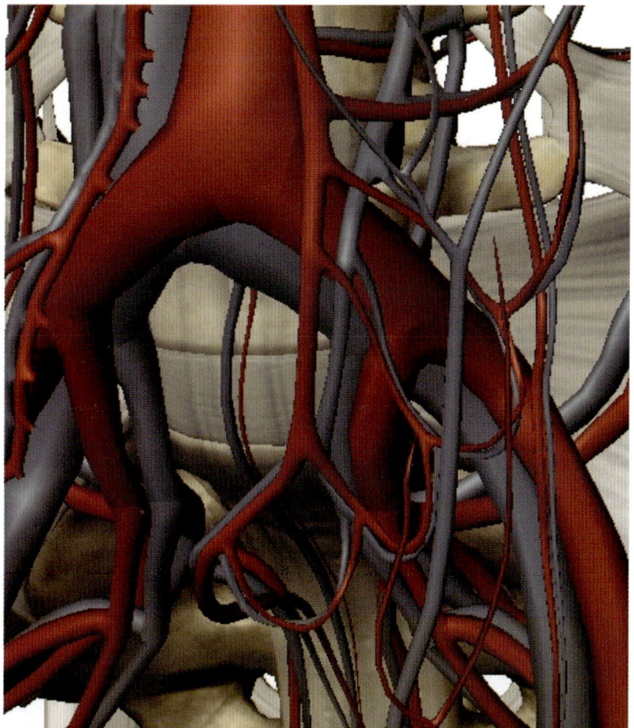

• **Fig. 13.1** Three-dimensional rendering of a lumbar spine showing the bifurcation of the abdominal aortic *(red)* and the anastomoses of the common iliac veins *(blue)* overlying the superior aspect of the L5 vertebral body. The L5-S1 disk can be seen immediately below with the internal iliac arteries and veins overlying the anterolateral margins of the disk space. (Reprinted with the permission of Medtronic, Inc., Memphis, TN, USA © 2016.)

the left common iliac vessel and vertically to the first vascular structure that crossed midline. They found sufficient anatomic access to the L5-S1 interspace in 69% of patients analyzed and observed that the lower the iliocaval junction was, the less probable it was that sufficient access was present. This study failed to take into account the additional space gained by intraoperative mobilization and retraction of the iliac vessels, but interestingly, they found that in 13% of patients with no anterior access to the L5-S1 disk, an oblique corridor could be delineated between the psoas and the iliac vessels similar to that previously described by Silvestre et al.[3]

The benefits of L5-S1 OLIF may be largely in contrast to other procedures. Some authors discuss the benefits of OLIF's oblique pre-psoas approach in contrast to a lateral transpsoas approach (lateral lumbar interbody fusion [LLIF] eXtreme LIF [XLIF]/DLIF), as OLIF does not require dissection or splitting of the psoas muscle. This may theoretically decrease postoperative pain and avoid injury to the psoas and lumbar plexus, which may obviate the need for intraoperative neuromonitoring.[2] Specifically, in regards to the L5-S1 level, a nonoblique lateral approach can be extremely difficult or impossible owing to obstruction by the iliac crests.[7]

In contrast to a traditional PLIF, OLIF avoids dissection of the paraspinal muscles, reduces the risk of incidental durotomies, and eliminates the need for nerve root retraction.[8] It also may have some benefit over a direct ALIF, which can lead to injury to abdominal viscera, retrograde ejaculation, and prolonged ileus,[8] while still potentially offering the similar benefits in sagittal balance and restoration of disk height associated with these other interbody approaches.

Surgical Indications

The L5-S1 OLIF has similar indications as other interbody fusion techniques. These include a number of symptomatic pathologies including, but not limited to, degenerative disk disease with disk collapse, spondylolisthesis, discitis, and scoliosis. OLIF at other levels has been reported in the literature for revision of a pseudoarthrosis[9] because it affords good disk space visualization. It may be chosen over other approaches to the L5-S1 disk space for reasons previously discussed, including the ability to access multiple levels through one incision without having to reposition the patient.

Limitations

A number of potential limitations of L5-S1 OLIF exist. Vascular anatomy may in some cases make L5-S1 access a challenge, if not impossible. As previously discussed, a low-lying iliocaval junction may prohibit access to the L5-S1 interspace and can be evaluated with preoperative imaging at the surgeon's discretion. In trauma patients with substantial pelvic injuries, a lateral decubitus position may be prohibited. A posterior approach which avoids peritoneal manipulation may be preferred in patients with an ostomy or significant abdominal or retroperitoneal pathology. Similarly, an alternative approach that avoids iliac vessel retraction may be preferred in vasculopathic patients with lower extremity arterial insufficiency.

The surgeon may have difficulty using this approach in a morbidly obese patient if the retractor system is not long enough to accommodate the extra depth from the skin to the spine. However, it may also be argued that access and exposure for this approach is often easier in the morbidly obese patient than a traditional posterior approach, or a direct anterior transabdominal approach, owing to the tendency of the abdominal pannus to "fall away" anteriorly when the patient is placed in the lateral position. In the authors' experience, this has been the case in the moderately and morbidly obese, but begins to lose its advantage in the supermorbidly obese (BMI >50). We recommend measuring along the planned approach trajectory on the preoperative imaging, and comparing the expected depth with the retractor system's available lengths to minimize the chance of access problems. Accommodation should be made, in a "best guess" manner, for expected shifting of the tissues between intraoperative positioning and the typical supine position in which preoperative imaging is obtained.

Although one might reasonably assume that all aspects of the surgery would be easier in very thin patients, the more extreme end of this spectrum can pose some challenge in the sense that the normal retroperitoneal fat planes used to help proceed with the exposure may be more difficult to identify and stay safely within, potentially increasing the risk of inadvertent entry into the peritoneum or injury to other retroperitoneal structures.

Although spondylolisthesis is an approved indication for the OLIF procedure, surgeon discretion should be used in selecting appropriate cases for OLIF, especially in the early part of the surgeon's learning curve. The authors advise against attempting to treat Meyerding grade III or higher spondylolisthesis with this technique. Additionally, when approaching L5-S1, we suggest that a dysplastic/congenital spondylolisthesis, with associated anatomic variations (such as domed or rounded S1 superior endplate) should be avoided unless the surgeon has both significant experience treating these types of spondylolisthesis with other techniques and significant experience with OLIF in more conventional cases.

As discussed previously, OLIF may offer the opportunity to complete interbody fusions at multiple levels through a single incision. However, if supplemental fixation beyond what can be achieved through an anterior approach is necessary, then additional incisions, possibly requiring repositioning of the patient, may still be necessary.

Surgeons more familiar with a direct anterior and/or direct lateral approach may find that working in the disk space from an oblique angle can be disorienting. The use of intraoperative image guidance and/or extensive fluoroscopy may be necessary, particularly early in the learning curve, to avoid inadvertent entry into the spinal canal. However, both image guidance and extensive use of fluoroscopy carry well documented risks and costs associated with them.

Another prohibitive factor may be the cost of the procedure or availability of necessary equipment. A specialized retractor system is only available at this time through one device manufacturer and may have limited availability or be expensive to purchase or lease for individual cases. Similarly, if anterior plating systems or specialized cages are desired they present the same challenges.

Surgical Technique (Videos 13.1 and 13.2)

- Place the patient in the right lateral decubitus (left side up) position. The upper hip is extended to facilitate access to the L5-S1 disk space. This is in direct contradistinction to a typical transpsoas approach in which the upper hip is usually flexed to relax the psoas muscle. The patient is secured to the radiolucent

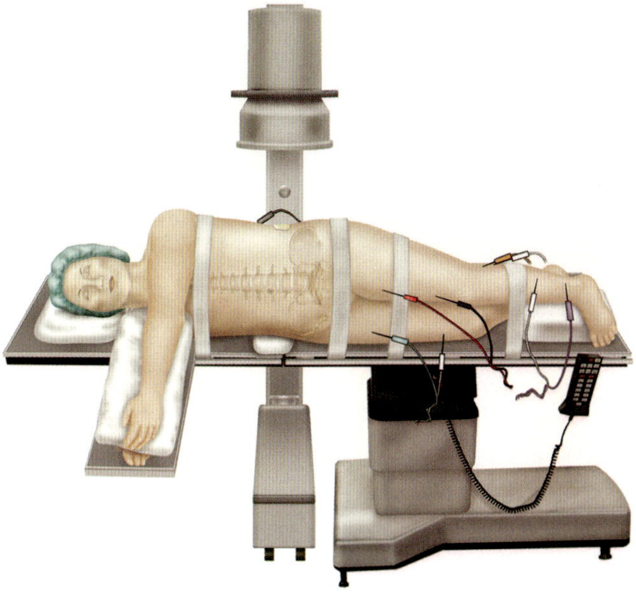

• **Fig. 13.2** Patient positioned in a right lateral decubitus position with upper hip extended. Use of neuromonitoring leads as depicted is optional. (Reprinted with the permission of Medtronic, Inc. © 2016.)

operating table and padded appropriately (Fig. 13.2). The surgeon should approach the patient from the abdominal side with the base of the fluoroscopy unit behind the patient. It has been noted, however, that when rotating the C-arm into the anteroposterior (AP) projection, the radiation source in this configuration will be on the surgeon's side; we highly recommend standing away from the operative field when shooting these views owing to scatter radiation. Pulse oximeters are placed on both feet and monitored throughout the case to ensure that retraction of the iliac vessels does not result in unrecognized lower limb ischemia.

- Under fluoroscopy the L5-S1 disk is localized and a line is drawn on the patient's skin over and perpendicular to the disk space. This line is extended anteriorly onto the patient's abdomen. A 3 cm incision is then made, extending rostral from this line beginning at a point approximately 3 cm anterior to the anterior superior iliac spine (Fig. 13.3). This incision may need to be extended further rostrally if additional levels are being treated.
- The external oblique muscle (Fig. 13.4) or its fascia will be encountered, depending on patient anatomy, and is swept anteriorly with the surgeon's finger (Fig. 13.5A). After confirming that the peritoneum is released by sweeping a finger under the ASIS and iliac crest, retroperitoneal exposure is performed using blunt dissection with two fingers to facilitate exposure of a wide rostral-caudal plane (Fig. 13.5B). The ureter is attached to the posterior peritoneum and should be carefully mobilized anteriorly with the peritoneum.
- Dissection is continued anterior to the psoas while palpating the pulsations of the common iliac artery. The artery is utilized as a landmark to identify the common iliac vein, which is located immediately medial to it on the L5-S1 disk space (Fig. 13.5C).
- Once the disk space is encountered, the adventitial layer overlying it should be mobilized using gentle blunt dissection as it is adherent to the common iliac vein as well as the annulus. This

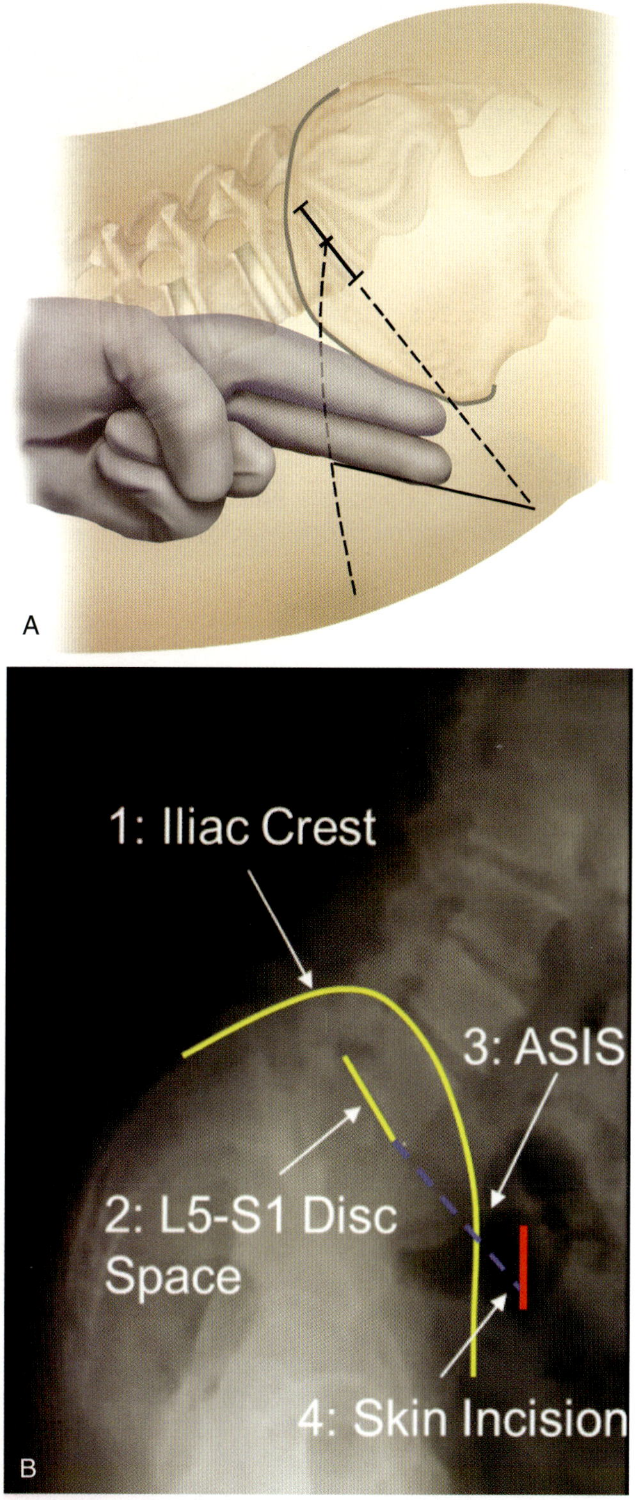

• **Fig. 13.3 A.** Mapping and marking of the skin incision. A line is marked over the L5-S1 disk space using fluoroscopy (*solid hashed line*). The line is extended anteriorly (*dashed straight line*) onto the abdomen. The incision (*solid line*) is then marked extending rostrally from this line approximately two finger breadths anterior to the anterior superior iliac spine. **B.** The described markings superimposed over a lateral plain film of the lumbar spine. (Reprinted with the permission of Medtronic, Inc. © 2016.)

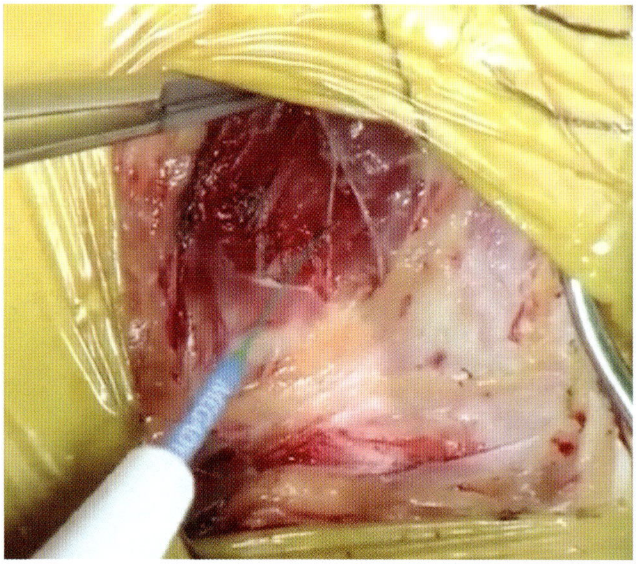

• **Fig. 13.4** Intraoperative photograph demonstrating the incision with external oblique muscle exposed. (Reprinted with the permission of Medtronic, Inc. © 2016.)

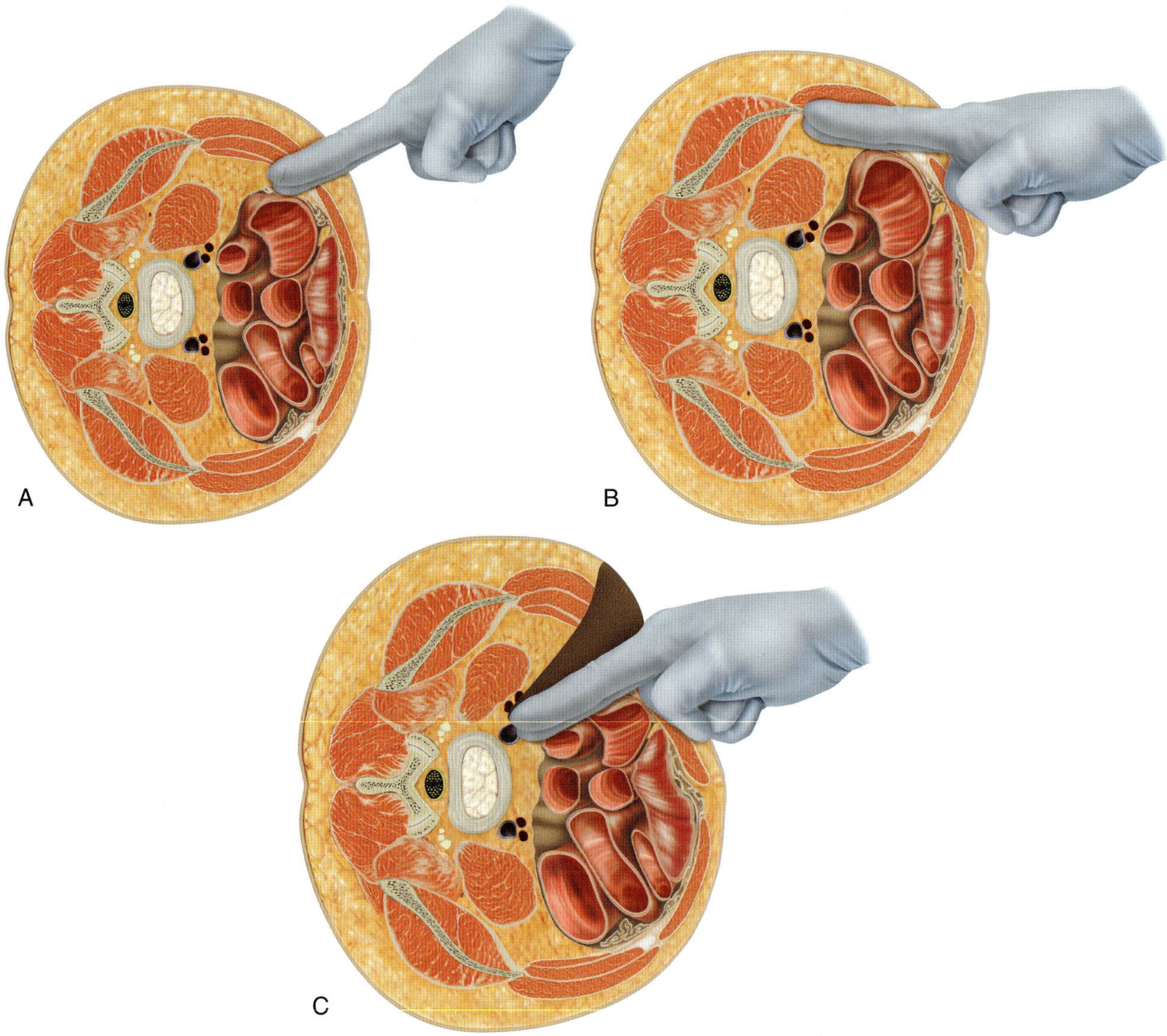

• **Fig. 13.5** Developing the retroperitoneal dissection. **A.** The plane deep to the external oblique muscle and its fascia is entered. **B.** A finger is swept under the anterior superior iliac spine to confirm that the peritoneum is released. **C.** The retroperitoneal plane is developed while palpating for the common iliac artery and vein. (Reprinted with the permission of Medtronic, Inc. © 2016.)

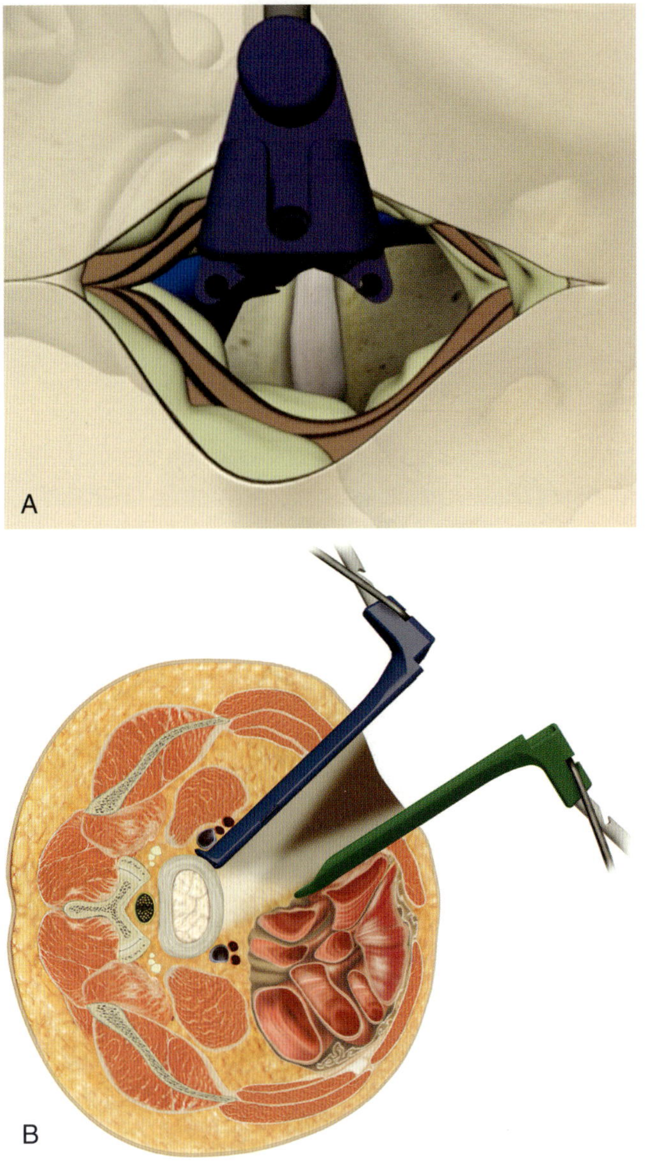

• **Fig. 13.6** A. The lateral *(blue)* retractor blade is inserted medial to the common iliac vein after release of the adventitial layer. **B.** The medial retractor blade *(green)* may be used to visualize the vessels directly during its placement. (Reprinted with the permission of Medtronic, Inc. © 2016.)

layer can also contain portions of the sympathetic chain and superior hypogastric plexus. Great care should be taken during this dissection to avoid injury to the vein, which is much more susceptible to minor trauma than the artery. Nevertheless, both vessels must be diligently protected throughout the dissection and subsequent interbody work.

- Medial and lateral retractor blades are then inserted with the lateral blade protecting the common iliac vessels and the medial blade wrapping around to the contralateral side of the disk space (Fig. 13.6). Overzealous retraction with this medial blade can result in injury to the contralateral iliac vein and/or artery and should be avoided. Per surgeon's preference, the lateral blade can be pinned to the L5 body or sacrum to stabilize the retractor (Fig. 13.7). Finally, a third blade is placed rostrally and can be pinned to the L5 body to protect the bifurcation of the great vessels. Of particular note, this retractor blade

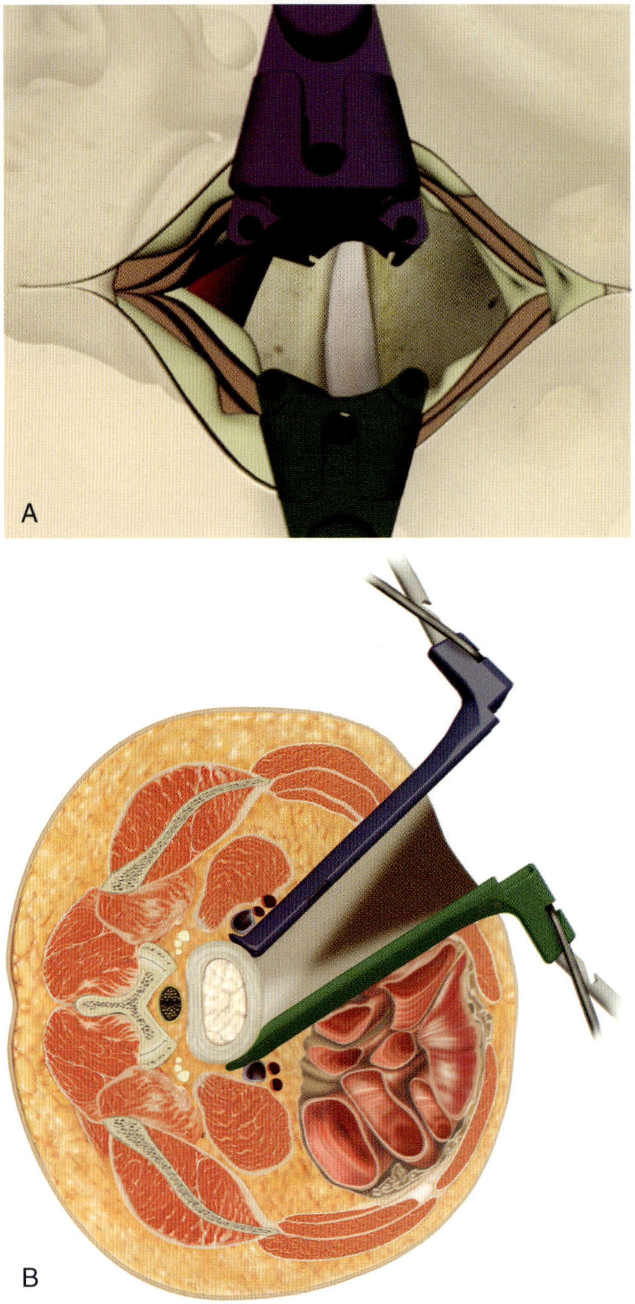

• **Fig. 13.7** A and **B.** The medial *(green)* retractor blade is positioned on the contralateral side of the disk space. The lateral *(blue)* retractor blade may be secured to the body of L5 as per the surgeon's preference. (Reprinted with the permission of Medtronic, Inc. © 2016.)

configuration is in contradistinction to the typical cranial-caudal retractor blades associated with standard lateral transpsoas and OLIF approaches above L5 where one is working entirely lateral to the vasculature.

- Once the disk is well visualized (Fig. 13.8), the midline of the disk space can be identified and marked using AP fluoroscopy to help maintain orientation. An annulotomy (Fig. 13.9) and diskectomy (Fig. 13.10) are then performed in a standard fashion with lateral fluoroscopy available to determine the depth of instruments relative to the posterior annulus and epidural space.[10]

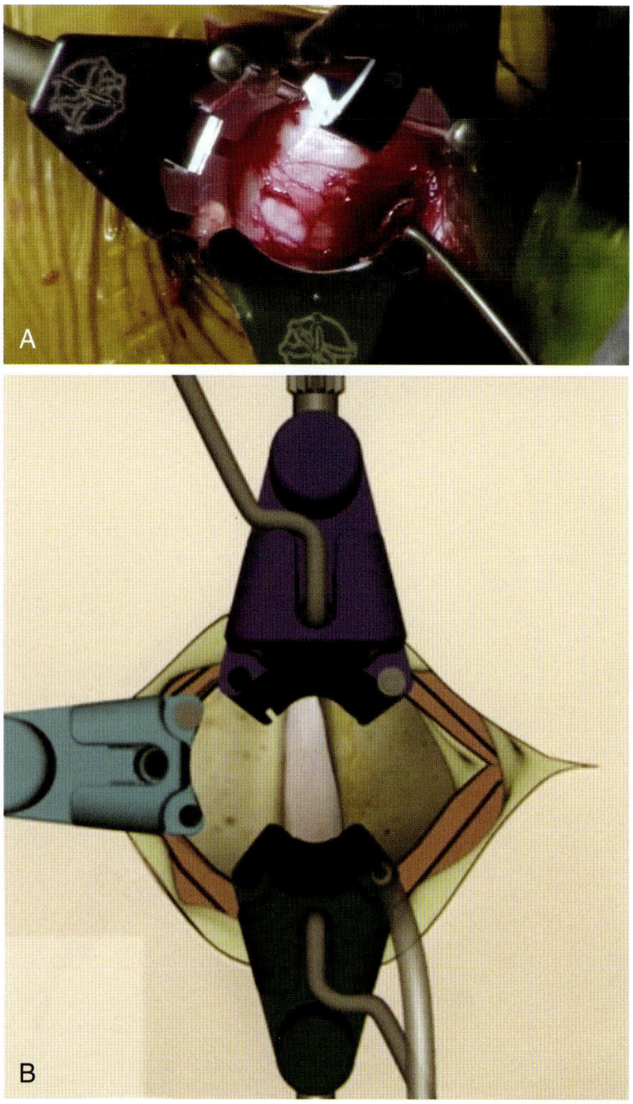

• **Fig. 13.8** With all retractors in place, the disk space is well visualized. (A) Intraoperative photograph and (B) corresponding illustration. (Reprinted with the permission of Medtronic, Inc. © 2016.)

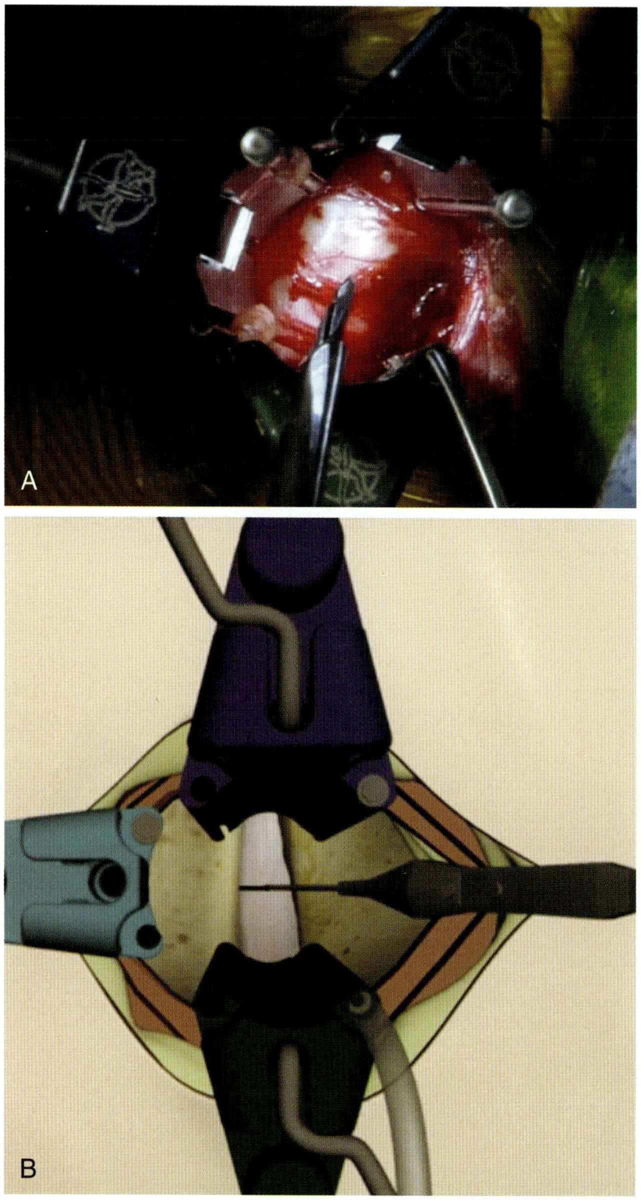

• **Fig. 13.9** After appropriately identifying the midline of the disk, an annulotomy is performed. (A) Intraoperative photograph and (B) corresponding illustration. (Reprinted with the permission of Medtronic, Inc. © 2016.)

- Once the diskectomy is completed, the surgeon's choice of interbody device is appropriately trialed (Fig. 13.11) prior to implantation (Fig. 13.12). Choice of biologics/bone graft materials to be packed into the OLIF spacer is per surgeon's discretion, and should mirror the same considerations as that of any other interbody fusion construct, including different considerations of product cost as well as each patient's biology and risk profile for possible pseudoarthrosis. The authors typically use an allograft bone product with autologous bone marrow. In recent years we have avoided use of high-potency, off-label osteoinductive agents except in rare cases considered exceptionally high risk for pseudoarthrosis. Use of a device with self-retaining screws may avoid the need for supplemental fixation in select cases, but at the surgeon's discretion a supplemental anterior plating system may be implanted at this stage, or a variety of posterior stabilization options may be utilized after completion of the OLIF. Posterior stabilization may be performed in the lateral decubitus position or after turning the patient prone. After completing all work on the anterolateral spine, the rostral blade is then cautiously removed prior to the removal of the lateral blade, followed by the medial blade in order to identify any potential bleeding.

Closure

Once retractors are withdrawn and hemostasis obtained, the surgeon may proceed with wound closure. Any inadvertent entry into the peritoneum, if not already closed during the initial approach, can be repaired at this stage. We typically close the fascia of the external oblique muscle with absorbable suture. Depending on the patient's body habitus, closure of any additional dead space between the fascia and skin may be performed at the surgeon's discretion. The surgeon may then proceed to close the skin according to his/her preference. In the majority of our cases we typically utilize a subcuticular skin closure with topical skin adhesive applied over the incision.

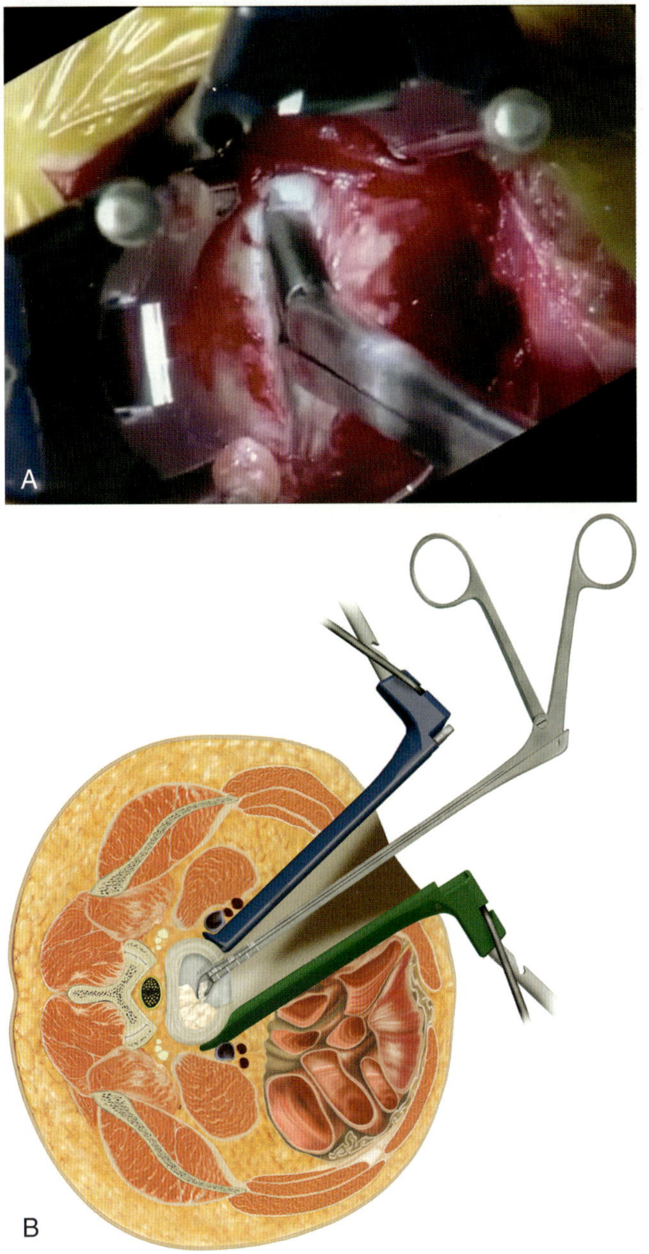

• **Fig. 13.10** A and B. Annulotomy and diskectomy are performed in a standard fashion with direct visualization of the disk space facilitated by the retractor blades. (Reprinted with the permission of Medtronic, Inc. © 2016.)

Postoperative Care

We recommend obtaining postoperative x-rays (Fig. 13.13) after surgery to serve as a baseline for future comparison. Particularly in patients with deformity (e.g., those with degenerative scoliosis), plain x-rays can be difficult to interpret as to accuracy of implant placement and we recommend considering routine postoperative computed tomography scans to better evaluate these patients. Despite the retroperitoneal approach, ileus is a common concern and patients should be maintained on bowel rest with intravenous fluids until return of bowel sounds. Owing to the mobilization and retraction of the iliac arteries, we have nursing perform bilateral lower extremity pulse checks with gradually decreasing frequency over the first

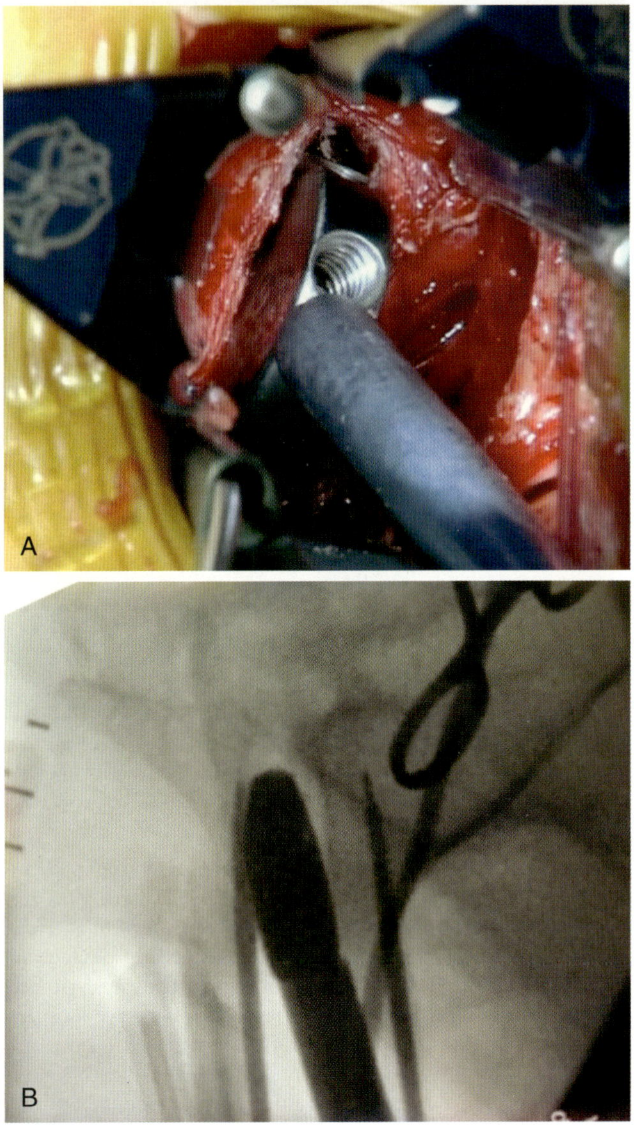

• **Fig. 13.11 A.** Intraoperative photograph demonstrating placement of a device trial for appropriate sizing. **B.** Corresponding lateral radiograph showing the same. Note the pins present in L5 and the sacrum for retaining the medial and lateral retractors. (Reprinted with the permission of Medtronic, Inc. © 2016.)

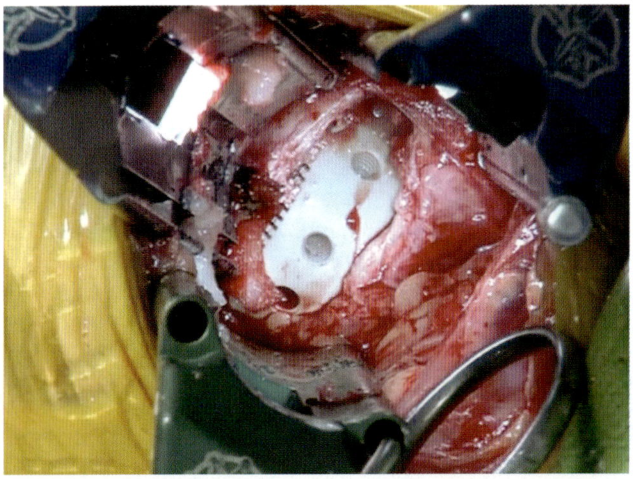

• **Fig. 13.12** Intraoperative photograph showing final placement of interbody device prior to placement of plating system. (Reprinted with the permission of Medtronic, Inc. © 2016.)

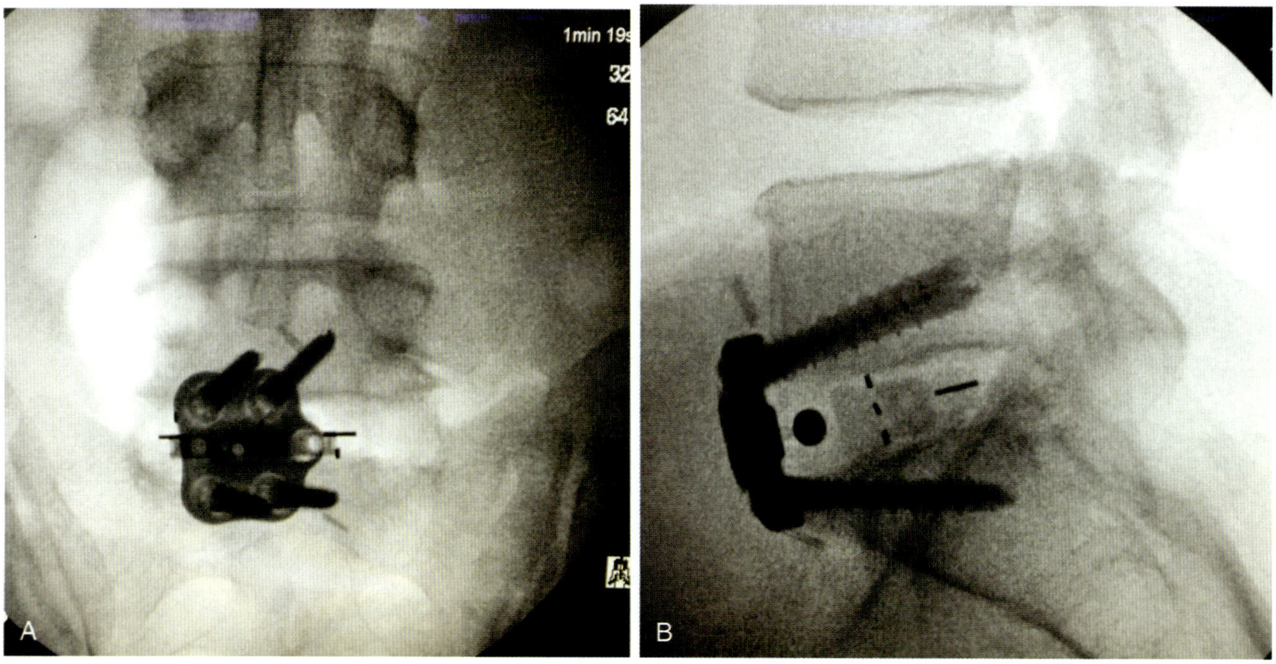

• **Fig. 13.13** Postoperative anteroposterior (A) and lateral (B) radiographs of a patient who underwent L5-S1 OLIF demonstrating final placement of the interbody device and anterior plating system. (Reprinted with the permission of Medtronic, Inc. © 2016.)

24 hours after surgery, based on a standardized vascular protocol at our institution. Complaints of excessive flank pain may be a sign of hydronephrosis from ureteral dysfunction and warrant further investigation. Sequential compression devices and early mobilization should be used as prophylaxis against deep vein thrombosis and at 24 hours postoperatively we augment them with subcutaneous heparin if not otherwise contraindicated. We require patients to meet the usual postoperative milestones prior to discharge, including independent ambulation, adequate pain control, voiding, a bowel movement, and tolerating a regular diet. If necessary, in-house physical therapy consultation may be obtained to assist with early ambulation. Unless the patient has poor bone quality or other extenuating circumstances, we do not typically prescribe a brace. As with all of our patients having fusion, we suggest light activity for 12 weeks postoperatively at which point we will obtain repeat x-rays before releasing any restrictions.

Complications/Side Effects

Many of the potential complications of OLIF at L5-S1 have yet to be reported in the literature. These include complications common to any interbody fusion procedure or spine surgery in general such as infection, excessive blood loss, pseudoarthrosis, risks of anesthesia, development of adjacent level disease, injury to neural elements, graft subsidence, and graft migration/extrusion. A number of complications that are already established in the literature for retroperitoneal surgery will likely prove to be shared with OLIF as well. Ileus may result from manipulation of the peritoneum and lumbosacral plexus. Retroperitoneal dissection or retraction may result in ureteral injury and hydronephrosis or vascular injury (with resultant deep vein thrombosis, arterial insufficiency, or retroperitoneal hematoma). Abdominal wall pseudohernia may present in a delayed fashion owing to nerve injury (most commonly the iliohypogastric nerve) of the abdominal wall. Whereas some of these complications have been reported to us through personal communication from colleagues or observed through personal experience, there have been no systematic studies in the literature regarding complication rates associated with OLIF in general, nor has there been any specific literature regarding complications associated with OLIF specifically at the L5-S1 level.

Outcomes in a Nutshell

Outcomes of the L5-S1 OLIF procedure are largely unknown owing to the recent development of the technique and the paucity of reported cases. It seems likely that outcomes will be comparable to other anterior or lateral interbody techniques with similar fusion rates, degrees of lumbar and segmental lordosis obtained, and impact on quality of life. Clinical, radiographic, and socioeconomic outcomes all remain areas ripe for future study.

Conclusion

The oblique lateral approach for interbody fusion at L5-S1 is a relatively new technique with only a handful of published cases. It appears likely to have many of the advantages of an anterior or lateral approach while potentially minimizing the complications of a transabdominal or transpsoas approach. Most notably, it may be unique among lumbar approaches in facilitating interbody fusion at multiple levels through a single incision.

References

1. Mayer HM. A new microsurgical technique for minimally invasive anterior lumbar interbody fusion. *Spine (Phila Pa 1976).* 1997;22(6):691–699; discussion 700.
2. Molinares DM, Davis TT, Fung DA. Retroperitoneal oblique corridor to the L2-S1 intervertebral discs: an MRI study. *J Neurosurg Spine.* 2015;9:1–8.
3. Silvestre C, Mac-Thiong J-M, Hilmi R, et al. Complications and morbidities of mini-open anterior retroperitoneal lumbar interbody fusion: oblique lumbar interbody fusion in 179 patients. *Asian Spine J.* 2012;6(2):89–97.
4. Davis TT, Hynes RA, Fung DA, et al. Retroperitoneal oblique corridor to the L2-S1 intervertebral discs in the lateral position: an anatomic study. *J Neurosurg Spine.* 2014;21(5):785–793.
5. Kanno K, Ohtori S, Orita S, et al. Miniopen oblique lateral L5-s1 interbody fusion: a report of 2 cases. *Case Rep Orthop.* 2014;2014:603531.
6. Wakita H, Shiga Y, Ohtori S, et al. Less invasive corrective surgery using oblique lateral interbody fusion (OLIF) including L5-S1 fusion for severe lumbar kyphoscoliosis due to L4 compression fracture in a patient with Parkinson's disease: a case report. *BMC Res Notes.* 2015;8(1):126.
7. Molloy S, Butler JS, Benton A, et al. A new extensile anterolateral retroperitoneal approach for lumbar interbody fusion from L1 to S1: a prospective series with clinical outcomes. *Spine J.* 2016;16:786–791.
8. Phan K, Rao PJ, Scherman DB, et al. Lateral lumbar interbody fusion for sagittal balance correction and spinal deformity. *J Clin Neurosci.* 2015;22(11):1714–1721.
9. Phan K, Mobbs RJ. Oblique lumbar interbody fusion for revision of non-union following prior posterior surgery: a case report. *Orthop Surg.* 2015;7(4):364–367.
10. *Medtronic OLIF51 Procedure [Internet].* Memphis, TN: Medtronic Sofamor Danek USA, Inc; 2015.

14

Interlaminar Lumbar Instrumented Fusions (ILIF)

VINCENT J. ALENTADO AND MICHAEL P. STEINMETZ

Introduction

As the population ages, the incidence of lumbar spinal stenosis and the number of available surgical options for its treatment continue to increase. To date, posterolateral spinal fusion via pedicle screw and rod fixation has been regarded as the mainstay surgical treatment option for stabilization of a degenerative spinal segment. The intended benefits of this treatment include reduced back pain and prevention of continued degeneration of the segment through stabilization and development of bony fusion. However, pedicle screw and rod constructs carry significant morbidity, such as cerebrospinal fluid leaks, neural injury from misplacement of pedicle screws, adjacent segment degeneration and disease, and instrumentation-related complications. In addition, this procedure often injures the unfused rostral facet joints and its musculotendinous attachments. Furthermore, pedicle screw and rod fusion constructs require greater operative times, which may be difficult for elderly patients to tolerate.

In many patients, pedicle screw and rod fixation may be an overtreatment. In the degenerative spine in which there is mechanical back pain and the presence of neurologic symptoms with or without grade I spondylolisthesis, the unfavorable adverse outcomes and increased morbidity of instrumented fusion may not be worth the risks. In contrast, decompression without fusion may fail to address all of the patients' symptoms and may fail to slow the progression of degenerative changes. The interlaminar lumbar instrumented fusion (ILIF) technique was developed to overcome the potential shortcomings of these current treatment standards by avoiding pedicle screw fixation while creating stabilization in a minimally disruptive surgical technique.

Indications

The ILIF procedure is indicated in cases where decompression and spinal stabilization is required. The most common indication is grade I degenerative spondylolisthesis and spinal stenosis. The authors typically choose this procedure in a patient with advanced age where a more aggressive pedicle screw construct is less desirable.

Limitations

There are a number of limitations of ILIF. The patient's site of spinal compression must be located at the interspinous space. If the compression is significant in the craniocaudal direction and the spinous process and significant portions of the laminae will have to be resected to perform an adequate decompression, the ILIF procedure will not be possible. The procedure is not possible in revision cases in which the spinous processes have previously been resected. Care must be taken in patients with severe osteoporosis. In these patients it may be easy to fracture the spinous process during plate placement. This procedure is not ideal for those patients with high-grade instability. Lastly, there is limited bony surface area for bony fusion during this procedure. The facets may be packed with auto or allogenic bone; many of the implants also permit the placement of fusion material within the device.

Operative Technique

1. The patient is placed on the operative table in the prone position. It is possible to perform this procedure in the lateral decubitus position, but the authors do not prefer this. The authors prefer to use a radiolucent Jackson table, but any table is appropriate as long as it can accommodate imaging modalities (Fig. 14.1).
2. Following preparing and draping of the lumbar region, the incision is planned. The incision is typically slightly caudal to a standard incision planned for a laminectomy; specifically, it only is required to expose the interspinous space, which is typically slightly caudal to the disk space on lateral imaging. An approximately 2.5- to 4-cm incision is made, the subcutaneous fat and lumbodorsal fascia are then divided and retracted. After dividing the fascia, electrocautery is used to perform a subperiosteal dissection so that the bilateral erector spinae muscles can be mobilized off of the cranial and caudal spinous processes to the spinolaminar junction (Fig. 14.2).
3. Many surgeons believe that the ILIF procedure is best performed with distraction laminoplasty.[1,2] The distraction laminoplasty technique, as first described by O'Leary and McCance,[3] allows for robust distraction and greater access to the spinal canal, while minimizing the risk of spinous process fracture during device implantation. Furthermore, this technique has the advantage of minimizing bony resection, including maintenance of the bilateral facet joints. At this point, a Kerrison rongeur is used to excise the supraspinous and interspinous ligaments at the index level (Fig. 14.3). If required based on bony overgrowth, the Kerrison

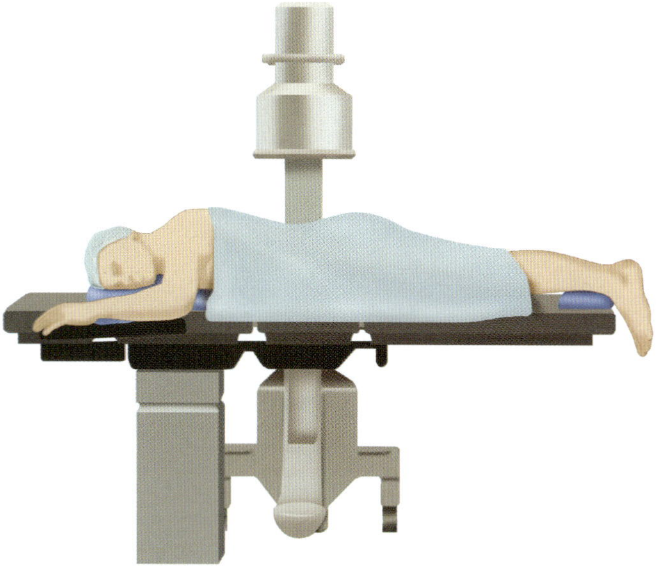

• **Fig. 14.1** The patient is positioned prone on a radiolucent spine table. The authors prefer a Jackson table, but this is not required. Fluoroscopy is helpful when performing interlaminal lumbar instrument fusions (ILIF). (With permission from ZimmerBiomet.)

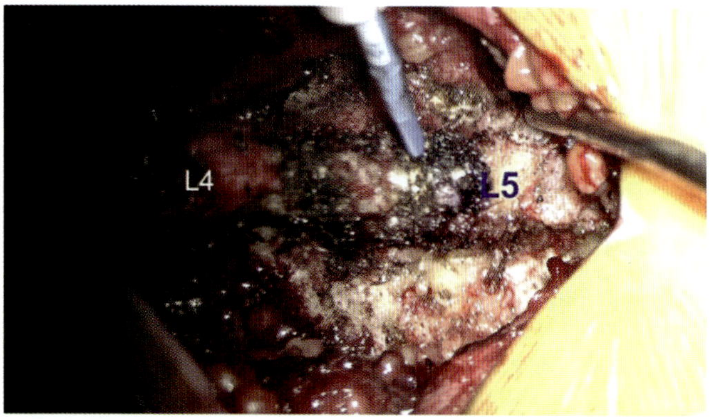

• **Fig. 14.2** Following skin incision. The fascia is incised and the paraspinal muscles reflected off the spinous processes to expose the lamina and the medical one-third of the facet joint. The authors typically clear all soft tissue off the index spinous processes at this point. It is often critical to clearly delineate the dorsal aspect of the process to plan optimal placement of the caspar posts as to avoid fracture during placement. L4 and L5 spinous processes are labeled. The cautery is touching the interspinous space. (With permission from ZimmerBiomet.)

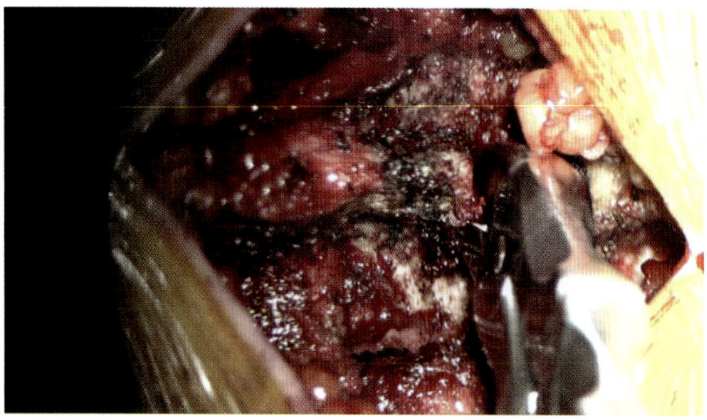

• **Fig. 14.3** The interspinous and supraspinous ligaments may be removed by a thin rongeur. One can remove a small caudal portion of the cranial spinous process (L4 in this example) at this point. This will aid in visualization of the interspinous space (With permission from ZimmerBiomet.)

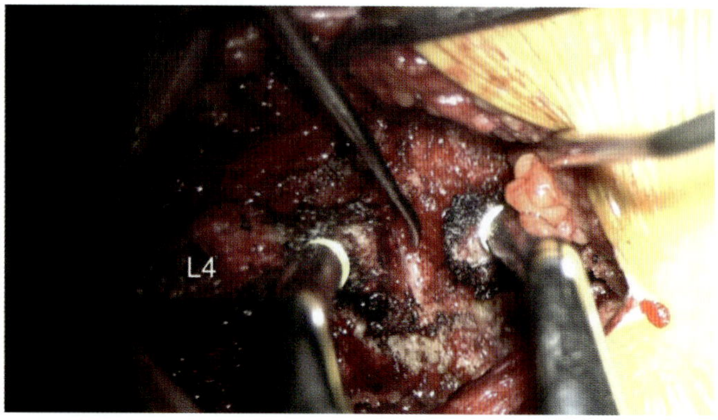

• **Fig. 14.4** Caspar posts have been placed in the rostral and caudal spinous processes. The supra- and intraspinous process ligaments have been resected. Distraction across the posts permits visualization of the intralaminar space and ligamentum flavum (Penfield elevator). (With permission from ZimmerBiomet.)

rongeur is used to remove the caudal one-third of the superior spinous process and laminae, as well as the cranial edge of the inferior spinous process. This step is not required in all patients and if not needed should be avoided because the spinous process may be fractured and the procedure aborted for a standard laminectomy and pedicle fixation and fusion. The facet joint capsules should be spared as much as possible. If significant facet hypertrophy is present, the spinolaminar junction between the cranial and caudal vertebrae is then thinned down with a high-speed burr in order to create a surface to accept an interlaminar distractor.

4. Surgeon preference and implant choice will determine how spinous process distraction is next performed. This step is required to provide adequate visualization of the intralaminar space, permit laminoplasty, and decompress the neural elements. The authors prefer to place Caspar posts in the top of the spinous processed to apply distraction with a post distractor as one would use during an anterior cervical diskectomy and fusion. Pilot holes are drilled into the cranial and caudal spinous processes and Caspar pins are inserted into the drill holes. These posts should be placed in the cranial portion of the spinous processes, which is the thickest portion of the spinous process. Distraction of the segment is then performed, enabling enhanced access to the interlaminar space without additional excision of the spinous processes (Fig. 14.4). It is important to insert the Caspar pins parallel to each other so that iatrogenic spinous fracture is avoided. Also, overly aggressive distraction should be avoided to minimize damage to the spinous process. As mentioned above, other tools for distraction are available. Bilateral hemilaminoties and medial facetectomies may next be performed to gain access to the compressed neural elements (Fig. 14.5). Next, curettes are used to mobilize the ligamentum flavum insertion from the laminae. Kerrison rongeurs are then used to remove soft tissue from the medial aspect of the facet joints just lateral to the ligamentum flavum. Again, care should be taken to leave the capsular tissues undisturbed. The ligamentum flavum insertion on the superior lamina is then released with angled curettes, and the ligamentum flavum is removed partially or completely at the stenotic segment (Fig. 14.6).

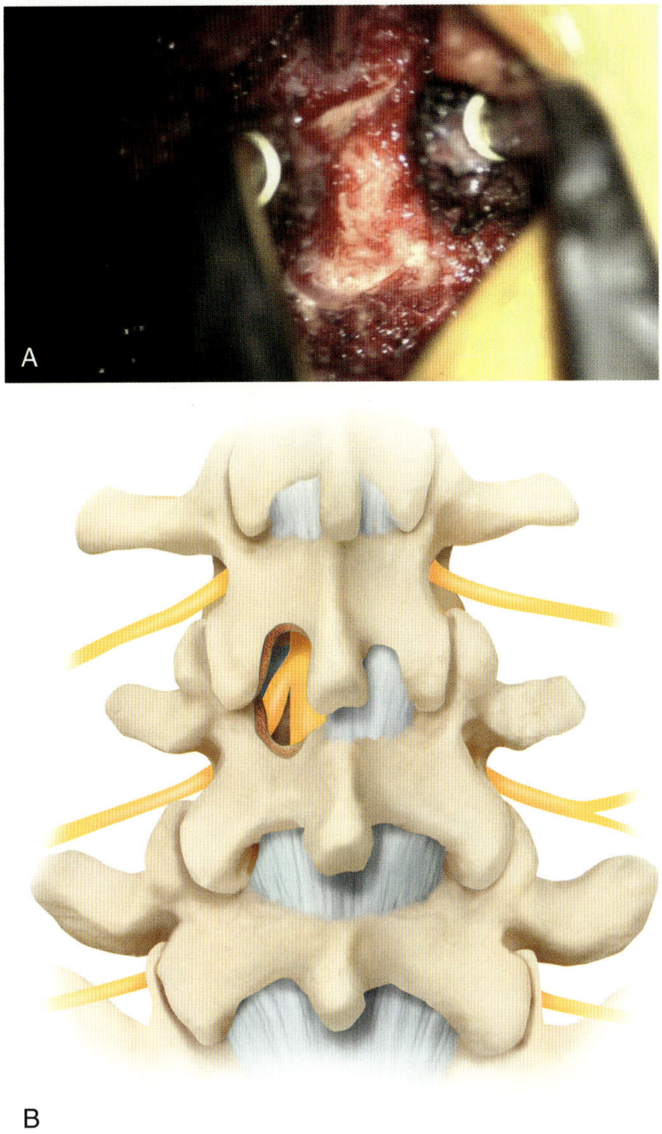

• **Fig. 14.5** A. Following distraction and exposure of the intralaminar space, bilateral hemilaminotomies and medical facetectomies are performed. With distraction, the undersurface of the cranial lamina is also carefully undercut. **B**. Bilateral hemilaminectomies and undercut laminoplasty have been performed at L4. One can visualize the ligamentum flavum. (With permission from ZimmerBiomet.)

5. After removal of the ligamentum flavum, decompression of the lateral recess and neuroforamen is performed. The more horizontal trajectory of the Kerrison rongeurs allows for better access to the contralateral lateral recess and neuroforamen with less inferior articular process excision than is possible from the ipsilateral side such as during traditional laminotomies and laminoforaminotomies. While using the Kerrison rongeur, the surgeon should avoid leaning against the spinous processes with excessive force to decrease the risk of fracture. This portion of the procedure is identical to the open or traditional equivalent.
6. At the completion of the distraction laminoplasty, the ligamentum flavum has been resected completely, the spinous processes are largely preserved, the posterior laminae are intact except for the small midline laminotomy defect, and the facet joints are functionally minimally disturbed

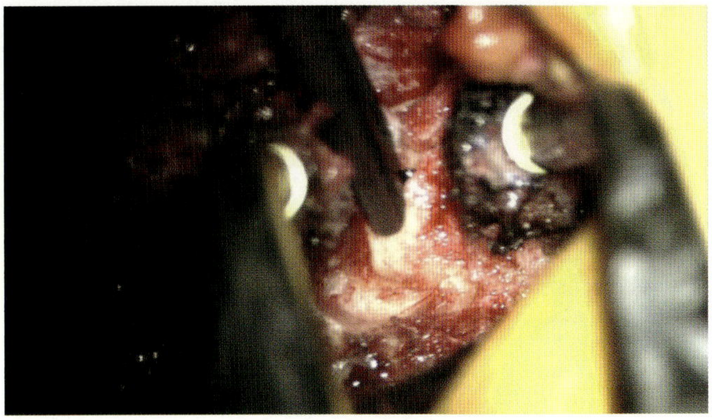

• **Fig. 14.6** The ligamentum flavum may now be removed with a Kerrison rongeur. The decompression is performed underneath the cranial fashion until all the ligament has been removed. One can then remove overgrown bone and ligament in the lateral recess to finish the central decompression prior to performing the index foraminotomies. (With permission from ZimmerBiomet.)

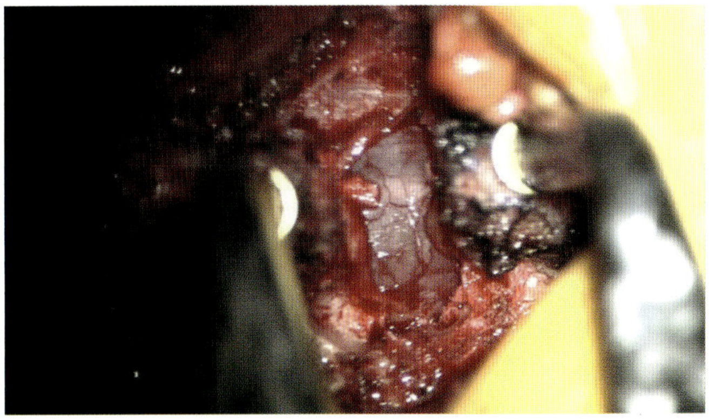

• **Fig. 14.7** The ligamentum flavum has been removed to expose the dura and decompressed spinal segment. (With permission from ZimmerBiomet.)

(Fig. 14.7). At this point, the laminae are decorticated with a high-speed burr in preparation for fusion. The facets may be cleared of soft tissue and a facet fusion performed as well.
7. The interlaminar and spinous space is next prepared for fusion and implant placement. The technique outline is for placement of the ASPEN system (Zimmer Biomet, Denver, CO), but is similar to those offered from others including Nuvasive and Globus. There are slight variances, but the technique presented may be broadly applied across systems. A rasp may be used to clear the bone of any soft tissue (Fig. 14.8). Distraction is fully released on the spinous processes followed by the placement of a spreader. The spreader is used to mobilize the segment and measure the size of the implant. The spreader is opened, distracting the spinous processes with care not to over distract and fracture the bone (Fig. 14.9). The spreader's ratchet is kept up at this point; when proper distraction is achieved, it is dropped down and a measurement may be made.
8. The appropriate size post plate is next chosen. The diameter is based on prior sizing with the spreader and rasp. It is desired to place the intralaminar space in a mild degree of distraction. The barrel of the ASPEN implant holds this distraction (Fig. 14.10). Other systems have similar features such as polyetheretherketone (PEEK) inserts or even machined allograft. The length is based on local

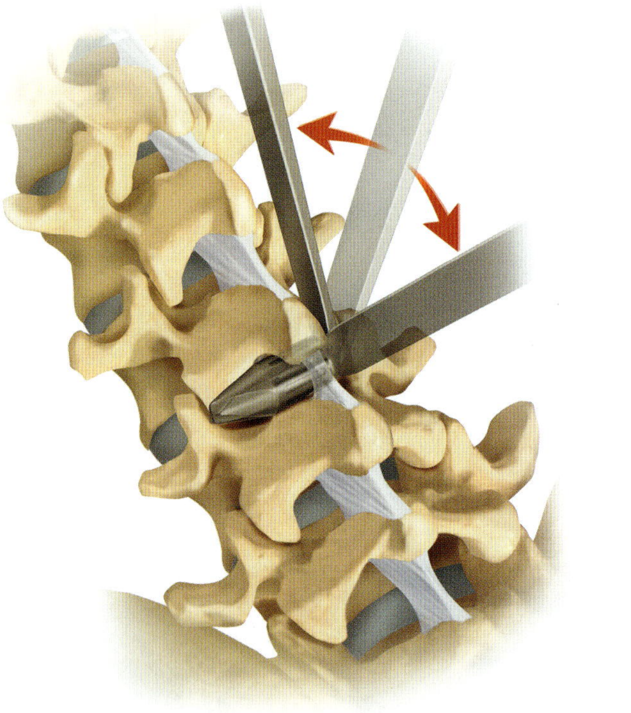

• **Fig. 14.8** Following decompression, the facing surfaces of the spinous processes are cleaned of all soft tissue and prepared for either an implant or bone graft, utilizing a rasp. (With permission from ZimmerBiomet.)

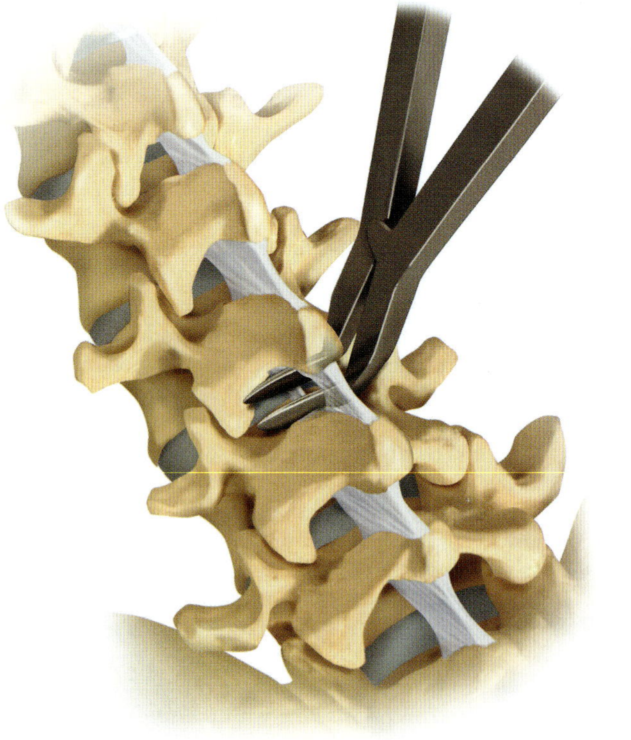

• **Fig. 14.9** A spreader is placed in the intraspinous space. The authors release all distraction at this point in the procedure. The spreader is opened until resistance is met. A reading then is used to size the barrel of the interspinous device. (With permission from ZimmerBiomet.)

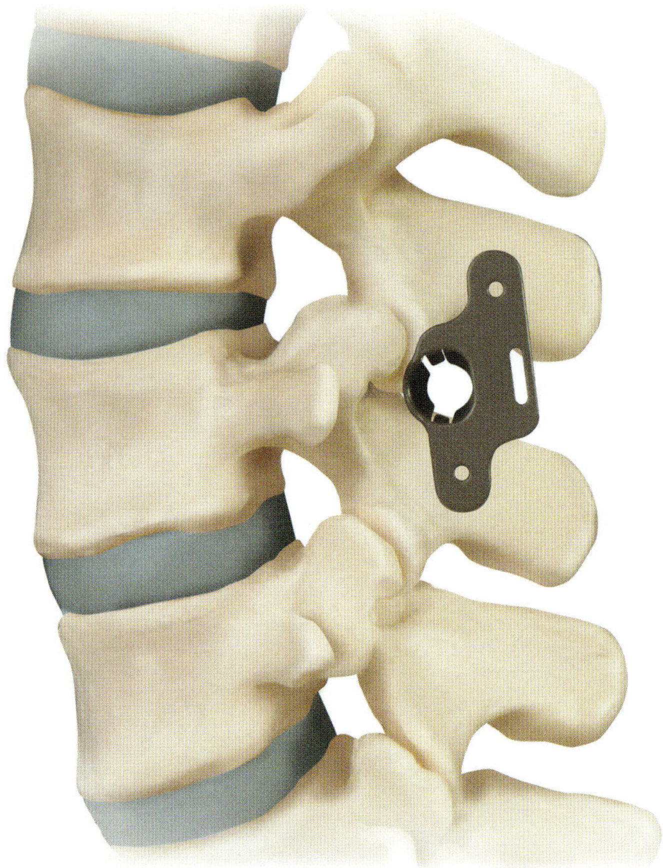

• **Fig. 14.10** The barrel size as determined by the spreader, which is then is used to pick the post plate. As seen in the illustration, the barrel of the device holds distraction. (With permission from ZimmerBiomet.)

anatomy. The standard barrel length is typically appropriate; however, if there is significant facet hypertrophy limiting anterior placement, a medium barrel length may be chosen. The chosen plate must engage an appropriate amount of spinous process without extending beyond the bone cranially and caudally; it must be anterior (Fig. 14.11). The ASPEN system offers a flared design, which may allow fixation at S1, but also offers anterior placement at all levels. Because the supraspinous ligament has been resected, the barrel of the post plate may be placed directly into the intralaminar space. It may be pushed directly into the space in the midline or pushed into place from a paramedican direction. Distraction may be placed against the spinous processes at this point to aid placement. If placed from a paramedian approach, the implant may be rotated 45 degrees in the sagittal plane and then in the intralaminar space rotated back to normal position. The barrel of the post plate will ensure a degree of distraction of the spinous processes. If distraction was again placed, it should be fully removed at this point. The locking plate is then slid in place over the barrel engaging the opposite side of the spinous process (Fig. 14.12). Once in place, compression is placed on the cranial and caudal portions of the device, driving the spikes of the plates into the spinous processes (Fig. 14.13). They should be fully driven in with care not to apply too great of a force, which may fracture the bone. Once adequate compression is achieved, final

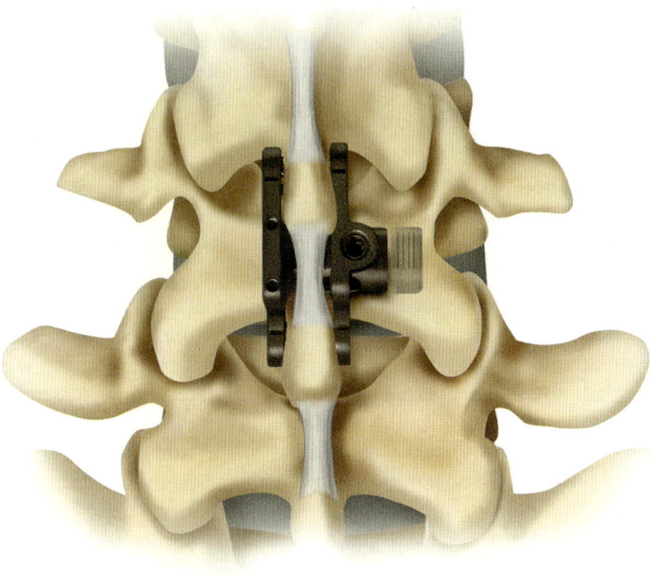

• **Fig. 14.11** It is important to choose the optimal size of spinous process plate. The device must be as anterior as possible and the plate must cover the maximal amount of rostral and caudal spinous process. It should not extend beyond either spinous process. (With permission from ZimmerBiomet.)

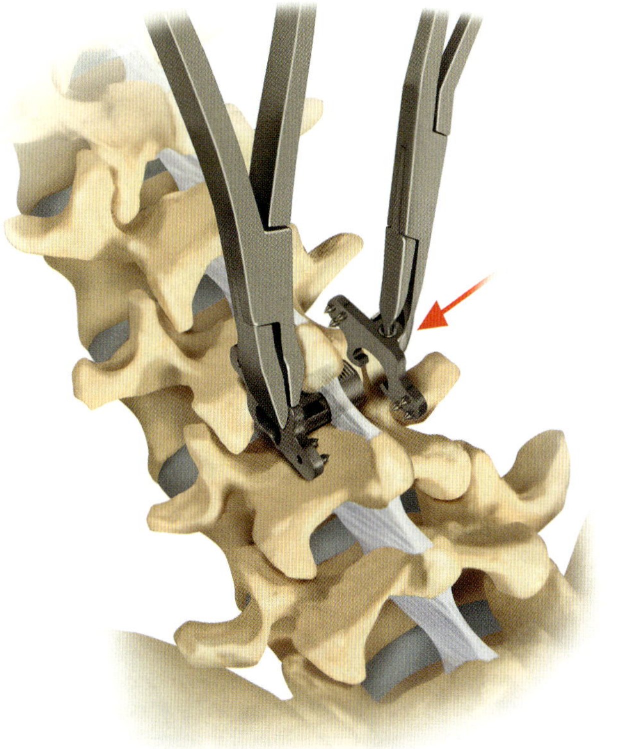

• **Fig. 14.12** Once the appropriate size device has been chosen and the post plate placed, the locking plate is slid over the barrel. (With permission from ZimmerBiomet.)

tightening is placed across the locking screw. The authors utilize fluoroscopy at this point to ensure appropriate placement.

9. Bone graft is then placed within the barrel of the implant and along the decorticated laminae and facet joints. The authors prefer to use local bone autograft obtained during the laminotomies and foraminotomies. This may be supplemented with allograft if required.

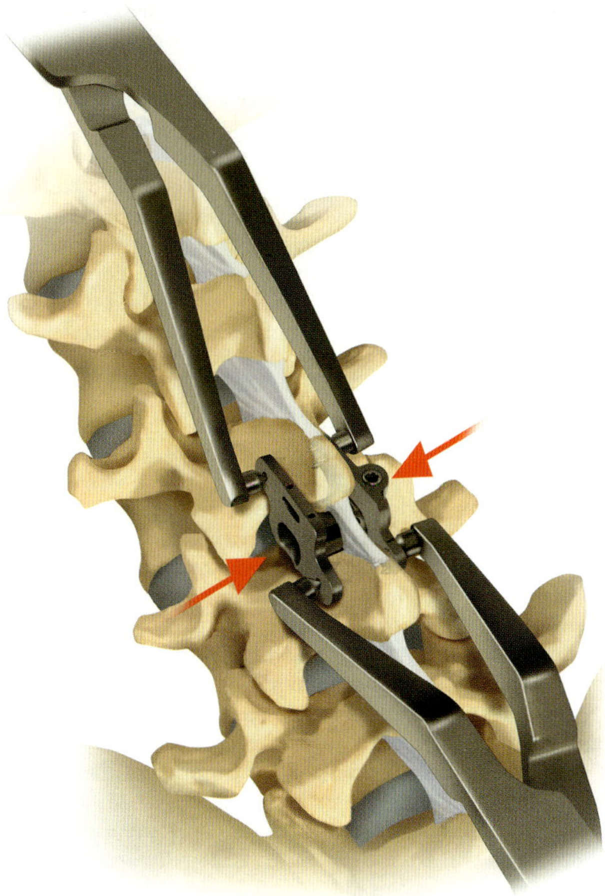

• **Fig. 14.13** Compression is applied across the cranial and caudal portions of the implant to drive the spikes of the plate completely into the spinous processes. (With permission from ZimmerBiomet.)

Closure

The wound is closed in multiple layers. The fascia is closed with 1-0 Vicryl or alternative resorbable suture. This is followed by 2-0 Vicryl in the subcutaneous and dermis. The authors close the skin with 4-0 monocryl in a subcuticular fashion followed by skin glue or Steri-Strips.

Postoperative Care

Patients are allowed to mobilize immediately. They typically are discharged from the hospital the following day. Postoperative restrictions are surgeon specific, but typically consist of limited bending and lifting for the first 4 to 6 weeks, followed by physical therapy for core conditioning.

Complications

There are complications specifically for spinous process plating. Most may be avoided with meticulous surgical technique. Fracture of the spinous process may occur by over distraction during sizing, overzealous bone removal of the spinous process or midline lamina, placement of too large implant, over compression of the plates, and lastly dorsal placement of the device. Following proper surgical technique as outlined above should mitigate this complication.

Inadequate fixation may result from improper sizing of the implant (i.e., too large or too small), dorsal placement, or inadequate compression. The appropriate barrel size is chosen based on tactile feel during spreading. The plate length is chosen to fully cover the spinous process bone. The plate must be placed anterior; if too posterior, fracture of the spinous process may occur.

Cuellar et al.[2] in their series, reported complications including one dural tear, one new neuro deficit that resolved by 6 weeks, one implant failure, one seroma, and one case of cancer diagnosis.

Outcomes

Clinical Utility

The ILIF implant provides several important functions and advantages over traditional posterolateral instrumented lumbar fusion. The implant acts as an extension block that functions to maintain foraminal height in a similar manner to an interbody cage. Moreover, the implant provides a protective covering over the spinal canal and dura, which theoretically limits dura adhesions and reduces the risk of durotomy during any necessary revision operations. If the implant is composed of prefabricated bone, the large mass of bone enables fusion between the bone block and the adjacent spinous processes and the laminae. Furthermore, the laminae and spinous processes provide a greater surface area of bone for fusion compared with traditional posterolateral fusion that often relies on extensively excised facet joints and small transverse processes for fusion nidus. This is especially true for those techniques which utilize a large "H" allograft placed between the lamina under compression. The graft buttress placed between the lamina and spinous process adds a greater degree of stability to the spine with the addition of the spinous process place, but not as biomechanically sound as a pedicle screw construct. Postacchini et al.[4] demonstrated an overall fusion rate of 84% across the spinous process and lamina in their series of 25 patients.

Despite the many advantages of the ILIF procedure, this technique is not optimal for every patient. Contraindications to ILIF include patients with grade II spondylolisthesis or pars interarticularis defects, as the currently available devices are not intended to treat these larger instabilities. Furthermore, patients with osteopenia or osteoporosis should not receive an ILIF because of the increased risk of spinous process fractures in these patients.

Preliminary Results

Owing to the relatively recent advancements and increased interest in the ILIF technique, studies reporting outcomes with the device are sparse. However, Pradhan et al.[1] performed a biomechanical investigation of the ExtenSure H2 (NuVasive, Inc., San Diego, CA, USA) ILIF device. This device is a prefabricated allograft bone-block that is paired with a separate spinous process plate. The authors found that in flexion-extension, decompression with bilateral pedicle screw fixation was more rigid than ILIF, but the two constructs provided statistically similar rigidity. In lateral bending, the ILIF device was similarly rigid to decompression with unilateral pedicle screws, which were both stiffer than an intact spine. However, decompression with bilateral pedicle screw fixation resulted in increased rigidity compared with the ILIF construct. Furthermore, decompression with bilateral pedicle screws resulted in more rigidity than the ILIF construct, which was found to be similarly rigid to an intact spine. Notably, bilateral pedicle screws resulted in more motion in the rostral and caudal segments than the ILIF construct in all ranges of motion other than the rostral segment motion in flexion-extension.

Postacchini et al.[4] also investigated the ExtenSure H2 ILIF device with an Affix (NuVasive, Inc.) spinous process plate as a stand-alone configuration in 25 patients with grade I degenerative spondylolisthesis with dynamic instability. The authors implanted a PEEK interspinous device and utilized local bone autograft for fusion substrate. The authors reported a mean operative time for implantation of the ILIF device and bone grafting of 21 minutes with an average estimated blood loss of 19.7 mL. In cases where iliac grafting was needed, the mean operative time and estimated blood loss were 37.4 minutes and 46.2 mL, respectively. At a 7-month follow-up, 21 of the 25 (84%) patients included in the study demonstrated bony fusion based on computed tomography scanning. Of the four cases of nonunion, one patient demonstrated an increase in spondylolisthesis with severe dynamic instability and moderate angular instability, two patients had continued mild dynamic instability, and one patient had moderate dynamic instability. At 7 months, the mean visual analogue scale (VAS) score decreased by 64.5% for low back pain and 80.4% for leg pain. Moreover, the mean Oswestry Disability Index (ODI) score diminished by 52.6% and the mean Short Form-36 (SF-36) bodily pain and physical function scores improved by 53.7% and 58.9%, respectively. However, for patients who developed pseudarthrosis, only the VAS score for leg pain improved from preoperative scores. At final average follow-up of 34.4 months, the authors noted that no intraoperative complications and no implant disassembly, migration, or dislocation; and no patient required revision operation.

Cuellar et al.[2] also studied clinical results of patients treated with the ExtenSure H2 ILIF construct with the Affix spinous process plate. Preshaped allograft was utilized as the fusion substrate. The study was a prospective, multicenter study of 37 patients over the age of 40 with single-level degenerative disk disease between the levels of L1 and L5, with evidence of disk collapse and spinal stenosis causing symptomatic neurogenic claudication unresponsive to conservative treatment for greater than 6 months, or progressive neurologic symptoms while receiving conservative treatment. The authors reported a mean operating time (including time spent performing distraction laminoplasty) of 84 minutes. The mean hospital length of stay was 2 days. Perioperative complications included one incidental durotomy, one prolonged hospitalization secondary to perioperative pain, one implant failure, one seroma, and one mild postoperative neurologic sensory deficit that resolved within 6 weeks. The number of patients exceeding a minimum clinically important difference (MCID) of 2 points for VAS improvement was 23/34 (68%) for back and 22/34 (65%) for worst leg pain at 12 months and 22/33 (67%) for back and 22/33 (67%) for worst leg pain at 24 months. The number of patients meeting the MCID of ≥12.8% improvement for ODI scores was 20/33 (59%) at 12 months and 24/33 (73%) at 24 months. Furthermore, 25/34 (74%) and 24/34 (71%) met the MCID of ≥0.5 for Zurich Claudication Questionnaire-Symptom Severity (ZCQ-SS) and ZCQ-Physical Function (ZCQ-PF) scores at 12 months, respectively. At 24 months, 25/34 (74%) and 24/34 (73%) met the MCID for ZCQ-SS and ZCQ-PF, respectively. Moreover, at 24-month follow-up 94% of patients were no longer consuming opiates; 94% of patients stated they were satisfied with the procedure; and 88% said they would repeat the surgery. In addition, 52% of patients reported an increase in their activity level compared with only 12%

reporting a decreased activity level. Of the 17 patients who presented with a neurologic deficit, 14 (82%) patients had resolution of preoperative symptoms within 6 weeks of operation, whereas 2 had continued deficit at 24-month follow-up. With regard to radiographic analysis, 23/32 (72%) of patients had solid fusion at 24 months with 97% of patients meeting criteria for stability.

Conclusions

The preliminary biomechanical and clinical data presented herein demonstrate the relatively low complication rates and high fusion rates achieved with ILIF. Furthermore, the biomechanical data demonstrate the high rigidity offered by ILIF prior to development of bony fusion. With good operative technique, this treatment option can be used successfully in patients with low-grade instability causing spinal stenosis. As the use of these devices gains popularity, future studies will assess the stability and outcomes of these constructs over longer periods of follow-up and in larger patient cohorts.

References

1. Pradhan BB, Turner AWL, Zatushevsky MA, et al. Biomechanical analysis in a human cadaveric model of spinous process fixation with an interlaminar allograft spacer for lumbar spinal stenosis: laboratory investigation. *J Neurosurg Spine*. 2012;16(6):585–593. https://doi.org/10.3171/2012.3.SPINE11631.
2. Cuéllar JM, Field JS, Bae HW. Distraction laminoplasty with interlaminar lumbar instrumented fusion (ILIF) for lumbar stenosis with or without grade 1 spondylolisthesis: technique and 2-year outcomes. *Spine (Phila Pa 1976)*. 2016;41(suppl 8):S97–S105. https://doi.org/10.1097/BRS.0000000000001484.
3. O'Leary PF, McCance SE. Distraction laminoplasty for decompression of lumbar spinal stenosis. *Clin Orthop*. 2001;384:26–34.
4. Postacchini F, Postacchini R, Menchetti PPM, et al. Lumbar interspinous process fixation and fusion with stand-alone interlaminar lumbar instrumented fusion implant in patients with degenerative spondylolisthesis undergoing decompression for spinal stenosis. *Asian Spine J*. 2016;10(1):27–37. https://doi.org/10.4184/asj.2016.10.1.27.

15 Endoscopic Lumbar Interbody Fusion

PENG-YUAN CHANG, HSUAN-KAN CHANG, JOHN PAUL G. KOLCUN, AND MICHAEL Y. WANG

Introduction

Since the early 20th century, spinal fusion has been performed as a therapy for both traumatic and degenerative disorders of the spine. Lumbar interbody fusion (LIF) in particular has proved an effective therapy for a variety of conditions, improving patients' activity and quality of life.[1] As the field of neurosurgery advanced, new and better surgical approaches were developed to reduce the morbidity and complications associated with this procedure. Of the major LIF approaches today, the transforaminal lumbar interbody fusion (TLIF) is one of the least invasive paths to the spine, avoiding several potential pitfalls of other LIF techniques.[2]

The TLIF has enjoyed increasing popularity since the 1990s, in particular as a minimally invasive surgery (MIS) procedure. However, even though the MIS-TLIF bypasses the abdominal structures at risk with an anterior approach (ALIF) and the neural stress seen in a posterior approach (PLIF), it still requires an open muscular dissection, and thus faces the complications of any open procedure.[3] Therefore, there have been efforts to further reduce the surgical trauma and exposure of the MIS-TLIF.

To this end, an endoscopic lumbar interbody fusion (endoLIF) protocol is described here. This chapter details the indications/contraindications, surgical technique, outcomes, and postoperative care of patients undergoing this procedure.

Indications

The indications for the endoscopic fusion are largely those of a typical open or MIS-TLIF, but there are subtle variations (Table 15.1). Major indications include degenerative disease of one or two levels, spondylolisthesis, recurrent herniation, and spondylosis.[4,5] The reduced blood loss, reliance on anesthesia, and recovery time also widen the patient population to include the elderly, and those with severe comorbid conditions that might otherwise preclude surgery.[6] As the TLIF approach involves less neural retraction, these procedures can be performed at or above the level of L2, the site of the conus medullaris. This approach is also useful for revision of a prior PLIF, as there will be limited involvement of the previous entry site and scar tissue.[2]

Relative contraindications include severe bilateral or central canal stenosis, osteoporosis, and anomalous congenital nerve root fusion. Each patient's unique anatomy and pathology must also be weighed in choosing a procedure, including considerations of neuroforaminal size, the geometry of any disk abnormality or herniation, and the size and location of the iliac crest relative to the target level.[7] These anatomic factors can limit the surgical access of the endoLIF approach.

Limitations

The development of modern endoscopic instruments and the continuous demand by patients for improved postoperative recovery have resulted in a robust advancement in the realm of endoscopic spinal surgery. To date, established experiences in the literature include far lateral disk herniation, lumbar reherniation, spondylolisthesis (no more than grade II), discogenic pain, and spinal tumors. Some surgeons have found that the merits of endoscopic surgery in the lumbar spine could be better appreciated in the treatment of patients with severe obesity and advanced age.

The endoscopic lumbar spinal procedure adopted by most surgeons is the oblique transforaminal approach. Given that the greatest difference between endoscopic surgery and nonendoscopic surgery is the method of visualization (i.e., 2D vs. 3D); more deformed or degenerative changes in Kambin's area increase the difficulty and technical demand of the procedure. Even though there has not been an established contraindication to this procedure, it has been generally agreed that patients with spondylolisthesis more than grade II, and patients with severe scoliotic changes or rotatory deformity at the indicated levels may not be good candidates to undergo endoscopic spinal fusion surgery.

Limitations also exist when the surgical neuroanatomy contradicts the accessibility created by the utmost minimally invasive spinal procedure. With the transforaminal approach, removing a centrally located pathology is more challenging, but can be managed with an interlaminar approach. However, this may not be the case if the herniated disk has significant cranial or caudal migration. It has been suggested that the herniated disk may not be managed with an endoscopic procedure if it extends below the mid-pedicle level caudally, or up to the inferior edge of the pedicle cranially.[7]

Another challenging condition is advanced spondylosis. At any level, an enlarged facet or superiorly deformed superior articular process may block the placement of endoscopic instruments to the disk. Sometimes this can be managed by using endoscopic drills, osteotomes, or adjusting the entering angle. In extreme cases, however, deformity of the structure in the foramen and facet above the 2D visualization may lead to less optimal surgical outcomes.

High rising iliac wings can also be problematic, especially when targeting lower lumbar disk levels. In a publication by Yue and Long,[7] it is suggested that the superior border of the iliac shadow should not be more proximal than the middle level of the pedicle above the indicated disk on lateral fluoroscopy. Male patients undergoing endoscopic procedures at the level of L4-5 or L5-S1 deserve special consideration, as male anatomy tends toward a more steep and upright pelvic structure.

TABLE 15.1 Indications and Contraindications for Endoscopic Fusion

Indications	Contraindications
1. Major indications: • Degenerative disk disease • Spondylolisthesis • Recurrent disk herniation • Spondylosis • Lumbar deformity 2. Specific indications: Can be performed at or above L2 Revision of prior PLIF 3. MIS benefits: • Reduced blood loss • Reduced anesthesia • Reduced recovery time	1. Relative contraindications: • Conjoined nerve root • Severe canal stenosis • Severe osteoporosis 2. Anatomic considerations: • Neuroforamen size • Geometry of disk herniation • Iliac crest orientation

MIS, Minimally invasive surgery; *PLIF*, posterior lumbar interbody fusion.

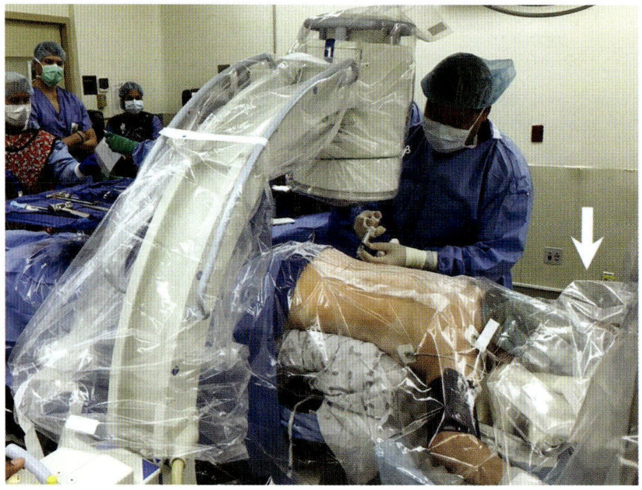

• **Fig. 15.1** Surgical positioning of an awake endoscopic lumbar interbody fusion surgery. Notice the relative location of the surgeon, the patient, and the fluoroscope. Transparent draping *(arrow)* is used in the setting of an awake procedure to facilitate better patient communication and monitoring.

Surgical Procedure

Anesthesia

The minimally invasive endoscopic LIF can be done when the patient is under general anesthesia or local analgesia with conscious sedation. The main advantages of general anesthesia include a better protection of the airway and less restriction of operative time. Conscious sedation offers greater interactive feedback from the patient, thus reducing the risk of jeopardizing neural structures.

Positioning

The patient can be in the prone position, although some surgeons prefer to use lateral positioning. There are a few advantages in utilizing lateral positioning, including reduced abdominal and venous pressures, less airway stress for the patient, and better interaction with the patient in case of an awake procedure. The downsides of lateral positioning are less familiarity of anatomic orientation and increased operative time for positioning.

It is recommended to utilize an operating room table that contains a four-point support system (e.g., Jackson table, Allen table) if the procedure is done with general anesthesia. The purpose is to obtain a better lumbar lordotic curvature once the fusion is completed. However, for patients undergoing awake procedures, the four-point support frame commonly leads to patient insecurity with less comfort. In that case, an arched frame (e.g., Wilson frame) may be utilized. In the setting of an awake procedure, transparent surgical draping is very useful for better monitoring and communication with the patient (Fig. 15.1). Care should be taken to lower the Wilson frame to minimize lumbar flexion.

Skin Incision

In the transforaminal approach, the goal is to access the indicated disk through the Kambin's triangle from the lateral aspect of the facet (Fig. 15.2). The skin incision is marked 6 to 12 cm paramedian to the midline. The Kambin's triangle is formed by the three borders: the exiting nerve root (the lateral border), the lateral margin of the traversing nerve root (the medial border), and the upper endplate of the lower vertebra (the caudal border). It has been generally agreed that the safety triangle ranges from L1-2 to L4-5 levels, based on cadaveric measurements. There are several ways to determine the paramedian length between the incision and the midline. Arbitrarily, it is suggested to make the incision 9 to 11 cm lateral to the midline, although several methods have been proposed in the literature. Some surgeons prefer to measure the length on preoperative computed tomography (CT) scans or magnetic resonance imaging,[8] others advocate more specific intraoperative measurement based on fluoroscopy, in which they measure the distance from the center of the indicated disk to the skin surface on lateral view and adopt this distance as the paramedian length.[9] Whatever method is utilized, it is generally recommended that the skin incision should not exceed ventrally to the posterior facet line shown on lateral fluoroscopic view, to avoid jeopardizing the peritoneal structures.[7] The angle of surgical trajectory in the coronal plane ranges from 25 degrees to 35 degrees, depending on the procedure level and the anatomic location of the pathology (i.e., intraforaminal vs. extraforaminal; central, lateral vs. far-lateral).[7,9–11]

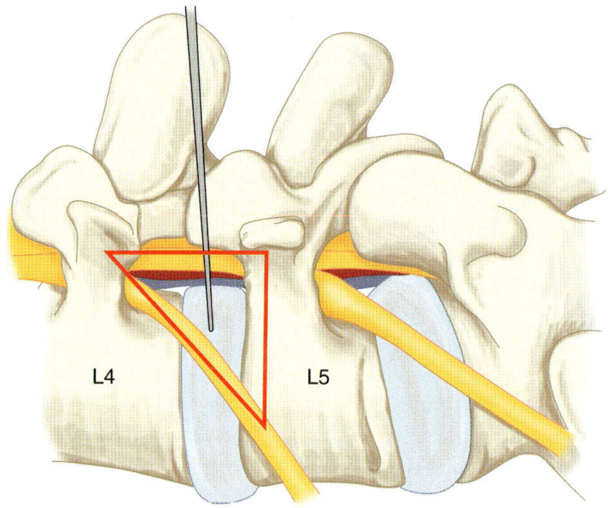

• **Fig. 15.2** Illustration of the transforaminal approach to the Kambin's triangle. The boundaries of the Kambin's triangle are formed by the exiting nerve root (laterally), the lateral margin of the traversing nerve root (medially), and the upper endplate of the lower vertebrae (caudally).

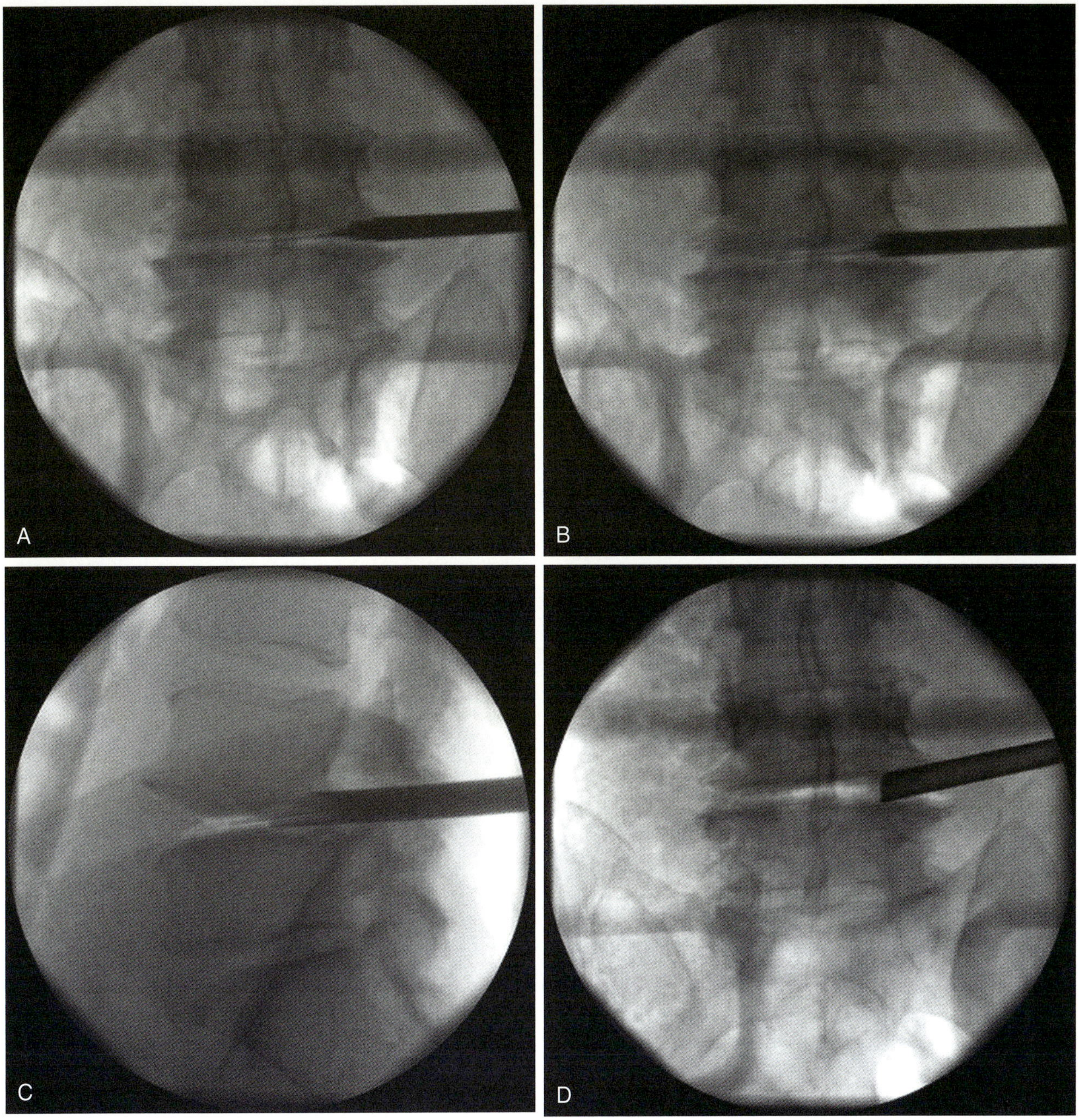

• **Fig. 15.3** Intraoperative fluoroscopy to demonstrate the process of establishing the endoscopic port. A–C, different sizes of dilators are used in sequence, finalized by removing all the dilators (D).

The skin, subcutaneous tissue, trajectory tract, and the peri-facet soft tissues are infiltrated with 1% lidocaine. An 18-gauge spinal needle is a useful tool for initial localization and estimation of the trajectory, as well as for delivery of lidocaine. After the administration of local anesthetic, a stab incision is made. The length of the incision should be just large enough for passage of the working port, which is usually 7 to 8 mm in diameter. The 18-gauge needle is then adjusted and advanced to the desired location for docking, which is above the pedicle at the disk level, and just outside of the facet. At this point, some surgeons use indigo carmine and radiopaque agents for an intraoperative diskogram for better differentiation of nervous tissue and degenerated nucleus.[11]

Working Port Placement

A Nitinol wire stylet is placed through the needle, followed by removal of the needle (Fig. 15.3). Serial dilators are then introduced along the guidewire, and finally this step is completed by introduction of the working endoscope. During the process of establishing surgical access, some tools (e.g., reamer, drills, and osteotomes) may be necessary in the face of hypertrophied facet or spurs.

There are two common methods for positioning the endoscope. One is to place it into the disk space (intradiscal method). The other method is to dock the endoscope in the caudal aspect of the foramen and work outside the annulus (extradiscal method). The intradiscal method allows for decompression of

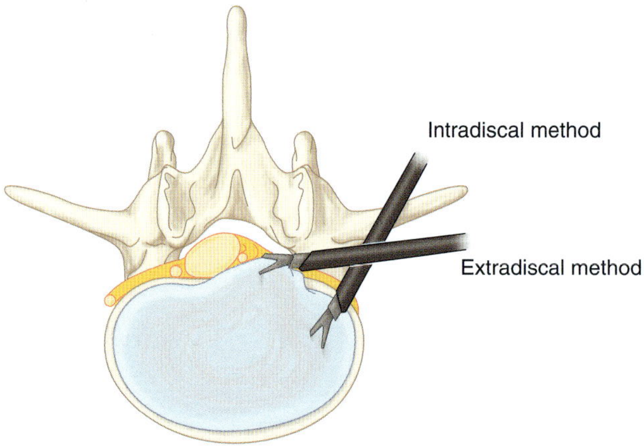

• **Fig. 15.4** Illustration of different methods of transforaminal endoscopic diskectomy.

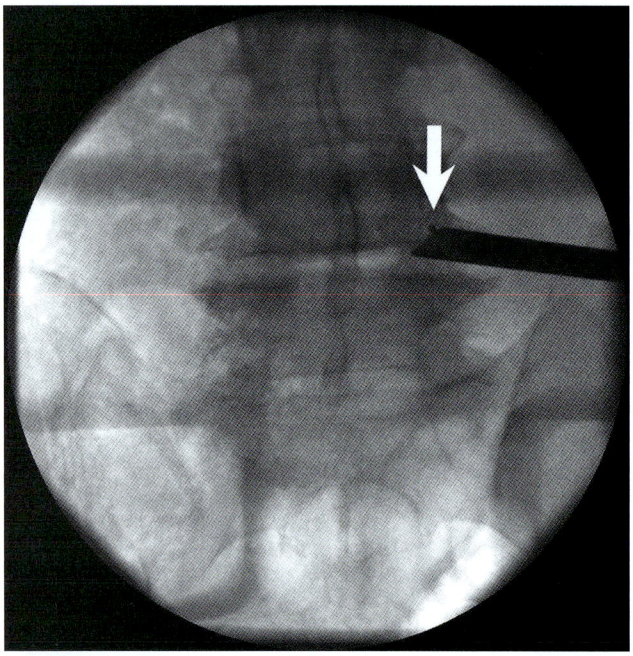

• **Fig. 15.5** Intraoperative fluoroscopy showing the surgeon using a probe for palpation.

more medialized pathology, but damages the normal disk structure. The extradiscal method avoids such trauma, but grants less access to the spinal canal (Fig. 15.4). Abundant vasculature around the disk space must be anticipated. Hemostasis can be managed by endoscopic electrocautery, quantitative irrigation, and/or hemostatic agents.

It is very important for the surgeon to be aware that once the endoscopic port is established, most of the maneuvers are limited within the linear trajectory of the endoscope, and the most efficient means of manipulation is by rotation of the working port. However, the bevel tip of the port and scope (mostly ranging from 30 degrees to 60 degrees) enables the surgeon to see the surrounding environment. Curved instruments (probe) allows the surgeon to "feel" the structures outside the tube (Figs. 15.5 and 15.6). This feedback may be especially useful to determine the thoroughness of the diskectomy.

Neural Decompression

The majority of neural decompression is achieved via removal of any disk herniations and through indirect decompression with expansion of the intervertebral space. "Traditional" removal of laminar bone, facet bone, and ligamentum flavum is more difficult and can be considered an advanced technique. This is partly owing to difficulties in manipulating tissues in multiple planes, challenges with neural retraction, and difficulties with resecting bone or soft tissue. Thus, severe central canal stenosis can be a relative contraindication.

Diskectomy and Interbody Device Placement

Removal of the disk material is usually accomplished with micropituitary rongeurs. During the removal process, the volume of the cartilage can be reduced by cauterization. In order to have a decent fusion surface, the efficiency of diskectomy can be enhanced by utilizing large drills, sharpers with expanding blades (to extend the drill track up to 15 mm), and back-biting instruments (Fig. 15.7). Endplate preparation can be finalized by electrically powered disk brushes to remove residual and loose disk material. At this point, a balloon can be inflated with radiopaque agent to evaluate the cavity size and degree of endplate preparation (Fig. 15.8).

An expandable cage for interbody fusion is necessary, as the working channel through an endoscopic port is too restrictive for the introduction of a traditional cage. Osteobiologic adjuvants are commonly used to promote bone fusion.

Percutaneous Pedicle Screw Placement

The fusion is completed by placement of percutaneous screws. Anteroposterior (AP) only fluoroscopic technique is one of those most commonly used. A "true AP" view on each vertebrae to be instrumented is crucial in this technique. Under this AP view, the skin incision location is marked and the stab incision is made. The Jamshidi needle is percutaneously inserted and docked over the base of the transverse process. With a proper trajectory (parallel to the upper endplate, 10 degrees to 12 degrees of medialization), the Jamshidi needle is advanced for about 2 cm to a point where the tip of the Jamshidi needle is at the base of the pedicle. On AP view, this should be within half or two-thirds of pedicle shadow laterally to medially (Fig. 15.9). Once the Jamshidi needle is in place, a guidewire can replace the obturator of the Jamshidi needle and be advanced for another 1.5 to 2 cm. This step is also important for the surgeon to palpate the cancellous bone to confirm the trajectory. After this, the pedicle can then be tapped and prepared for screw and rod placement (Fig. 15.10).

Closure and Postoperative Care

After the instrumentation is completed and confirmed by fluoroscope, the wounds (the stab incisions where the endoscopic port and screws were introduced) are irrigated, and can be easily closed in figure-of-eight fashion. Owing to the extremely minimal invasiveness of this procedure, surgical drain or Foley catheterization is generally not recommended to avoid the risk of postoperative urinary retention. Gabapentin, tramadol, and acetaminophen are frequently used in favor of bone fusion. Effective pain management is important for the patient to reduce anxiety and promote early mobilization. Lumbar bracing is recommended.

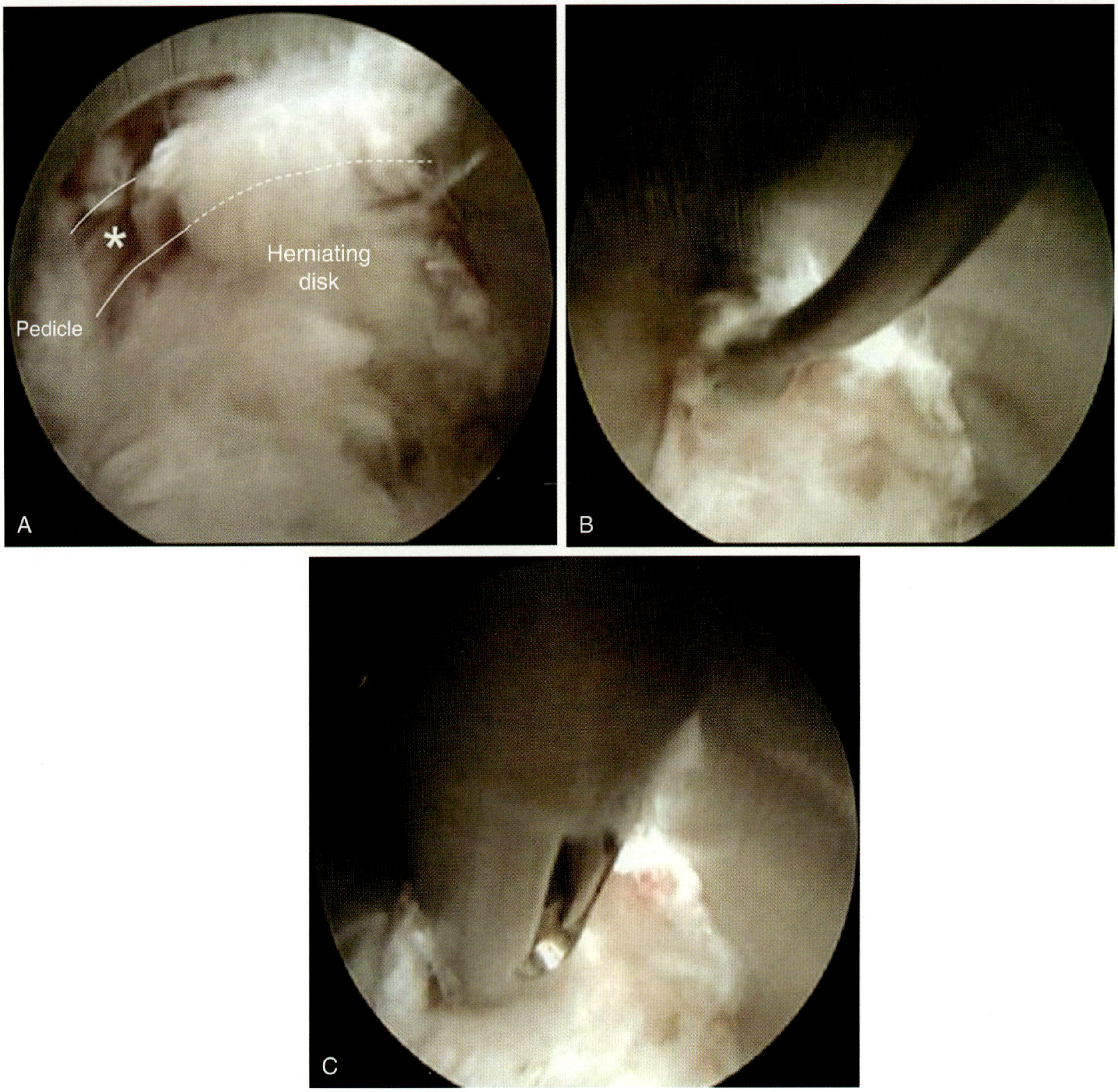

• **Fig. 15.6** Endoscopic view of the process of decompression. **A.** An overview of the anatomic landmarks under the endoscope. The traversing nerve root *(asterisk)* can be identified and palpated with a curved probe. **B.** A snapshot demonstrating the curved probe palpating the pedicle and the nerve root. Often times the sequestrated disk material can be poked out with this maneuver. **C.** An endoscopic forceps is used to grasp the disk material.

The patient should be warned to avoid bending or weight lifting. Regular follow-up with x-ray study should be conducted. Any sign of acute symptoms or neurologic deterioration should raise an alert. In that case, emergent examination, such as CT or magnetic resonance imaging, should be performed for evaluation.

Outcomes

The advantages of endoscopic procedures have been described in many studies. These include a local anesthetic setting, which avoids the risk of general anesthesia, smaller incisions and tissue damage than even microscopy-assisted minimal invasive surgery, shorter hospital stays, early ambulation, less blood loss, reduced operative time in an experienced surgeon's hand, no canal scar tissue, and a low risk of systemic complications. Disadvantages include a steep learning curve for surgeons new to these techniques, difficult intraoperative hemostasis, and—in the case of damage—difficulty in repairing the dura.[3,6,12] Overall, 85% to 93% of patients who underwent an endoscopic procedure were satisfied.[12–14]

Although there is a lack of head-to-head comparisons with standard MIS or open lumbar disk surgery in the literature, several single-armed case series have already shown promising outcomes after endoscopic-assisted LIF, including significant improvement in clinical parameters, and favorable demographic and

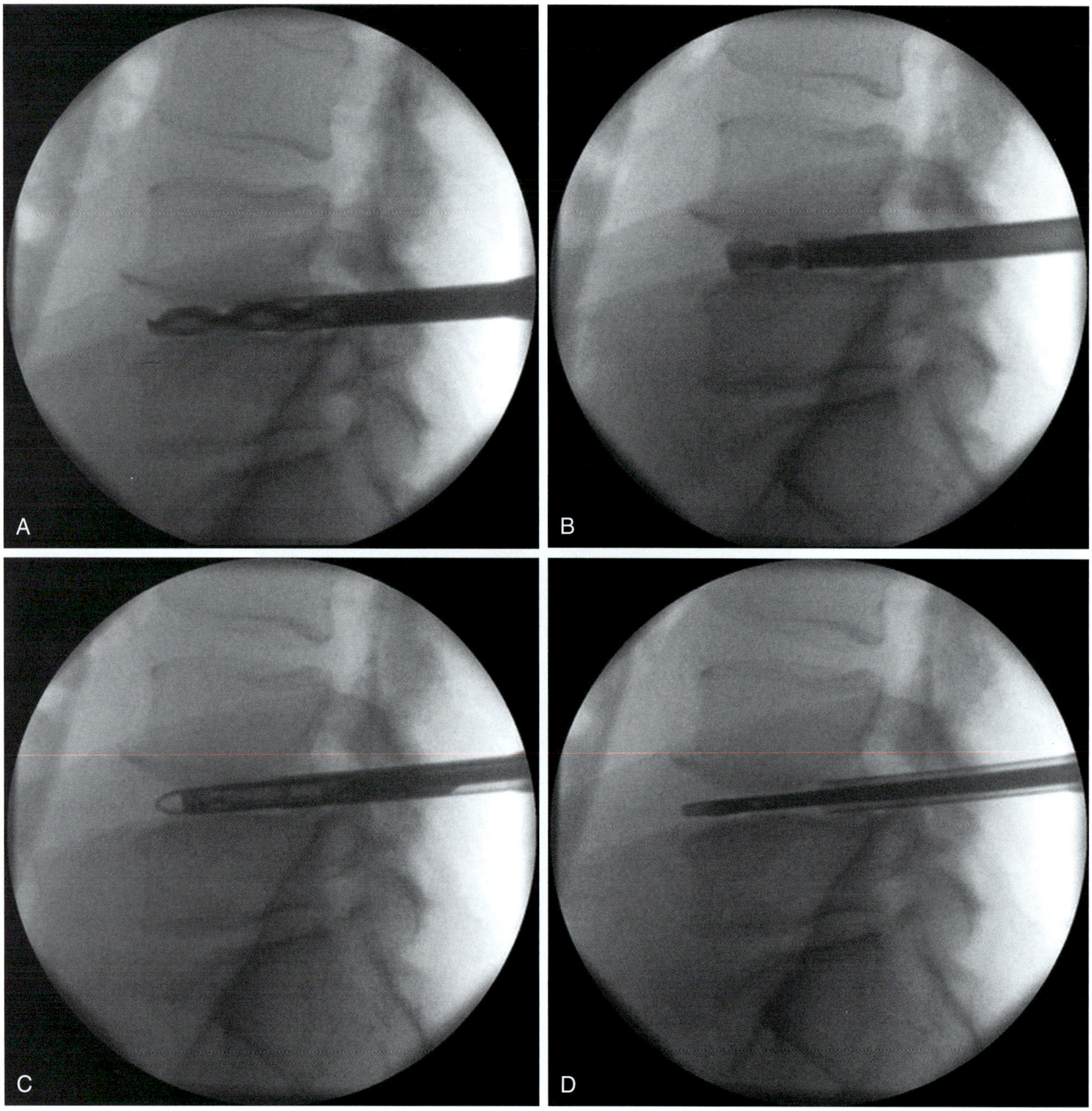

• **Fig. 15.7** Intraoperative fluoroscopy in the process of diskectomy. **A.** A drill is used for gross resection of the disk material. **B.** A sharper with expanding blades is used for extension of diskectomy. **C.** Shredded disk material is removed with an endoscopic rongeur. **D.** A back-biting rongeur is used for further removal of remaining cartilage.

radiographic results. Remarkable relief of leg pain and lower back disability were demonstrated in these case series, with improvement of visual analog scale (VAS) and Oswestry Disability Index (ODI) score after surgery.[3,13–15] Postoperatively, patients' reported quality of life was typically improved.[3] Intraoperative findings included minimal blood loss, less operative time, and a short hospital stay. The majority of patients will be discharged from hospital after one day.[3,14] Radiographic outcomes also showed promising results, in that fusions were solid (95.8% to 100% in reported series).[3,13–15]

Complications/Side-effects

Perioperative complications may be encountered with percutaneous endoscopic TLIF, and are generally seen in procedures such as endoscopic diskectomy, interbody cage fusion, or percutaneous screw fixation. In a nationwide retrospective study from Japan, the incidence of surgery-related complications for endoscopic spinal surgery, including diskectomy, laminectomy, fenestration, and fusion, was 2.1%.[16] These complications included dural tear (75% of all complications), injury of the cauda equina or a nerve

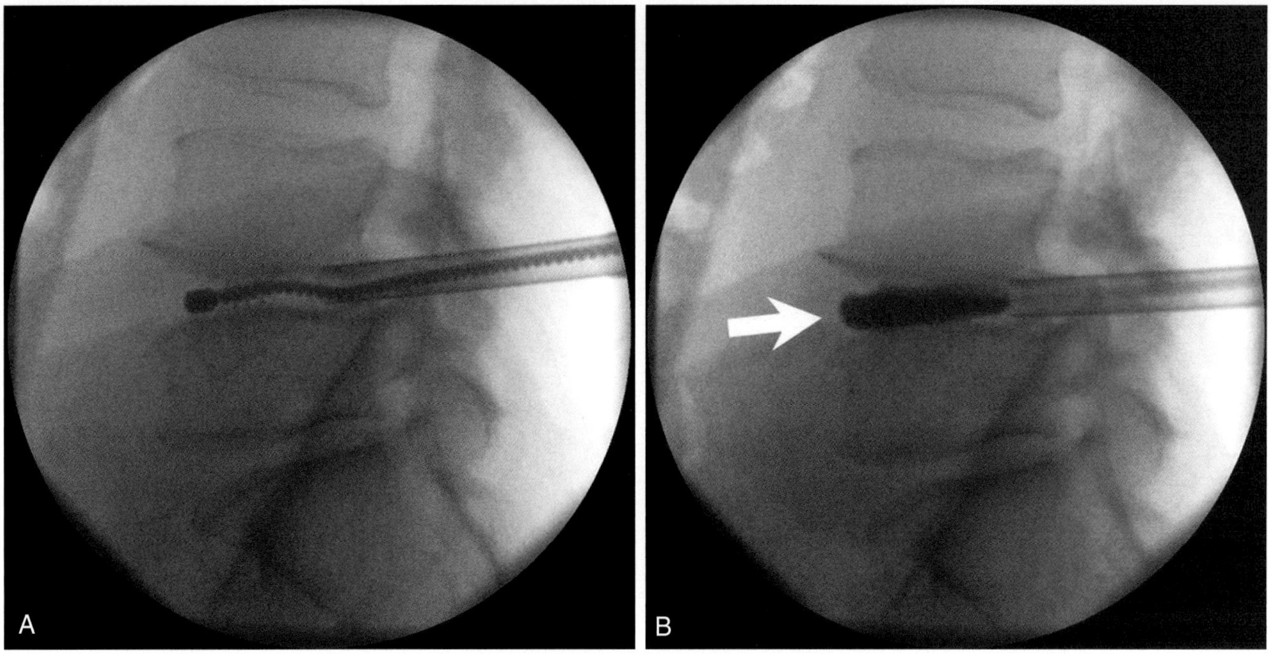

• **Fig. 15.8** **A.** An electrically powered disk brush is utilized for endplate preparation. **B.** After the diskectomy is completed, a balloon with radiopaque dye can be inflated to estimate the extent of diskectomy and endplate condition.

root (5.3%), facet fracture (5.3%), hematoma (4.5%), wrong level (4.5%), and wrong side (0.8%). However, the total risk remained low.[16,17]

Conversion to open surgery or microscopy-assisted MIS surgery is also a possible intraoperative complication, but has never been reported in literature. Conversion of local anesthesia to general anesthesia with the requirement of tracheal intubation is also a potential risk during endoscopic TLIF. In this case, airway management in the prone position is obviously difficult and may have severe consequences. To avoid this major risk, an expeditious surgery should be carried out within a fixed limit of time.[3]

Other systemic perioperative complications may include stroke, acute coronary events, pulmonary embolism, deep vein thrombosis (DVT), respiratory complications (e.g., pneumonia, postoperative respiratory disorders, or respiratory failure), urinary tract infection, acute renal failure, sepsis, and so forth. Wound infection is also possible after endoscopic procedures. However, patients undergoing endoscopic diskectomy were reported to have a significant lower systemic complication rate (0.8% vs. 1.3%, $P = .01$) and wound infection rate (0.1% vs. 0.2%, $P = .02$) compared with traditional open diskectomy.[18]

Recurrence of disk herniation, revision surgery, and cage subsidence after endoscopic LIF has been reported in the literature.[6,13,19] Recurrence of disk herniation after percutaneous endoscopic lumbar diskectomy is a not uncommon complication, but only one Chinese study has reported recurrence of disk herniation 4 months after endoscopic interbody fusion in a single case of L4-5 fusion, which was subsequently corrected by laminectomy plus diskectomy.[19] Revision is necessary in cases of adjacent segment degeneration, pseudoarthrodesis, or cage migration. Since a small-diameter working channel and extremely minimal invasion are the hallmark of endoscopic LIF, cage sizing has come into serious consideration intraoperatively. Jacquot and Gastambide operated on 57 patients with endoscopic LIF. Asymptomatic migration of the cages occurred in 2 cases, and there were symptomatic migrations requiring a conventional secondary reoperation in 13 cases (22.8% in this series). Further, perioperative radicular trauma with postoperative paresia and painful syndromes was encountered in 8 additional patients (14 % in this series). Given that 36% of the patients in this series had a complication related to the endoscopic technique, the authors did not recommend this approach. The authors specifically considered the high percentage of cage migration in their series, as other case series have not shown similar results.[6] They concluded the rigid standalone percutaneous titanium cage introduced through the endoscopic tube and filled with calcium phosphate substitute in this series may be the cause.

Recent series have adopted an expandable cage, such as the expandable mesh cage[3] (OptiMesh cage, Spineology), the titanium expandable cage[15] (Opticage, Interventional Spine Inc., Irvine, CA, USA) and the B-twin expandable spinal spacer[13,19,20] (Disc-O-Tech Medical Technologies Ltd., Herzliya, Israel) for interbody fusion. Most cases in these series reported no cage migration after the mean follow-up period of 12 to 38 months, with the exception of one case with cage migration following fusion failure.[13] Cage subsidence has been reported in series using the B-twin expandable spinal spacer.[13,20] Four cases of a total of 147 patients in two series using the B-twin expandable spinal spacer have been documented.

Minimally invasive technique, such as MIS-TLIF, DLIF, or XLIF, percutaneous screw fixation, and endoscopic techniques mainly proceed under the guidance of intraoperative fluoroscopy. Radiation exposure has always been a concern for both patients and medical staff. There are studies focusing on radiation exposure for both minimally invasive and endoscopic procedures. Based on two studies for endoscopic lumbar diskectomy, patient radiation exposure during surgery is

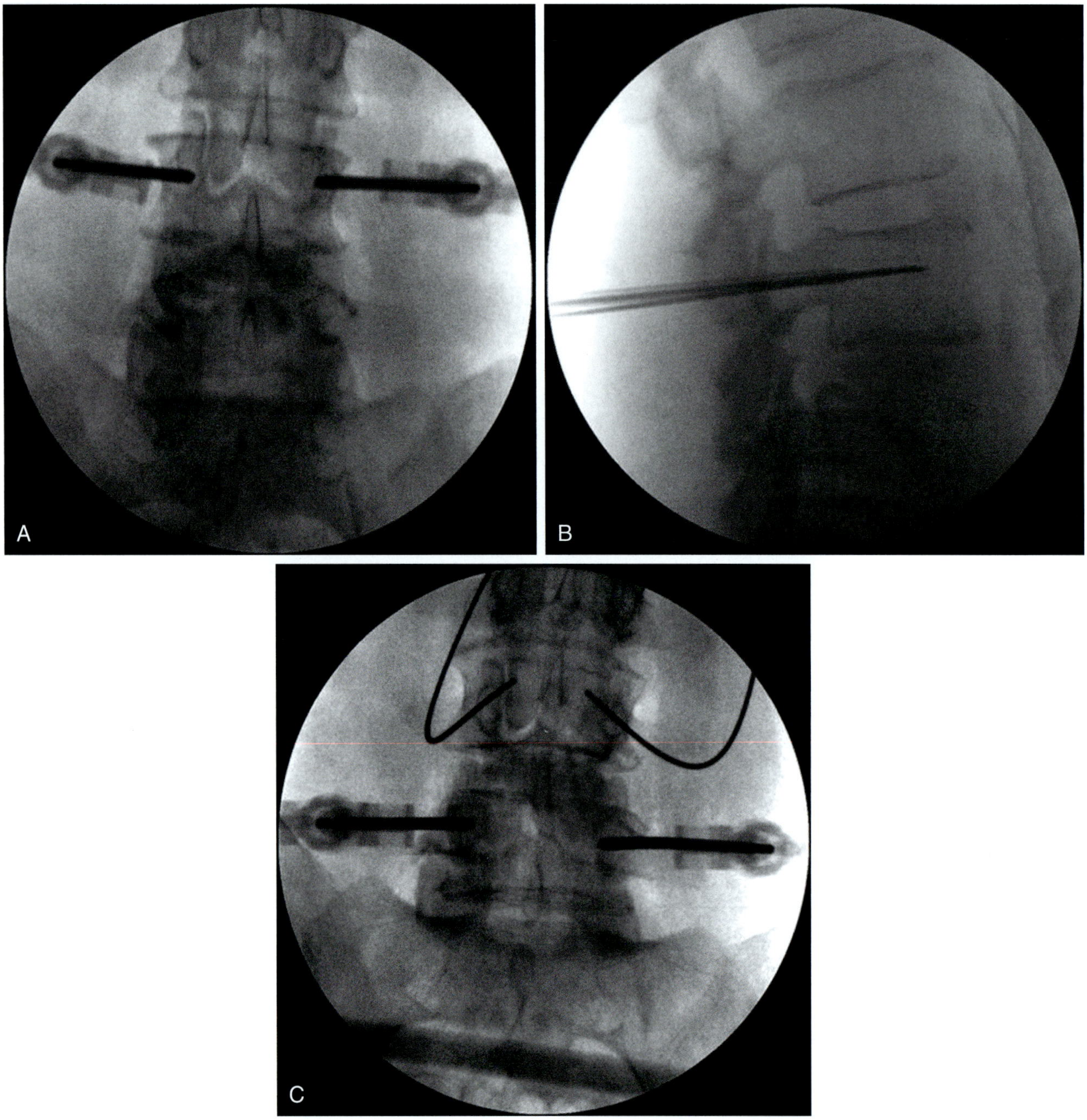

• **Fig. 15.9** Intraoperative fluoroscopy showing the process of percutaneous screw placement. (A) Jamshidi needles are adjusted to desired locations, followed by replacement of the obturator with guidewires (B) and the same procedure in the subsequent segment (C). Tapping, and placement of the screws can be done after all guidewires are placed for the purpose of efficiency.

small, similar to a fulltime airline crewmember (about 2 mSv per year) and less than the average American exposed annually (6 mSv). However, the exposure may increase in L5-S1 level cases and in initial cases. As of now, there has been no report on the radiation exposure of medical staff during endoscopic lumbar procedures.

Although this endoscopic approach has proved its short-term feasibility, future analysis of long-term complications is mandatory to assure its safety, as it is a new and developing technique. In addition to the above-listed complications, certain off-label uses of specific instruments or bio-materials, such as expandable mesh cages, recombinant human bone morphogenetic protein-2, and liposomal long-acting local anesthetics,[3] require long-term observation for side effects.

Conclusion

Endoscopic LIF has been evolving, and continues to demonstrate its unique advantages over traditional microscopic fusion procedures, including the ability to achieve interbody fusion without general anesthesia, fast recovery surgery, and even less invasiveness of lumbar surgery. It is a truly minimally invasive procedure which can also be incorporated with ongoing researches and technologies, including intraoperative CT scan, ergonomic designs of the long surgical

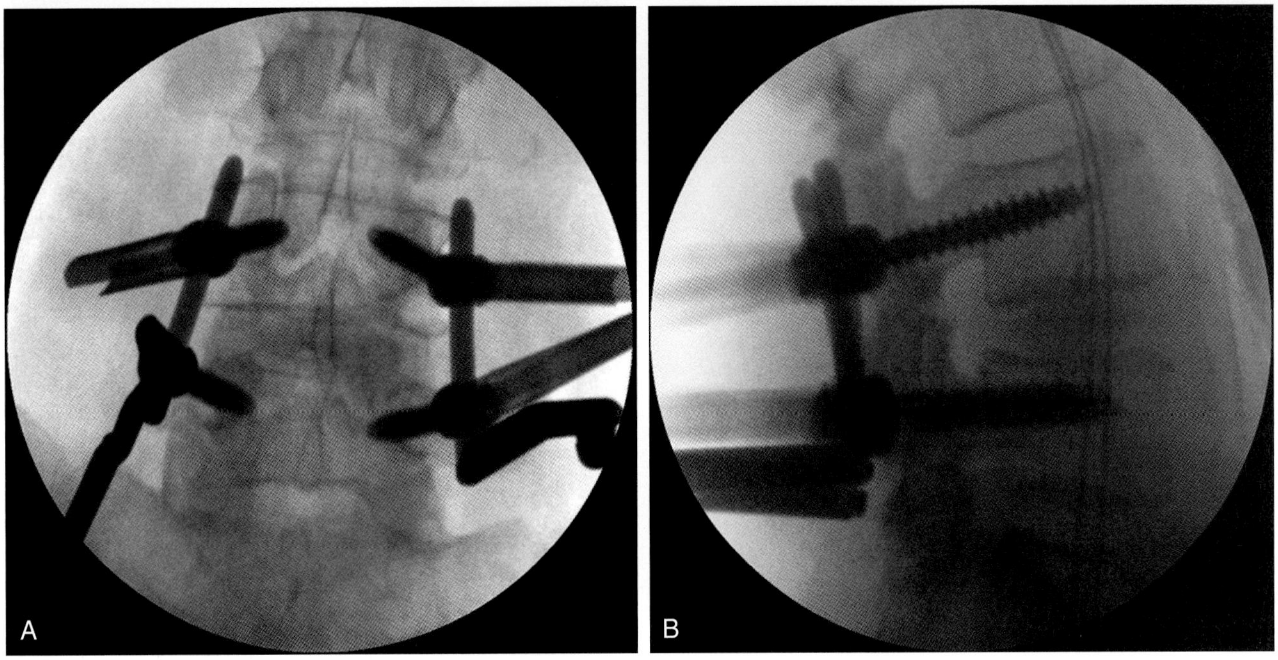

• **Fig. 15.10** AP (A) and lateral (B) intraoperative fluoroscopy demonstrating the final position of the hardware.

instruments through the same shaft, as well as spinal robotic technology. Despite that the available outcomes and future development of the endoscopic surgery seem very promising, it should always be known to the surgeon that difficulties and risks can never be ruled out, especially during the learning curve.

References

1. Eck JC, Sharan A, Ghogawala Z, et al. Guideline update for the performance of fusion procedures for degenerative disease of the lumbar spine. Part 7: lumbar fusion for intractable low-back pain without stenosis or spondylolisthesis. *J Neurosurg Spine*. 2014;21(1):42–47.
2. Talia AJ, Wong ML, Lau HC, et al. Comparison of the different surgical approaches for lumbar interbody fusion. *J Clin Neurosci*. 2015;22(2):243–251.
3. Wang MY, Grossman J. Endoscopic minimally invasive transforaminal interbody fusion without general anesthesia: initial clinical experience with 1-year follow-up. *Neurosurg Focus*. 2016;40(2):E13.
4. Wang MY. Minimally invasive transforaminal lumbar interbody fusion (MIS TLIF). In: Baaj AA, Mummaneni PV, Uribe JS, et al., eds. *Handbook of Spine Surgery*. New York: Thieme; 2012:341–347.
5. Wang YT, Wu XT, Chen H, et al. Endoscopy-assisted posterior lumbar interbody fusion in a single segment. *J Clin Neurosci*. 2014;21(2):287–292.
6. Jacquot F, Gastambide D. Percutaneous endoscopic transforaminal lumbar interbody fusion: is it worth it? *Int Orthop*. 2013;37(8):1507–1510.
7. Yue JJ, Long W. Full endoscopic spinal surgery techniques: advancements, indications, and outcomes. *Int J Spine Surg*. 2015;9:17.
8. Ruetten S, Komp M, Merk H, et al. A new full-endoscopic technique for cervical posterior foraminotomy in the treatment of lateral disc herniations using 6.9-mm endoscopes: prospective 2-year results of 87 patients. *Minim Invasive Neurosurg*. 2007;50(4):219–226.
9. Yeung AT, Tsou PM. Posterolateral endoscopic excision for lumbar disc herniation: surgical technique, outcome, and complications in 307 consecutive cases. *Spine (Phila Pa 1976)*. 2002;27(7):722–731.
10. Ahn Y. Transforaminal percutaneous endoscopic lumbar discectomy: technical tips to prevent complications. *Expert Rev Med Devices*. 2012;9(4):361–366.
11. Tsou PM, Alan Yeung C, Yeung AT. Posterolateral transforaminal selective endoscopic discectomy and thermal annuloplasty for chronic lumbar discogenic pain: a minimal access visualized intradiscal surgical procedure. *Spine J*. 2004;4(5):564–573.
12. Cong L, Zhu Y, Tu G. A meta-analysis of endoscopic discectomy versus open discectomy for symptomatic lumbar disk herniation. *Eur Spine J*. 2016;25(1):134–143.
13. Yao N, Wang W, Liu Y. Percutaneous endoscopic lumbar discectomy and interbody fusion with B-Twin expandable spinal spacer. *Arch Orthop Trauma Surg*. 2011;131(6):791–796.
14. Osman SG. Endoscopic transforaminal decompression, interbody fusion, and percutaneous pedicle screw implantation of the lumbar spine: a case series report. *Int J Spine Surg*. 2012;6:157–166.
15. Morgenstern R, Morgenstern C. Percutaneous transforaminal lumbar interbody fusion (pTLIF) with a posterolateral approach for the treatment of degenerative disk disease: feasibility and preliminary results. *Int J Spine Surg*. 2015;9:41.
16. Matsumoto M, Hasegawa T, Ito M, et al. Incidence of complications associated with spinal endoscopic surgery: nationwide survey in 2007 by the Committee on Spinal Endoscopic Surgical Skill Qualification of Japanese Orthopaedic Association. *J Orthop Sci*. 2010;15(1):92–96.
17. Gadjradj PS, van Tulder MW, Dirven CM, et al. Clinical outcomes after percutaneous transforaminal endoscopic discectomy for lumbar disc herniation: a prospective case series. *Neurosurg Focus*. 2016;40(2):E3.
18. Ohya J, Oshima Y, Chikuda H, et al. Does the microendoscopic technique reduce mortality and major complications in patients undergoing lumbar discectomy? A propensity score-matched analysis using a nationwide administrative database. *Neurosurg Focus*. 2016;40(2):E5.
19. Zhang X, Wang Y, Xiao S, et al. [Preliminary clinical results of endoscopic discectomy followed by interbody fusion using B-Twin expandable spinal spacer]. *Zhongguo Xiu Fu Chong Jian Wai Ke Za Zhi*. 2011;25(10):1153–1157.
20. Morgenstern R, Morgenstern C, Jane R, et al. Usefulness of an expandable interbody spacer for the treatment of foraminal stenosis in extremely collapsed disks: preliminary clinical experience with endoscopic posterolateral transforaminal approach. *J Spinal Disord Tech*. 2011;24:485–491.

16

Interbody Implant Options in Interbody Fusion

VINCENT J. ALENTADO AND MICHAEL P. STEINMETZ

Introduction

Lumbar fusion procedures have become increasingly common for the treatment of various degenerative lumbar spinal conditions.[1] Along with this upsurge is the increased utilization of interbody implants with or without traditional posterolateral instrumentation. The increasing usage of interbody cages is owing to the proposed advantages that interbody fusion offers, including higher fusion rates and improved clinical outcomes. Additionally, interbody grafts significantly decrease the strain of posterior spinal instrumentation during compression or flexion loading, which are the common modes of failure of these constructs.[1,2]

However, to achieve any theoretic advantages, interbody implants must provide early stability to the spinal segment, while also limiting any impact of the cage on the spine once bony fusion develops. Moreover, there is a balance to how much rigidity an interbody cage should offer. Too much stiffness may lead to stress shielding, increased subsidence, and subsequent revision operations, whereas too little stiffness may lead to biomechanical failure and/or pseudarthrosis. These important characteristics are affected by many cage-specific factors including size, shape, and implant material. Therefore, the goal of this chapter is to provide the reader with information on interbody implant options and describe the optimal implant properties to achieve the best fusion rates and clinical outcomes.

General Principles

To achieve a solid fusion, it is generally accepted that intervertebral motion should be restricted as much as possible. Therefore, the goal of any interbody device is to provide anterior column mechanical rigidity while a bony fusion develops. In addition, the interbody implants serve to directly maintain the increased disk space and neuroforaminal height that is achieved during the surgery, which may relieve compression on the nerve roots. Moreover, many constructs are designed to increase segmental lordosis, which improves overall sagittal balance.

Biomechanically, the most effective means of eliminating motion between two vertebrae is through the disk space rather than through the facet joints, as occurs during posterolateral fusion. As Wolff's law indicates, fusion potential is enhanced if grafts are placed under compression. Interbody fusions place the bone graft in the load-bearing position of the anterior and middle spinal columns, which support 80% of spinal loads and provide 90% of the osseous surface area, thereby maximally enhancing the potential for fusion.[2] In contrast, posterolateral construct grafts are compressed by 20% of spinal loads and occupy 10% of the osseous surface area. In addition, the interbody space is more vascular than the posterolateral space, increasing chances for fusion.

Implant Subsidence

Subsidence is a normal occurrence during the interbody fusion process owing to the early, normal, osteolytic phase of osteogenesis. Over time, settling of the cage into the vertebral endplates can occur if there is excessive subsidence. If significant subsidence occurs, it may result in loss of anterior column support and segmental lordosis, and loss of the indirect foraminal decompression achieved during surgery. These changes may result in an unfavorable biomechanical environment, which may contribute to the development of pseudarthrosis and possible compression of the neural elements. This is especially evident in flexion of the lumbar spine, as implant subsidence will reduce anterior wedging and decrease construct rigidity in this range of motion.[3]

Subsidence depends, in part, on regional strength of the endplate, vertebral bone quality, cage design, degree of endplate removal during endplate preparation, and the addition of supplemental fixation. Indeed, pedicle screw instrumentation has been shown to decrease the subsidence rate associated with interbody implants.[4] Ideally, the cage should be placed in contact with the apophyseal ring and with the largest surface area possible.[5] This is especially important during transforaminal lumbar interbody fusion (TLIF) and posterior lumbar interbody fusion (PLIF) where only a smaller cage can be inserted, allowing a lower surface area for distribution of force between the implant and vertebral endplates.

Additionally, endplate failure has a linear correlation with decreased bone density. Therefore, osteoporosis is considered to be a relative contraindication to interbody fusion because of the risk of endplate collapse and subsidence. However, attempts to maximize surface area contact are important when interbody implants are placed in osteopenic or osteoporotic patients. This helps to dissipate the axial loading forces over a broader area, and lessens the chance of endplate fracture and subsidence.

Implant Size

Implant size has many implications on the biomechanics of the spinal segment where it is placed. Annular tension is an important component of segmental stability and is primarily influenced by the vertical height of the cage. Oversizing the height of the implant leads to increased annular tension, which may improve the rigidity of the construct. Taller cages have been found to increase stiffness in torsion and lateral bending compared with smaller cages.[6] However, larger cages do not increase stiffness in flexion or extension. This is likely owing to the maintenance of contact with the cage surfaces in taller cage designs compared with shorter ones. However, larger cages may not always allow for optimal placement, such that the largest cage that can be placed suitably in a given segment is warranted.

Cage diameter also plays an important role in segmental stability. A smaller diameter cage applies more direct load to the portion of the endplate where it is placed, such that it is more important to place these cages where the endplate is strongest to decrease the chance of subsidence.[5] This may be owing to the inability of these cages to distribute the load across a larger endplate surface area. The widest cages may be placed only anteriorly through an anterior lumbar interbody fusion (ALIF) approach, whereas narrower cages are all that can be placed during PLIF and TLIF, demonstrating the importance of implant placement in these posterior approaches.

Implant Design

A variety of lumbar interbody implant designs are available from a number of manufacturers. Cages come in various shapes, including circular, cylindrical, tapered, and rectangular, with or without curvature to match the endplate. Some devices have design features such as radiolucency, projections for endplate interdigitation, integrated screws, or spikes. Others are modular so that they can be customized to fit a patient's unique intervertebral anatomy. In addition, most implants on the market today are created to allow for increased segmental lordosis. A description of common cage designs, along with their inherent benefits and shortcomings, are described below.

Shape of Interbody Cage

The shape of an interbody cage has important biomechanical implications on the intervertebral segment where it is placed. Early cage designs were rectangular in shape and tended to force the vertebral endplates into parallel alignment, thereby limiting segmental lordosis and improvements to sagittal balance. To obtain segmental lordosis with these cages, the posterior bone would be resected or the posterior disk space would be compressed to induce subsidence of the posterior cage. A disadvantage to these designs is that decreased posterior disk space height can lead to foraminal narrowing. Therefore, more modern implants incorporate a tapered design to facilitate insertion, and achieve segmental lordosis while maintaining distraction of the neuroforaminal space.

The interbody cage designs, as described by Bagby,[7] Ray,[8] and Brantigan et al.,[9] are examples of early interbody cage designs. The BAK (Spine-Tech, Inc., Minneapolis, MN) cage is a hollow, porous, squared, threaded cylindrical, titanium alloy device. It is similar in design to another cylindrical threaded titanium interbody cage, the RTFC (Surgical Dynamics, Norwalk, CT) cage. Cylindrical threaded fusion cages enjoyed brief popularity as stand-alone PLIF devices. However, high complication rates associated with their use, including segmental loss of lordosis, resulted in their virtual disappearance as a stand-alone posterior spinal implant. Moreover, recent studies have demonstrated that threaded fusion cages have statistically similar construct rigidity to nonthreaded cages, and they also create more stress-shielding compared with nonthreaded cages.[10] In addition, the degree of lordosis is limited by their design. In the modern era of interbody implants, the main improvement to these cages has been the incorporation of a tapered design. The first tapered cage on the market was the LT (Medtronic, Memphis, TN) cage for ALIF surgery.

Alternatives to cylindrical threaded cages include vertical interbody rings or boxes, such as the Harms (DePuy-Acromed, Cleveland, OH) titanium-mesh cage, Brantigan (DePuy-Acromed) carbon fiber cage, and the femoral ring allograft (FRA) (Synthes, Paoli, PA) allograft spacer. With vertical cage designs, the cage shape and endplate coverage significantly affects failure load and construct rigidity. Cage designs that optimize contact with the strongest portions of the endplate are desirable and include cloverleaf designs and large round cages, both of which have peripheral endplate contact. Biomechanical studies have demonstrated that with the same amount of endplate coverage, a cloverleaf shape provides a higher mean failure load compared with a kidney or elliptical shape.[11] In addition, a cloverleaf shape provides higher construct stiffness compared with the other cage designs. Moreover, a cloverleaf design that provides 40% endplate coverage has a higher load to failure compared with a cloverleaf design with only 20% endplate coverage.[11] However, amount of endplate coverage does not affect construct stiffness. Furthermore, cage shape does not affect rotational stiffness, as this is more affected by interdigitation of the endplate by the interbody implant.[3,11]

Kettler et al.[3] investigated biomechanical differences between various interbody cage shapes. They compared a cuboid titanium cage with two fixation hooks, a bullet-shaped polyetheretherketone (PEEK) cage, and a cylindrical threaded titanium cage. They found that the cuboid and cylindrical cages were stabilizing compared with an intact spine in flexion-extension and lateral bending ranges of motion, whereas the bullet-shaped cage was destabilizing compared with intact.[3] In addition, the authors noted that only the threaded cylindrical cage was stabilizing in axial rotation, as interdigitation of the endplate is the main stabilizer in this range of motion. After 40,000 axial compression cycles, a median subsidence of 0.9 mm was observed in the cuboid implant compared with 1.2 mm in the bullet-shaped implants and 1.4 mm in the threaded cylindrical implant. The initial stability decreased in all cages after cyclical loading. The greatest loss of stability occurred in the threaded cylindrical implant, likely owing to the higher subsidence seen with this cage. Cyclic loading causes nondestructive compression in combination with a penetration of the surface structures of the cages such as the cage threads. Therefore, cyclical loading may have destroyed the threads of the Ray cages, causing the cage to loosen.

Hollow versus Solid Cages

Interbody implants are designed such that the osteogenic potential for fusion comes from graft substrate that is packed into a hollow cage or packed tightly around a solid cage. For porous implants, a larger pore size is desirable as long as the design of the cage provides adequate structural support for the endplate. A solid spacer results in a higher mean maximal load to failure compared with a similarly sized hollow spacer.[5] Therefore, the maximal diameter hollow cage allowable should be utilized to decrease the risk of endplate subsidence while also maximizing fusion potential by allowing more space for bone graft material.

There are options currently available that allow improved "steering" of the implant as it is placed from a posterior approach. This maneuverability is owing to the adjustable cage—inserter articulation that the surgeon can change during placement of the cage into the disk space. For example, during TLIF, this added versatility allows more precise placement to the desire region of the interbody space. Expandable cages provide versatility in optimizing the interference fit of the cage. These can be particularly useful in cases of exaggerated segmental lordosis wherein the posterior disk space is much more narrow than the anterior disk space. Although expandable cages can be helpful, they are also typically more expensive. Furthermore, it is difficult, if not impossible, to fully pack the cage with substrate to completion as it is inserted in the collapsed position and expanded inside the disk space where no further substrate can be added to the cage itself.

Implant Material

In the standing position, 80% of spinal loads are transmitted through the anterior column.[2] An interbody implant must be able to withstand these loads to allow fusion to occur. Initially, bicortical iliac crest autograft supplemented with a screw and washer was the gold standard for interbody implants. However, high rates of pseudarthrosis, graft collapse and migration, and loss of stability were observed with the use of autologous iliac crest alone. In contrast, an interbody cage provides immediate mechanical support and stability postoperatively, allowing the graft material inside the cage to form a solid fusion mass.

There are a number of implant materials available, including cortical allograft, vascularized autograft, synthetic bone, vertical mesh cages, carbon fiber cages, cylindrical threaded cages, titanium, and PEEK cages. The stiffness of a cage has been shown to influence fusion rates. The ideal cage has a modulus of elasticity that is similar to that of vertebral bone in order to optimize the load transfer between the cage and the adjacent vertebral bodies, as well as to reduce the effects of stress shielding on the graft material within the cage.

Bone Grafts

Early interbody grafting incorporated the use of bicortical or tricortical spacers harvested from iliac crests. The safety and efficacy of iliac crest grafts have been well demonstrated. However, when used alone, these grafts are associated with significant rates of mechanical failure, loss of biomechanical correction, and pseudarthrosis.[12] Additionally, iliac autograft is associated with significant harvest site morbidity in up to 25% of patients.[12]

Owing to the shortcomings associated with iliac crest autograft, tricortical bone allograft gained popularity. The proposed benefits of allograft included the fact that allograft is stronger than fresh, autologous bone, and no morbidity accompanies autograft harvest. FRA obviates the need for cortical autograft and provides a strut with significant compressive strength that eventually incorporates into host bone. FRAs come in many machine-made sizes, which allows for selection of the most appropriately sized graft to fit a given intervertebral space. Additionally, cancellous allograft or autograft can be placed in the center of the cortical ring to augment fusion. Unfortunately, some of these grafts were unable to provide sufficient structural support, thus leading to the metal and polymer constructs that are more routinely used for circumferential fusions in the modern era.

Metallic Cages

Until the end of the 1990s, most cages were made of titanium. There is a long history of success with titanium implants as this metal offers excellent promotion of both bony ongrowth and ingrowth. Previous animal studies have demonstrated that porous titanium-mesh blocks exhibit ingrowth of bony trabeculae as early as 14 days after implantation.[13] Furthermore, after 3 weeks, there is deep bony penetration with intimate contact between bone and metallic fibers. In addition, clinical studies have also demonstrated a high rate of incorporation of titanium implants into local bone, even without the incorporation of supplementary autogenous bone chips.[14]

Metal cages significantly exceed the stiffness of vertebral bone. The Young's modulus of elasticity of stainless steel and titanium implants is 200 GPa and 110 GPa, respectively, compared with 2.1 GPa and 2.4 GPa for trabecular and cortical vertebral bone, respectfully.[15] This difference in elasticity may facilitate subsidence through the vertebral endplates in patients with osteoporosis. Furthermore, micromotion may cause cages to dislodge debris through the fusion segment, which may result in a cellular reaction with subsequent loosening of the bone and implant interface.[16] In addition to the aforementioned limitations, dense metal implants create imaging artifacts secondary to their opacity and scatter potential, thus limiting postoperative evaluation of fusion development.

There has been a recent influx of various metallic interbody cages into the spine market over the past several years. These include 3D-printed titanium cages (e.g., Styker Tritanium interbody cages) of varying densities, reductive titanium processing surface technology (e.g., Titan Spine Endoskeleton interbody cages) as well as titanium coated-PEEK cages (e.g., Nanovis FortiCore). The benefits of these types of cages include better compatibility with computed tomography and magnetic resonance imaging owing to a decrease in cage density, as well as heightened osseous integration. Materials that contribute to the latter provide certain benefit over other cages, such as PEEK, that have no potential of bone ongrowth or ingrowth. This, in theory, should promote higher initial and late stability at the cage/endplate interface, and thus, higher fusion rates.

Purported benefits of the 3D-printed titanium cages include close approximation of pore size to allograft bone and randomization of pore size, both of which are thought to promote cellular attachment, cellular and vascular proliferation, and ingrowth. In a similar vein, porous titanium surfaces formed through reductive processing are also purported to promote bone ingrowth without the concern of delamination that has been shown with titanium-coated PEEK. Extensive research is also being performed on hydroxyapatite (calcium phosphate) nanocoating (spray-painted at less than 100 nm) technologies that can promote tissue ingrowth and bony integration.

Polymer Cages

Polymer cages such as those made from carbon fiber and PEEK more closely approximate the elasticity of bone. These materials are also available in unlimited supply. By having a similar elastic modulus to bone, these cages prevent changes in load distribution and subsequent undesired remodeling of bone at the interface between the vertebral endplate and interbody implant. In addition, these cages are radiolucent to allow for improved visualization of bony fusion. A previously noted disadvantage of PEEK and other synthetic cages is that they do not participate in the fusion process. Specifically, such cages are not osteoconductive and only act as a spacer.

Carbon fiber cages may be made completely out of carbon fiber or carbon fiber embedded in a composite material such as PEEK to prevent their breakdown and release. The biomechanical drawback of carbon fiber implants is their relative brittleness, which allows for splintering, micromotion, and composite material failure.[17] To circumvent this, newer carbon fiber implant designs have incorporated threaded or ridged interfaces, thus minimizing slippage and migration.

Radiolucent PEEK cages were first introduced in the late 1990s. PEEK is a semicrystalline, aromatic hydrophobic polymer that offers structural support without osteogenesis. PEEK cages have gained popularity because of their similar modulus of elasticity of bone. The Young's modulus of elasticity of PEEK is 3.6 GPa compared with 2.4 GPa of cortical bone. Radiomarker dots are successfully used at the ventral and dorsal aspects of the cages so that the surgeon can see the implant on radiographs. Furthermore, PEEK is also magnetic resonance imaging and computed tomography compatible and does not create significant implant artifact on these imaging studies.

Vadapalli et al.[15] biomechanically investigated the amount of endplate stress and stress shielding seen when using titanium or PEEK cages. The stress on the endplates increased by 2.5-fold when using a titanium cage compared with a PEEK cage. The maximal amount of stress was seen during lateral bending, which was 48 MPa for a titanium spacer with supplemental posterior instrumentation compared with 20 MPa for the PEEK spacer with posterior instrumentation. The stress on the cancellous bone graft material in the PEEK cage was 9-fold higher in extension and axial rotation, 11-fold higher in flexion, and 15-fold higher in lateral bending compared with a titanium cage. These data demonstrate the lower risk of subsidence and stress shielding when using a PEEK cage compared with a titanium cage.

Surgical Approach

The unique benefits and risks of each specific lumbar interbody fusion technique are described in more detail in other chapters of this text. However, a brief overview of approach-specific implications for interbody implant designs is reviewed below.

PLIF Cages

The first interbody cages for lumbar fusion were threaded PLIF cages. The proposed benefits of the threaded PLIF cages included providing anterior column support, placement of the cage closer to the vertebral axis of rotation, and a reduced bone graft requirement. Modern PLIF cages are usually tapered with bullet-shaped noses for improved segmental lordosis and easier insertion into the disk space.

ALIF Cages

The ALIF technique was created in order to achieve an interbody fusion with a decreased complication profile compared with PLIF. It is easier to restore segmental lordosis from a ventral approach because circumferential release of the annulus fibrous allows more effective restoration of disk space height and a larger cage can be inserted in terms of both height and width.[2] Furthermore, these cages can have varying degrees of lordosis.

Anterior lumbar interbody fusion may be achieved with a stand-alone cage or supplemented with dorsal instrumentation. The stand-alone cage has the benefit of preserving dorsal elements, which avoids perioperative morbidity related to the dissection of the spinal muscles and complications of dorsal instrumentation. In contrast, dorsal instrumentation increases stabilization, creating an environment more conducive to fusion. However, integrated fixation devices have been developed to limit anterior exposure while maintaining the benefits of supplemental fixation.

TLIF Cages

Transforaminal lumbar interbody fusion was developed to reduce complication rates compared with PLIF while eliminating the need for both ventral and dorsal approaches during the same procedure. From the perspective of interbody implants, TLIF cages have similar limitations to PLIF implants. Positioning of TLIF cages dorsolaterally maximizes stability of the construct. The disadvantage of this position is that it may increase the likelihood of cage retropulsion into the canal.

LLIF Cages

Lateral lumbar interbody fusion is the most recent of these lumbar interbody fusion techniques. Cages inserted through this lateral approach provide superior compressive stability in comparison to the smaller cages that must be inserted through a dorsal approach because LLIF allows for the utilization of wider implants that are supported by the periphery of the endplate. Both ALIF and LLIF promote the placement of tall cages, but achieving segmental lordosis is easier if the ALL is released.

OLIF Cages

Oblique lateral interbody fusion (OLIF) was first described by Michael Mayer[18] in 1979. With the patient in the lateral decubitus position, the approach utilizes the retroperitoneal approach wherein a cage is placed obliquely into the disk space. The latter is entered just anterior to the psoas muscle and, as such, does not put the muscle or lumbar plexus at risk.

Axial LIF Cages

Axial lumbar interbody fusion (AxiaLIF) utilizes a small parasacral incision and a presacral approach to the L5-S1 and the L4-5 interspaces. A tubular portal is anchored into the anteroinferior S1 body, and a transosseous tunnel is developed to the disk space of interest. At this time a diskectomy tool is rotated in the disk space to remove the disk material and prepare the disk space. The same process at L4-5 can be repeated after the L5-S1 space. A threaded cage is then developed from caudal to cranial through the tubular access and anchored into the adjacent bodies and spanning the disk space(s) of interest.

Although there was some enthusiasm about the novelty of this technique, it has not become mainstream. Clearly, an axially placed implant compared with a typical interbody cage cannot provide the same resistance to axial physiologic loading. Further, preparation of the disk space is often difficult to achieve given the limited exposure. Finally, bowel perforation has been reported, which has subtracted further from the early appeal of this technique.

Conclusions

Size, shape, material, and overall design of interbody implants significantly affect their function during interbody fusion. The ideal features of an interbody cage include a hollow region of sufficient size to allow packing of bone graft or bone graft substitute. Moreover, the ideal implant should be structurally sturdy so that it can withstand the substantial loading forces applied to it in the immediate postoperative period. Furthermore, it should have a modulus of elasticity that is similar to that of vertebral bone to optimize fusion and avoid subsidence. Additionally, it should have ridges, teeth, or screw integration to resist ventral migration or retropulsion into the canal. It should be radiolucent to allow visualization of fusion on radiographs. If inserted from a dorsal approach, it should be tapered to allow improved segmental lordosis and insertion into the disk space. Future interbody implant devices will continue toward meeting these goals and improving clinical outcomes.

References

1. Weiner BK, Fraser RD. Spine update lumbar interbody cages. *Spine (Phila Pa 1976)*. 1998;23(5):634–640.
2. Mummaneni PV, Haid RW, Rodts GE. Lumbar interbody fusion: state-of-the-art technical advances. Invited submission from the Joint Section Meeting on Disorders of the Spine and Peripheral Nerves, March 2004. *J Neurosurg Spine*. 2004;1(1):24–30. https://doi.org/10.3171/spi.2004.1.1.0024.
3. Kettler A, Wilke HJ, Dietl R, et al. Stabilizing effect of posterior lumbar interbody fusion cages before and after cyclic loading. *J Neurosurg*. 2000;92(suppl 1):87–92.
4. Ambati DV, Wright EK, Lehman RA, et al. Bilateral pedicle screw fixation provides superior biomechanical stability in transforaminal lumbar interbody fusion: a finite element study. *Spine J*. 2015;15(8):1812–1822. https://doi.org/10.1016/j.spinee.2014.06.015.
5. Lowe TG, Hashim S, Wilson LA, et al. A biomechanical study of regional endplate strength and cage morphology as it relates to structural interbody support. *Spine (Phila Pa 1976)*. 2004;29(21):2389–2394.
6. Goh JC, Wong HK, Thambyah A, et al. Influence of PLIF cage size on lumbar spine stability. *Spine (Phila Pa 1976)*. 2000;25(1):35–39; discussion 40.
7. Bagby GW. Arthrodesis by the distraction-compression method using a stainless steel implant. *Orthopedics*. 1988;11(6):931–934.
8. Ray CD. Threaded titanium cages for lumbar interbody fusions. *Spine (Phila Pa 1976)*. 1997;22(6):667–679; discussion 679–680.
9. Brantigan JW, Steffee AD, Lewis ML, et al. Lumbar interbody fusion using the Brantigan I/F cage for posterior lumbar interbody fusion and the variable pedicle screw placement system: two-year results from a Food and Drug Administration investigational device exemption clinical trial. *Spine (Phila Pa 1976)*. 2000;25(11):1437–1446.
10. Kanayama M, Cunningham BW, Haggerty CJ, et al. In vitro biomechanical investigation of the stability and stress-shielding effect of lumbar interbody fusion devices. *J Neurosurg*. 2000;93(suppl 2):259–265.
11. Tan J-S, Bailey CS, Dvorak MF, et al. Interbody device shape and size are important to strengthen the vertebra-implant interface. *Spine (Phila Pa 1976)*. 2005;30(6):638–644.
12. Noshchenko A, Hoffecker L, Lindley EM, et al. Perioperative and long-term clinical outcomes for bone morphogenetic protein versus iliac crest bone graft for lumbar fusion in degenerative disk disease: systematic review with meta-analysis. *J Spinal Disord Tech*. 2014;27(3):117–135. https://doi.org/10.1097/01.bsd.0000446752.34233.ca.
13. Galante J, Rostoker W, Lueck R, et al. Sintered fiber metal composites as a basis for attachment of implants to bone. *J Bone Joint Surg Am*. 1971;53(1):101–114.
14. Leong JC, Chow SP, Yau AC. Titanium-mesh block replacement of the intervertebral disk. *Clin Orthop*. 1994;300:52–63.
15. Vadapalli S, Sairyo K, Goel VK, et al. Biomechanical rationale for using polyetheretherketone (PEEK) spacers for lumbar interbody fusion—a finite element study. *Spine (Phila Pa 1976)*. 2006;31(26):E992–E998. https://doi.org/10.1097/01.brs.0000250177.84168.ba.
16. Steffen T, Tsantrizos A, Fruth I, et al. Cages: designs and concepts. *Eur Spine J*. 2000;9(suppl 1):S89–S94.
17. Tullberg T. Failure of a carbon fiber implant. A case report. *Spine (Phila Pa 1976)*. 1998;23(16):1804–1806.
18. Mayer MH. A new microsurgical technique for minimally invasive anterior lumbar interbody fusion. *Spine*. 1997;22(6):691–699.

17

Biologic Options in Interbody Fusion

MARCO C. MENDOZA, BRETT D. ROSENTHAL, AND WELLINGTON K. HSU

Introduction

Interbody fusion devices aim to provide anterior column support as bony fusion between adjacent vertebral bodies progresses. Irrespective of the material utilized for structural support, depending on exact surgical technique, supplemental graft material should be placed within and/or around the allograft or cages in order to achieve a solid fusion. Achieving a solid arthrodesis can be directly correlated to long-term clinical outcomes and the durability of the procedure. Spine biologics can aid in facilitating arthrodesis by altering the existing environment by enhancing specific cellular and molecular activity. As a result, the field of biologics has expanded rapidly over recent years to include not only autogenous bone graft but also allograft, demineralized bone matrix, ceramic carriers, recombinant growth factors, and tissue engineering therapies.

The ideal bone graft substitute possesses three distinct properties: osteogenesis, osteoconduction, and osteoinduction. Osteogenic grafts contain osteoprogenitor or osteogenic precursor cells capable of directly forming bone. Osteoinduction is the mechanism whereby these precursor cells are stimulated to differentiate into mature osteoblasts, whereas osteoconductive materials provide a biocompatible physical structure or scaffold that supports the formation of new bone (Table 17.1). One additional feature of bone grafts, which is more commonly discussed in maxillofacial surgery, is that of osseointegration. This refers to an implant's ability to bind to bone without any intervening tissue.[1] Surgeons should assess the biologic requirements of the respective fusion site and select a bone graft strategy based on these properties.

Autograft

Iliac crest autograft contains all three properties for bone formation and remains the gold standard for fusion procedures as it has a number of advantages. Depending on the procedure, it can be obtained anteriorly or posteriorly as well as through the same incision versus a separate incision. It is cost effective, readily available, and is biocompatible without risk of antigenicity. The main drawback of its use is related to donor site morbidity, which can include pain, paresthesias, hematoma, and infection with an incidence rate as high as 50% in some series.[2] In one multicenter prospective study, Sasso et al. found that 31% of patients reported pain even at 2 years postoperatively, suggesting that the duration is not merely transient in many patients. Of note, there was no significant difference in pain scores when comparing posterior versus anterior harvest sites.[3]

One alternative to iliac crest bone graft (ICBG) and its potential harvest-related complications is local autograft. This can be harvested from the spinous processes, lamina, and facets during both open and minimally invasive procedures. A systematic review of clinical studies demonstrated similar fusion rates when comparing local bone autograft with ICBG, 79% and 89%, respectively.[4] One primary limitation of local autograft is the potential for volume constraints, particularly in single-level fusions. Sengupta et al. compared ICBG with local autograft in a retrospective review and found similar healing rates in one-level fusions; however, local bone autograft had a significantly lower fusion rate compared with ICBG in multilevel fusions, 20% vs. 66%, respectively ($P = .029$).[5] As a result, a number of bone graft extenders have subsequently been developed to remedy this volume-related limitation.

Allograft

Allograft, bone obtained from human donors, serves as an osteoconductive agent, providing a scaffold for bone formation. Allograft is processed and preserved through freeze-drying or freezing. The osteogenic potential of the graft is sacrificed as bone cells are eliminated during its processing which decreases the risk of disease transmission, antigenicity, and infection. Therefore, it is recommended that allograft should always be applied in conjunction with autograft or another osteoinductive agent in the lumbar

TABLE 17.1 Review of the Osteoinductive, Osteoconductive, and Osteogenic Properties of Various Bone Graft Substitutes and Extenders

Bone Graft	Osteoinductive	Osteoconductive	Osteogenic
Autograft	√	√	√
Allograft		√	
DBM	√	√	
Ceramic		√	
rhBMP	√		
Platelet		√	
MSCs			√

DBM, demineralized bone matrix; *MSCs*, mesenchymal stem cells; *rhBMP*, recombinant human bone morphogenetic protein.

spine. Nonetheless, allograft is incredibly versatile as it is available in multiple forms including powder, strips, bone chips, and cage-type formulations. Femoral ring allograft has historically been one of the most common materials utilized in anterior lumbar interbody fusions. Thalgott et al. compared freeze-dried with frozen allografts from a single manufacturer in a prospective, randomized study with a minimum follow-up of 24 months. Frozen grafts were cooled and stored at -70°C and dehydrated via lyophilization, whereas freeze-dried grafts were stored at room temperature. They found freeze-dried allografts more likely to break intraoperatively and were also more likely to require reoperation for pseudarthrosis (P = .026). Over 85% of the revision surgeries were performed in the freeze-dried group; however, most of these patients were noted to be smokers. Despite this disparity, there was no difference in Oswestry disability index (ODI), Short Form-36 (SF-36), and pain scale scores.[6]

Demineralized Bone Matrix

Demineralized bone matrix (DBM) is a bone graft extender developed from human cadaveric bone by means of acid extraction. This process results in a matrix containing a type I collagen framework in addition to a number of growth factors such as bone morphogenetic proteins, transforming growth factor-β (TGF-β), insulin-like growth factor, and fibroblast growth factor. These components make DBM both osteoinductive and osteoconductive. However, DBM comes in a variety of formulations with over 50 commercial DBM products available for use in the lumbar spine. Bae et al.[7] evaluated the quantity of bone morphogenetic protein (BMP) in different products in addition to the variability of BMP in varying lots from the same manufacturer. Utilizing enzyme-linked immunosorbent assay, they identified BMP-2, BMP-4, and BMP-7. Both BMP-2 and BMP-7 were found in all DBM products in low concentrations (~20 to 200 ng/g); however, BMP-4 was not detected in all samples. Additionally, the variability of BMP concentrations among different lots of the same DBM formulation was higher than the variability of concentrations among different DBM formulations.

Despite the questionable reliability of providing consistent osteoinduction, evidence in the literature supports the use of DBM as a bone graft extender in posterolateral lumbar spine fusion surgery.[8] However, it should be noted that DBM lacks the structural stability needed for lumbar interbody fusion procedures and, in this setting, should be used in combination with a structural spacer. Thalgott et al. reported a 96% fusion rate in their series of 50 patients who underwent anterior lumbar interbody fusion with the use of titanium mesh cages, coralline hydroxyapatite, and DBM as part of a circumferential fusion.[9]

Ceramics

Ceramic-based bone grafts are a type of synthetic graft with osteoconductive properties, supporting new bone ingrowth but lack any osteoinductive potential. They convey numerous advantages including nearly unlimited supply, easy sterilization, and lack immunogenicity as they are biologically inert and generally do not induce an inflammatory response. Drawbacks include their brittle structure and low tensile strength obviating the need for protection from excessive force until a solid fusion has occurred. Calcium sulfate is resorbed in only a few weeks after implantation and therefore should not be used as a scaffold in lumbar fusion surgery. Ideally, the scaffold should facilitate bony ingrowth and then resorb as the fusion develops. As a result, more commonly used compounds include β-tricalcium phosphate and hydroxyapatite. β-tricalcium phosphate is resorbed over a period of months, making it more suitable for use in lumbar spine fusions, whereas hydroxyapatite is resorbed over the course of years.[10] In a recent systematic review with a collective population of 1332 patients, ceramics demonstrated an overall fusion rate in the lumbar spine of 86.4%. All interbody fusion studies reviewed included posterior instrumentation and were subsequently grouped together as circumferential fusions, which included anterior, posterior, and transforaminal techniques. The overall fusion rate for interbody fusions was not statistically different from the posterolateral technique, 88.8% versus 85.6%, respectively (P = .64).[11] This review suggests that ceramic-based scaffolds are an effective bone graft extender in each of these techniques; however, variability in assessing fusion status and the number of included patients may have led to the lack of difference between the two groups.

Bone Morphogenetic Proteins

Bone morphogenetic proteins belong to the TGF-β superfamily of growth factors. They act through serine-threonine kinase receptors and transduce their signal via the SMAD pathway[12] (Fig. 17.1). This subsequently results in the induction of bone formation through the differentiation, maturation, and proliferation of mesenchymal precursor cells into osteogenic cells. More than 20 types are described; however, only 2 commercial forms are available for clinical use: recombinant human bone morphogenetic protein-2 (rhBMP-2; Infuse) and rhBMP-7 (OP-1). The family of proteins were first discovered by Dr. Marshall Urist in 1965, but not until 2002 did the US Food and Drug Administration (FDA) approve their utilization clinically. Specifically, the use of rhBMP-2 is currently approved as a component of a titanium cage for anterior lumbar interbody fusion. Despite this single FDA-approved indication, rhBMP-2 is frequently used for a number of off-label applications, including posterolateral spine fusions, posterior lumbar interbody fusions, transforaminal lumber interbody fusions, and cervical spine procedures. Only two commercial forms of recombinant BMP are available for clinical use: rhBMP-2 (Infuse) (Medtronic, Memphis, TN) and rhBMP-7 (OP-1) (Stryker, Kalamazoo, MI). These proteins are water-soluble and are rapidly diffused from the surgical site when used independently. As a result, matrix carriers or scaffolds are required to decrease diffusion away from the desired site of application. The most common carrier currently utilized is a type-1 absorbable collagen sponge. It is deformable and can be easily inserted into a cage for interbody fusions. In 2002, Burkus et al. reported their results in an FDA-regulated, multicenter prospective randomized study of 279 patients who underwent anterior lumbar interbody fusion using two tapered titanium threaded fusion cages.[13] The rhBMP-2 group showed a statistically significant improvement in clinical outcomes, including back and leg pain scores as well as the ODI. Additionally, 32% of patients in the ICBG group reported graft site discomfort at 2-year follow-up. In a systematic review, Galimberti et al. also echoed favorable results for rhBMP-2 in anterior lumbar interbody fusion procedures, showing a significant improvement in fusion rates. However, they did not find any statistically significant improvement in fusion rates in posterior lumbar interbody fusion and transforaminal lumbar interbody fusion procedures. It should be noted that these conclusions are limited by the heterogeneity of rhBMP-2 dosing and varying levels of evidence.[14]

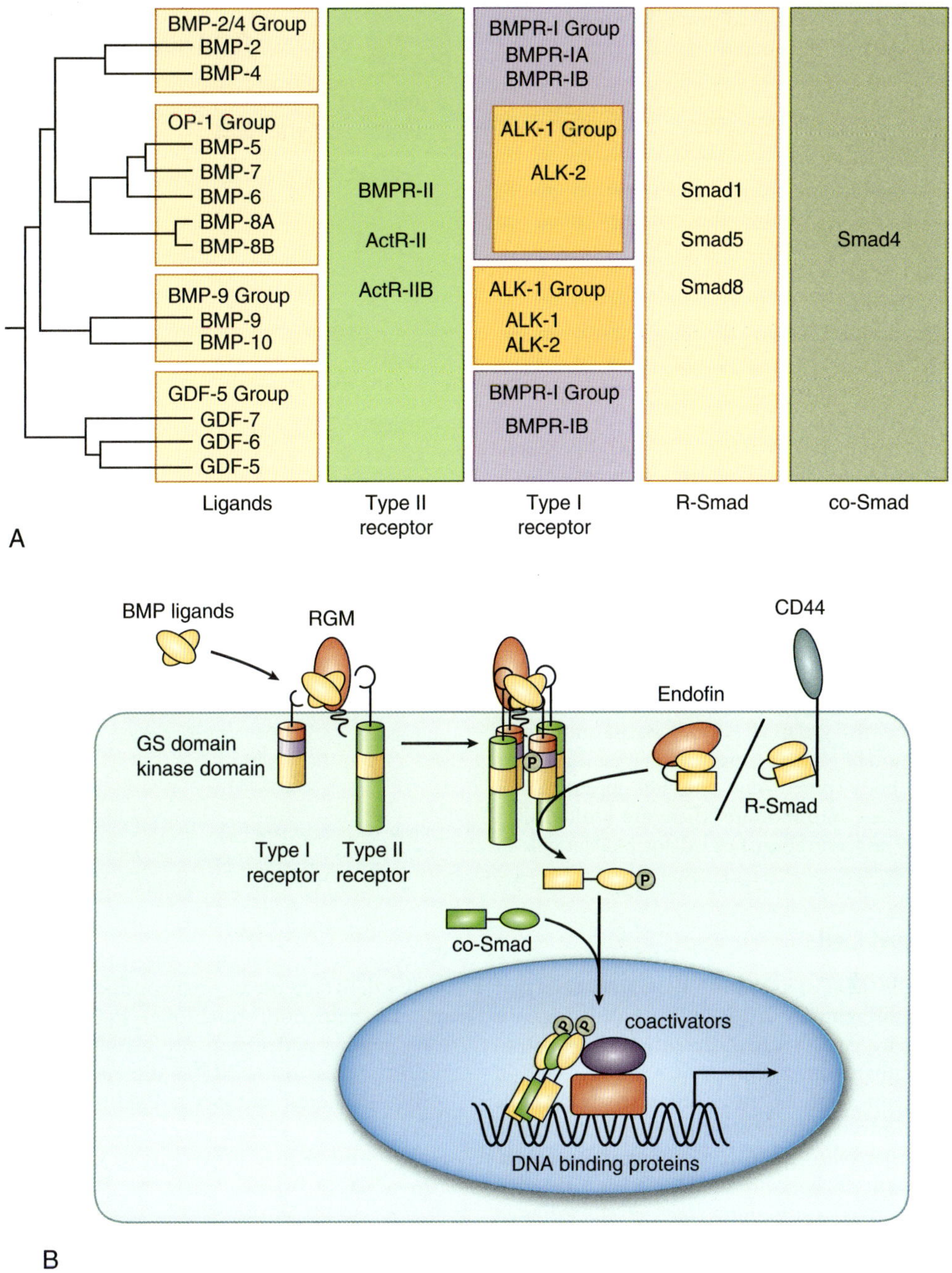

• **Fig. 17.1** Signal Transduction by BMP receptors and Smads12. **A.** Relationships between serine-threonine kinase receptors (type I and type II) and Smad proteins in signal transduction. **B.** Signaling from bone morphogenetic protein (BMP) receptors at the plasma membrane to the nucleus by Smads. *ActR,* activin receptor; *ALK,* activin receptor-like kinase; *BMPR,* bone morphogenetic protein receptor; *RGM,* receptor guidance molecule.

Early evidence demonstrated encouraging results, with increased arthrodesis rates and decreased reoperation rates when using rhBMP-2. This initial enthusiasm was subsequently tempered by a growing body of evidence elucidating potential adverse effects, including prevertebral swelling, hematoma formation, and increased cancer risk in patient exposed to rhBMP-2. Other described complications included radiculitis, heterotopic ossification, osteolysis, seroma, and retrograde ejaculation.[15] This ultimately led to an industry-sponsored clinical trial (the Yale Open Data Access project), which was led by two research groups at the University of York and Oregon Health and Science University.[16] Both groups concluded that rBMP-2 did result in high fusion rates in lumbar spine cases but demonstrated no significant difference in back pain and leg scores when compared to ICBG.

Currently, the cost-effectiveness and clinical indications for which BMP is most applicable are controversial. Identification of the proper carrier for various clinical scenarios is essential to reduce expenditures and potentially complications of recombinant proteins. Future investigations are currently underway in an effort to reduce the concentration of growth factors required for arthrodesis by improving carrier properties. Peptide amphiphile (PA) molecules, one promising alternative, are composed of nanofiber structures that mimic extracellular filaments and display biologic cues for cellular regeneration on its surface. Lee et al. developed a novel approach whereby a PA system was able to bind both endogenous and exogenous BMP-2. Using this technology in a rat model, PA with a binding affinity specific for BMP-2 led to successful fusion rates at a dose 10-fold lower than the required therapeutic dose. Moreover, a fusion rate of 42% was achieved even without the use of exogenous BMP-2.[17]

Platelet Concentrates

The release of growth factors, including platelet-derived growth factor (PDGF) and TGF-β, promote the differentiation and proliferation of mesenchymal stem cells, which can in turn enhance bone healing. As a result, methods have been developed to increase the concentrations of these growth factors from a patient's blood into autogenous growth factor (AGF) concentrates. AGFs are typically combined with thrombin and either ICBG, local autograft, or allograft. The osteoconductive capacity and lack of immunogenicity of AGFs make them an attractive option; however, harvesting does require a preoperative blood draw followed by processing, which potentially increases operative time.

Hee et al. performed a prospective study evaluating the efficacy of AGF in instrumented transforaminal lumber interbody fusions. They found no significant difference in pseudarthrosis rates between AGF/ICBG versus ICBG alone, 4% and 6%, respectively. However, they did note that AGF may facilitate faster fusions because 96% of patients in the AGF group demonstrated bony consolidation on radiographs at 6 months compared with 64% of patients in the control group ($P<.05$).[18] Based on the current evidence, the addition of platelet concentrates to autograft for posterolateral and interbody spine fusion does not appear to add any benefit to fusion rates. Furthermore, there are limited data regarding the necessary concentration needed for platelet gels to have an osteogenic effect.[19]

Mesenchymal Stem Cells

Mesenchymal stem cells (MSCs) are pluripotent stem cells that have the capacity to differentiate into multiple cell lines. In the proper environment, MSCs can differentiate into osteoblasts and promote lumbar spine fusion. MSCs can be found in bone marrow, periosteum, muscle, and adipose tissue. Autologous bone marrow aspirates (BMAs) can be harvested from the vertebral body or iliac crest. BMA lacks structural support, obviating the need for it to be combined with an appropriate carrier such as ceramics or allograft. Neen et al. evaluated the efficacy of bone marrow aspirate on a collagen/hyaluronic acid (HA) matrix compared with autograft in anterior and posterolateral spine fusions. They found equivalent fusion rates when the posterolateral approach was used, but noted BMA to be inferior to autograft for anterior interbody fusions.[20] Overall, as described by Khashan et al. in a systematic review, limited evidence exists to support the use of BMA or MSCs with synthetic or allograft materials as a substitute or as a supplement to autologous bone graft.[21]

In contrast to autogenous stem cells, data regarding the use of allogeneic mesenchymal precursor cells (MPCs) appear promising. Despite techniques that attempt to concentrate the cell component of bone marrow, producing adequate quantities of progenitor cells remains problematic. Recent advances in immunoselection have led to the isolation and purification of MPCs from donor bone marrow. In a recent ovine study, Wheeler et al. evaluated the fusion capacity of allogeneic MPCs delivered on an osteoconductive scaffold.[22] Results from manual palpation, functional radiographs, x-ray, computed tomography, and fusion site histologic analysis indicated that fusion success using MPCs did not differ from that achieved using iliac crest autograft. Additionally, regardless of dose, there was no evidence of adverse systemic or local responses. Future studies may prove this to be a viable option in spinal arthrodesis.

TABLE 17.2 Bone Graft Advantages/Disadvantages

Bone Graft	Advantages	Disadvantages
Autograft	Gold standard, biocompatible	Donor site morbidity, volume limitations
Allograft	Abundant supply, decreased antigenicity, multiple forms	Decreased osteogenic activity
DBM	Multiple forms, osteoconductive	Variable composition
rhBMP	Increased fusion rates, availability, osteoinductive	Cost, seroma, radiculitis, heterotopic ossification, osteolysis
Ceramics	Availability, lack of immunogenicity, compressive resistance	Potential brittle handling properties with low tensile strength, varying resorption
MSC	Osteogenic, easily accessible	No structural support, variability in bone marrow cellularity
Platelets	lack of immunogenicity, easily accessible	Preoperative blood draw, unclear dosing response for osteogenesis

DBM, demineralized bone matrix; *MSCs*, mesenchymal stem cells; *rhBMP*, recombinant human bone morphogenetic protein.

Conclusion

A successful spine fusion is a multifactorial process dependent on the type of bone graft selected in addition to a number of local and systemic factors that affect the healing response. Although autograft iliac crest is considered the gold standard, potential complications led to the development of a number of alternatives, each with their own advantages and disadvantages (Table 17.2). The efficacy of these materials varies widely in the literature and should be critically evaluated prior to implantation. Despite the potential added cost[23] and side effects (Table 17.3), bone graft substitutes may have a role in facilitating bony union, particularly in more stringent biologic environments such as smokers and osteoporotics. It is critical for surgeons to assess the host biologic environment and ensure that all necessary elements are present to promote bone healing.

TABLE 17.3 **Costs and Side Effects of Various Bone Grafts**

Biologic	Cost	Adverse Effects
Allograft		Infection, disease transmission, host rejection
Cancellous allograft (chips/freeze-dried)	$376/30 mL	
Cortical allograft (femoral shaft)	$530–$1,681/3–20 cm	
DBM (*Grafton/ Allomatrix*)	$726–$1,225/10 mL	Host rejection, variable composition
Ceramics		Varying resorption, potential brittle handling, low tensile strength, fracture
Calcium Sulfate (*Osteoset*)	$655/10 mL	
Calcium Phosphate (*CopiOs*)	$1520/10 mL	
Tricalcium Phosphate (*Vitoss, Orthovita*)	$875/10 mL	
rhBMPs (*Infuse*)	$3500–$4900, small-large	Ectopic bone formation, allergic reaction, prevertebral swelling, possible oncogenicity, retrograde ejaculation, seroma, osteolysis

DBM, Demineralized bone matrix; *rhBMPs*, recombinant human bone morphogenetic protein.

References

1. Branemark PI. Osseointegration and its experimental background. *J Prosthet Dent*. 1983;50:399–410.
2. Silber JS, Anderson DG, Daffner SD, et al. Donor site morbidity after anterior iliac crest bone harvest for single-level anterior cervical discectomy and fusion. *Spine (Phila Pa 1976)*. 2003;28:134–139.
3. Sasso RC, LeHuec JC, Shaffrey C, et al. Iliac crest bone graft donor site pain after anterior lumbar interbody fusion: a prospective patient satisfaction outcome assessment. *J Spinal Disord Tech*. 2005;18(suppl):S77–S81.
4. Hsu WK, Nickoli MS, Wang JC, et al. Improving the clinical evidence of bone graft substitute technology in lumbar spine surgery. *Global Spine J*. 2012;2:239–248.
5. Sengupta DK, Truumees E, Patel CK, et al. Outcome of local bone versus autogenous iliac crest bone graft in the instrumented posterolateral fusion of the lumbar spine. *Spine (Phila Pa 1976)*. 2006;31:985–991.
6. Thalgott JS, Fogarty ME, Giuffre JM, et al. A prospective, randomized, blinded, single-site study to evaluate the clinical and radiographic differences between frozen and freeze-dried allograft when used as part of a circumferential anterior lumbar interbody fusion procedure. *Spine (Phila Pa 1976)*. 2009;34:1251–1256.
7. Bae HW, Zhao L, Kanim LE, et al. Intervariability and intravariability of bone morphogenetic proteins in commercially available demineralized bone matrix products. *Spine (Phila Pa 1976)*. 2006;31:1299–1306; discussion 1307–1308.
8. Kang J, An H, Hilibrand A, et al. Grafton and local bone have comparable outcomes to iliac crest bone in instrumented single-level lumbar fusions. *Spine (Phila Pa 1976)*. 2012;37:1083–1091.
9. Thalgott JS, Giuffre JM, Klezl Z, et al. Anterior lumbar interbody fusion with titanium mesh cages, coralline hydroxyapatite, and demineralized bone matrix as part of a circumferential fusion. *Spine J*. 2002;2:63–69.
10. Jamali A, Hilpert A, Debes J, et al. Hydroxyapatite/calcium carbonate (HA/CC) vs. plaster of Paris: a histomorphometric and radiographic study in a rabbit tibial defect model. *Calcif Tissue Int*. 2002;71: 172–178.
11. Nickoli MS, Hsu WK. Ceramic-based bone grafts as a bone grafts extender for lumbar spine arthrodesis: a systematic review. *Global Spine J*. 2014;4:211–216.
12. Miyazono K, Kamiya Y, Morikawa M. Bone morphogenetic protein receptors and signal transduction. *J Biochem*. 2010;147:35–51.
13. Burkus JK, Gornet MF, Dickman CA, et al. Anterior lumbar interbody fusion using rhBMP-2 with tapered interbody cages. *J Spinal Disord Tech*. 2002;15:337–349.
14. Galimberti F, Lubelski D, Healy AT, et al. A systematic review of lumbar fusion rates with and without the use of rhBMP-2. *Spine (Phila Pa 1976)*. 2015;40:1132–1139.
15. Tannoury CA, An HS. Complications with the use of bone morphogenetic protein 2 (BMP-2) in spine surgery. *Spine J*. 2014;14: 552–559.
16. Fu R, Selph S, McDonagh M, et al. Effectiveness and harms of recombinant human bone morphogenetic protein-2 in spine fusion: a systematic review and meta-analysis. *Ann Intern Med*. 2013;158: 890–902.
17. Lee SS, Hsu EL, Mendoza M, et al. Gel scaffolds of BMP-2-binding peptide amphiphile nanofibers for spinal arthrodesis. *Adv Healthc Mater*. 2015;4:131–141.
18. Hee HT, Majd ME, Holt RT, et al. Do autologous growth factors enhance transforaminal lumbar interbody fusion? *Eur Spine J*. 2003;12:400–407.
19. Padilla S, Orive G, Sanchez M, et al. Platelet-rich plasma in orthopaedic applications: evidence-based recommendations for treatment. *J Am Acad Orthop Surg*. 2014;22:469–470.
20. Neen D, Noyes D, Shaw M, et al. Healos and bone marrow aspirate used for lumbar spine fusion: a case controlled study comparing healos with autograft. *Spine (Phila Pa 1976)*. 2006;31:E636–E640.
21. Khashan M, Inoue S, Berven SH. Cell based therapies as compared to autologous bone grafts for spinal arthrodesis. *Spine (Phila Pa 1976)*. 2013;38:1885–1891.
22. Wheeler DL, Fredericks DC, Dryer RF, et al. Allogeneic mesenchymal precursor cells (MPCs) combined with an osteoconductive scaffold to promote lumbar interbody spine fusion in an ovine model. *Spine J*. 2016;16:389–399.
23. Roberts TT, Rosenbaum AJ. Bone grafts, bone substitutes and orthobiologics: the bridge between basic science and clinical advancements in fracture healing. *Organogenesis*. 2012;8:114–124.

18

Integrated Screw/Plate Interbody Fusion Devices

VINCENT J. ALENTADO AND MICHAEL P. STEINMETZ

Introduction

The goals of an interbody fusion device is to restore disk height, create or maintain segmental lordosis, maintain sagittal balance, and restore weight bearing to the anterior column while bony fusion develops. Numerous cage options exist, including cages that require posterior fixation, stand-alone cages without integrated fixation devices, and stand-alone cages integrated with screws and/or anterior plates for fixation.

Interbody cages that require posterior fixation often result in higher fusion rates than stand-alone interbody cages, except those described with LT cages and bone morphogenetic protein-2 (BMP-2, Medtronic, Memphis, TN). However, the additional fixation may result in increased surgical morbidity and approach-related complications. Therefore, there has recently been an increased interest in stand-alone interbody cages.

Although stand-alone cages decrease the additional morbidity associated with additional posterior fixation, biomechanical studies have demonstrated that stand-alone interbody cages without any type of fixation are weakest in sheer strength and do not adequately increase stiffness in axial rotation or extension prior to the development of bony fusion. The absence of rigid fixation may impair fusion rates. Although additional anterior plating devices are effective, they require increased exposure and have a large anterior profile, which may result in soft tissue and vessel injury.

In order to obtain the benefits of a single-approach and negate the exposure necessary for additional plating devices, interbody devices with integrated bone fixation have been developed. These devices are generally composed of a polyetheretherketone (PEEK) interbody cage with three or four integrated locking screws that thread through the cage and into the adjacent inferior and superior vertebral bodies. This addition has minimized the occurrence of anterior migration and has increased biomechanical stiffness, theoretically increasing capacity for fusion.

In this chapter, we discuss the currently available integrated interbody devices from both a biomechanical and clinical perspective.

Anterior Lumbar Interbody Fusion

Most integrated interbody devices have been developed for the anterior lumbar interbody fusion (ALIF) technique. After surgery, both initial vertebral segment stability and loading transmission of the ALIF device play essential roles in the rate of fusion and development of adjacent level pathology. ALIF reinforces and stabilizes the anterior column, restores disk and foraminal height, and increases segmental lordosis.

Before the development of integrated interbody cages, stand-alone cages were kept in place by compressive forces of the spine. However, implantation of an interbody device during ALIF necessitates cutting the anterior longitudinal ligament, which is a major stabilizer in extension movements. Without this anterior tension band, the superior vertebral body may "lift off" of a nonintegrated interbody device in extension movements. The lack of rotational stiffness supplied by nonintegrated interbody devices allows for similar movements. To address the need for restoration of the anterior tension band, stand-alone cages with intrinsic plates and screws have been developed (Fig. 18.1)

The clinical summaries of stuides utilizing integrated ALIF are listed in Table 18.1.

SynFix-LR

The SynFix-LR (DePuy Synthes, West Chester, PA) integrated ALIF cage is the most studied integrated interbody cage to date. The device consists of a trapezoid PEEK interbody cage with an integrated anterior titanium alloy stabilization plate and four titanium alloy fix-angled screws that lock into the superior and inferior endplates. The device and integrated screws and plate are entirely within the disk space, minimizing the anterior footprint needed during exposure.

Several studies have investigated the biomechanical properties of the SynFix-LR device. Schleicher et al.[1] found that the SynFix-LR device significantly decreased range of motion (ROM) in extension, flexion, lateral bending, and axial rotation compared to an intact spine. Cain and colleagues[2] noted the same biomechanical advantages and also found a decreased neutral zone and elastic zone in the involved intervertebral segment in comparison to an intact spine. In contrast, the authors found that an anterior interbody cage without integrated screws, but with the addition of posterior transarticular facet screws, did not significantly reduce ROM, neutral zone, or elastic zone in extension or axial rotation. However, the authors did note that there was more stability in spines with the SynFix-LR device and transarticular facet screws compared with the SynFix-LR device only, but this was not statistically significant. Similarly, the SynFix-LR device was statistically equivalent to an anterior interbody cage with posterior pedicle

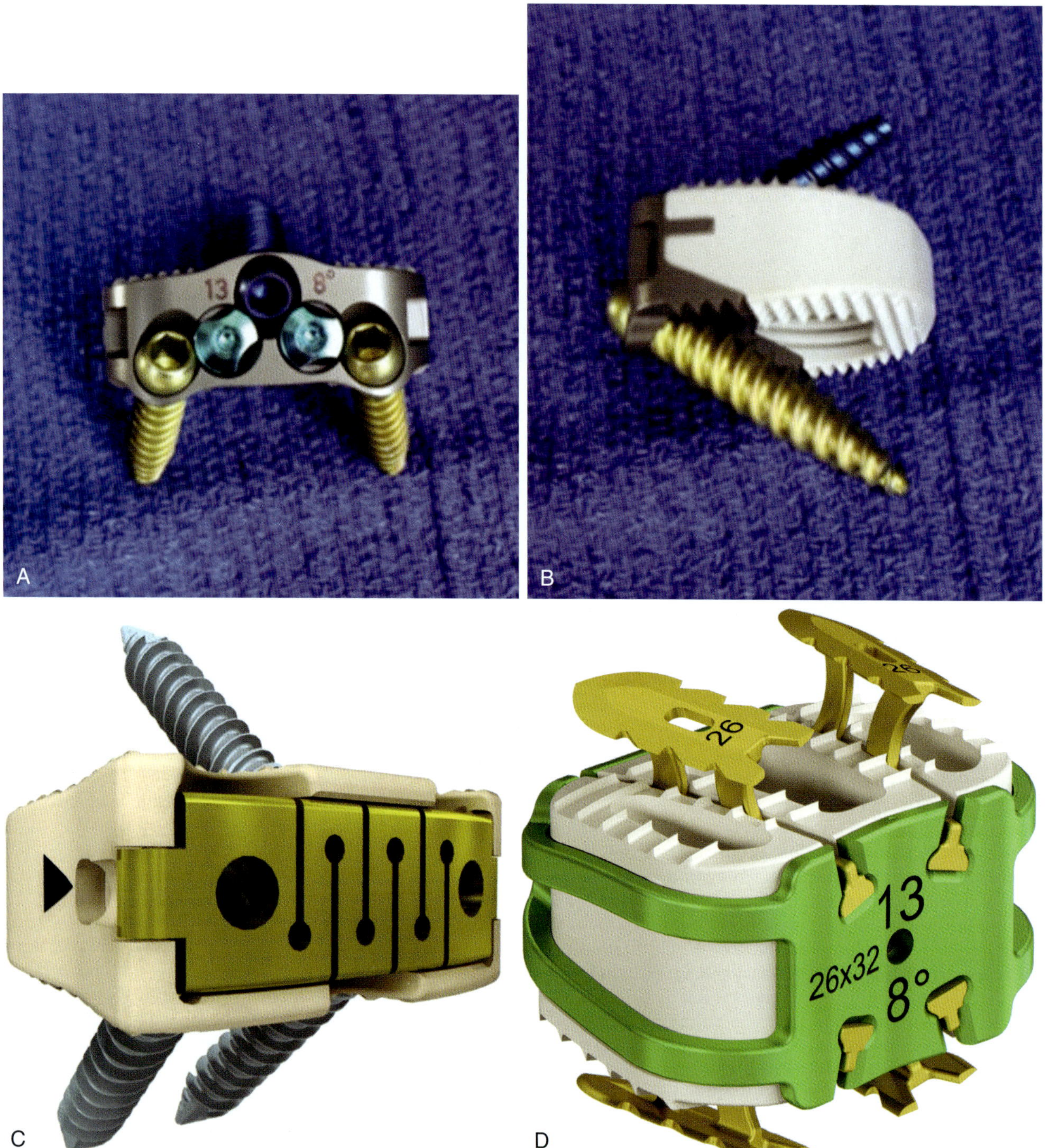

• **Fig. 18.1** **A.** The Globus Independence anterior lumbar interbody fusion implant permits the placement of three screws into the vertebral body. The device may be rotated 360 degrees to accommodate local anatomy. Specifically, one screw may be placed rostral and two caudal or it may be rotated for two to be placed rostral and one caudal. The screws are locked to the plate with locking screws. Parallel and lordotic implants are available. **B.** A large space is available for bone graft to be placed inside the device. **C.** Anchor L from Stryker Spine. Similar to Globus Independence, it was one screw rostral or caudal and two screws opposite. It may be rotated to accommodate either screw strategy. It too has an appropriate size hole in the middle of the polyetheretherketone (PEEK) to accommodate bone graft material; it comes in a number of lengths, widths, and parallel and lordotic implants. This implant offers a plate that locks across the front of the implant to prevent screw back out. **D.** Stryker Aero AL. This PEEK integrated implant is unique in its locking mechanism. Once the PEEK graft has been placed in the interbody space, four individual anchors are impacted through a groove in the graft and into the vertebral body.

TABLE 18.1 Clinical Studies Featuring Integrated ALIF Devices

Device	Author	Study Design	Patients (*N*)	Follow-up	Graft substrate	Fusion rate	Outcome	Pertinent Notes
SynFix-LR	Seipe et al.	Prospective	71	Minimum 12 months	PEEK	97.3%	Significant improvement in VAS and ODI	Segmental lordosis improvement 16.1 to 26.7 2 cases required revision surgery
	Cho et al.	Retrospective	28	Mean 27.3 months	PEEK	86.7%	Significant improvement in VAS back and Leg and ODI	SynFix vs. Stabilis Only SynFix-LR maintained disk and foraminal height over follow-up time
	Strube et al.	Prospective	80	Mean 47 months	PEEK	70.6%	Significant improvement in VAS, ODI	SynFix-LR compared to ALIF and pedicle screws Higher satisfaction rate, less blood loss and shorter OR time in SynFix LR
	Schimmel et al.	Retrospective	95	Mean 47.7 months	PEEK	76%	ODI improvement after initial surgery, but less improvement after revision	
	Behrbalk et al.	Retrospective	25	Mean 16.7 months	PEEK plus BMP-2	90.6%	None	15.6% graft subsidence at 16.7 months
STALIF	McCarthy et al.	Retrospective	85	Mean 19 months	PEEK	65%	None	STAFLIF vs. ALIF and pedicle screws 23% single level 60% dual level had nonunion
ROI-A								
	Allain et al.	Prospective	65	12 months	PEEK	96.3%	Significant improvement in VAS, ODI and SF-36	Cage subsidence, one requiring post instrumentation, one have persistent L5 paresthesia, one having migration of the superior plate
	Flouzat-Lachaniette	Retrospective	51	12 months	PEEK Iliac crest autograft vs. rhBMP-2	88.7% in ICAG; 71% in BMP-2	Not reported	
Hartshill Horshoe	Madan et al.	Retrospective	56	Mean 36 months	Titanium plus ICAG	100%	85.2% satisfied	No subsidence over 3 years 85.2% satisfied one patient with postoperative sciatica owing to screw impingement

BMP-2, bone morphogenetic protein-2; *ODI,* oswestry disability index; *PEEK,* polyetheretherketone; *VAS,* visual analogue score.

screws. In agreement with the aforementioned study, Choi et al.[3] also found that SynFix-LR had a similar ROM compared with an anterior interbody cage with posterior pedicle screw fixation. The authors noted that the SynFix-LR device also resulted in a similar decrease in ROM of superior and inferior vertebral segments, although the SynFix-LR did cause more same-level facet strain compared with the anterior cage with pedicle screws. Interestingly, the anterior cage with pedicle screws caused more facet strain at adjacent-level facet joints compared with the SynFix-LR device. Furthermore, SynFix-LR had a more anatomic load distribution, whereas the combined anterior-posterior approach resulted in a more posterior load distribution compared with an intact spine.

Multiple studies have compared SynFix-LR with the Stabilis (Stryker, Kalamazoo, MI) interbody device. Stabilis is an earlier, nonintegrated, stand-alone ALIF device consisting of a titanium cage shaped as a threaded cylinder that anchors to the adjacent vertebral bodies owing to the compressive forces of the spine. Chen et al.[4] found that the SynFix-LR device had more stability than Stabilis in flexion/ extension, lateral bending, and axial rotation in both osteoporotic and normal bone. Furthermore, SynFix-LR caused less stress and more even stress distribution on the annulus in all motions compared to Stabilis. Furthermore, SynFix-LR caused less facet joint contact force in extension and axial rotation. Notably, the authors determined that restriction of ROM was decreased by an average of 15.9% when using the SynFix-LR device in osteoporotic compared to normal bone, with most noticeable decreases occurring during extension. The authors stated that the device might be better suited for younger patients and those with a higher bone density.

In addition to the aforementioned biomechanical studies investigating SynFix-LR, multiple studies have examined clinical outcomes with the device. Siepe et al.[5] found that patients treated with stand-alone SynFix-LR had significantly improved visual analogue scale (VAS) and Oswestry Disability Index (ODI) scores at mean follow-up of 35.1 months. Overall, 77.5% (55/71) patients reported satisfaction with their procedure. The authors noted that segmental lordosis significantly increased from 16.1 degrees preoperatively to 26.7 degrees postoperatively. Fusion was achieved in 36/37 (97.3%) of cases with adequate radiographic follow-up. One patient required revision operation for back pain, two patients had a postoperative S1 radiculopathy, and one patient had a transient L5 radiculopathy.

Cho et al.[6] retrospectively studied 28 patients who received L5-S1 ALIF using Stabilis or SynFix-LR for the treatment of lumbar intervertebral foraminal stenosis. Clinical outcomes were similar between devices with both devices demonstrating improved ODI, VAS back, and VAS leg pain scores at average 27.3-month follow-up. However, the authors noted that, although both devices caused a significant increase in disk height and intervertebral foraminal height in the immediate postoperative period, only the SynFix-LR device maintained these improvements over the follow-up period.

Strube et al.[7] prospectively compared outcomes in 40 patients receiving stand-alone SynFix-LR with 40 patients receiving ALIF with transpedicular fixation. The authors found that VAS and ODI scores were significantly improved in both groups but significantly better in the SynFix-LR group at 12-month follow-up. Furthermore, the SynFix-LR group had a significantly higher satisfaction rate, less blood loss, and shorter operative time than the ALIF with transpedicular fixation group. Fusion rates were similar between groups.

In contrast to the excellent outcomes in the aforementioned studies, Schimmel et al.[8] investigated 95 patients treated with SynFix-LR and reported 26 (27%) patients required reoperation at average follow-up of 47.7 months. Most of the reoperations were for symptomatic pseudoarthrosis. The authors noted that the average ODI scores significantly improved after the initial operation, but that reoperation equated to worsened outcomes. The authors proposed that the lower stiffness and hydrophobic characteristics of PEEK lead to insufficient initial stability, thus creating suboptimal conditions for bony bridging with stand-alone SynFix-LR cages. In contrast, Behrbalk and colleages[9] investigated outcomes in patients operated on with SynFix-LR and supplemental recombinant human bone morphogenic protein-2 (rhBMP-2) and found a 90.6% fusion rate in 32 levels receiving stand-alone SynFix-LR. Five patients (15.6%) demonstrated graft subsidence at mean follow-up of 16.7 months. Of these, three resulted in nonunion that required revision operation. However, no patient had rhBMP-2-related complications.

Multiple studies have reported device-related complications with the SynFix-LR. Thaler et al.[10] reported two cases of postoperative bleeding from the right and left inferior epigastric arteries occurring from using SynFix-LR at the L5-S1 level. The authors stated that the divergent screws required more extensive mobilization, and thereby injury, of surrounding structures compared with standard ALIF without plate addition. Furthermore, Lastfogel et al.[11] reported three incidences of sacral fracture after L5-S1 ALIF with SynFix-LR for the treatment of isthmic spondylolisthesis. All three cases occurred within 45 days of the operation. The authors noted that there is an axial compression force perpendicular to the sacral endplate and a shear force parallel to it. Additionally, the sloping face of the sacral endplate results in the SynFix-LR implant being oriented such that the superior screws are in the coronal plane and the inferior screws lie in the axial plane. In this configuration, the inferior endplates take on an axial load perpendicular to the screw insertion, which may result in sacral fracture. Kwon et al.[12] reported a vertebral fracture of the L4 vertebral body after fusion of the L3-4 level for degenerative spondylolisthesis with the SynFix-LR device. The authors believed that instability from the degenerative facet joints led to excessive compression and shear load anteriorly, resulting in failure of the cage. The authors recommended additional pedicle screw fixation for patients requiring operation for degenerative spondylolisthesis.

Stalif

Two studies have investigated the Stalif (Surgicraft Ltd., Redditch, UK) ALIF interbody device. Stalif is composed of a PEEK interbody cage with spaces for nonintegrated screws. In a biomechanical study, Schleicher and colleagues[1] found that Stalif was statistically similar to SynFix-LR during extension, flexion, and axial rotation, but that SynFix-LR created more rigidity during these movements. Furthermore, the authors found that lateral bending was significantly more rigid with the SynFix-LR device.

McCarthy et al.[13] investigated 37 patients receiving ALIF with the Stabilis device and found that 5/22 (23%) patients receiving single-level and 9/15 (60%) patients receiving two-level ALIFs with the device had pseudoarthrosis, whereas fusion occurred in all 30 patients who received an ALIF cage with posterior pedicle screws.

ROI-A

Multiple studies have investigated the ROI-A (LDR Medical, Troyes, France) integrated ALIF device. The ROI-A device consists of a PEEK cage with an intracorporeal locking system (VerteBRDIGE, LDR Medical). The proposed advantage of this locking system is that it requires less exposure than cages with integrated bone screws, which necessitate high-angle trajectories for insertion.

Freeman et al.[14] investigated biomechanics of the ROI-A integrated cage and found that it significantly reduced motion in flexion-extension and lateral bending compared with an intact spine. However, there was no significant increase in rigidity in axial torsion. Additionally, the authors found that the deployment of the integrated plates did not significantly add to rigidity of the cage. Furthermore, addition of pedicle screws and rods decreased motion significantly in all planes compared with ROI-A alone.

Allain et al.[15] investigated the ROI-A and found that 52/54 (96.3%) of patients achieved fusion at 1 year. Furthermore, ODI scores improved significantly at 12-month follow-up with 88.7% of patients reporting satisfaction with their surgery and 80.4% stating that they would have the surgery again. Cage-related complications included one patient having migration of the superior plate, one demonstrating cage subsidence, one requiring additional posterior instrumentation, and one having persistent L5 parasthesias postoperatively.

Flouzat-Lachaniette et al.[16] investigated rhBMP-2 compared with autologous iliac crest bone graft in patients receiving ALIF with the ROI-A device and found that 88.7% of patients receiving iliac bone graft achieved fusion, whereas only 71.0% of patients receiving rhBMP-2 achieved fusion ($P = .001$). Furthermore, the bone quality was significantly better in patients receiving iliac bone graft, as there was a central void in 98.1% of fusions receiving rhBMP-2 compared with only 44.4% of fusions receiving iliac bone.

Other Integrated ALIF Devices

Multiple studies have reported on numerous other integrated ALIF devices. Most of these studies have investigated PEEK cages with integrated screws for fixation.

Voronov et al.[17] researched the PILLAR SA (Orthofix, Lewisville, TX) integrated PEEK ALIF device and found that the integrated cage decreased flexion, extension, lateral bending, and axial rotation compared with intact spinal segments with a physiologic preload of 400 N. However, the addition of bilateral pedicle screws and rods reduced the motion significantly more. Furthermore, the authors found that a 360-degree fusion consisting of an ALIF cage with posterior instrumentation was more rigid than the PILLAR SA device alone in flexion, extension, and lateral bending. However, axial rotation was similar between groups.

Similarly, Kornblum et al.[18] investigated an integrated PEEK ALIF cage, the Brigade Standalone ALIF System (NuVasive, Inc., San Diego, CA). Biomechanical testing determined that the addition of three integrated screws to the Brigade device provided more stability than the device without screws. A fourth screw did not add significant stiffness to the construct. Furthermore, the device demonstrated equivalent stability to an ALIF construct with supplemental posterior fixation in lateral bending and axial rotation. However, the Brigade system with integrated screw fixation allowed more flexion/extension than an ALIF cage with additional anterior plate fixation and an ALIF cage with additional pedicle screw fixation. In addition, the authors determined that adding a spinous process plate to the integrated cage provided the most rigid construct in flexion and extension, although this was statistically similar to a nonintegrated ALIF cage with bilateral pedicle screw fixation. Furthermore, ALIF with pedicle screw fixation decreased lateral bending more than the integrated cage with additional spinous process plating, although the two groups had a statistically similar decrease in axial rotation.

In another biomechanical study of an integrated PEEK ALIF device, Drazin et al.[19] demonstrated that the Independence (Globus Medical, Inc., Audubon, PA) integrated device was superior to an anterior spacer with posterior pedicle screws and an anterior graft with anterior tension band plate and screws. The integrated spacers demonstrated no subsidence, but rather at the bone-screw interface. The authors believed this superior outcome was owing to the angulation of the screws that were inserted at 30 degrees to 45 degrees of the endplate as opposed to parallel. Therefore, these screws must actually tear bone to fail. The authors noted a decreased stiffness with increasing sacral slope and suggested a stand-alone not be used for sacral slopes greater than 40 degrees.

Beaubien et al.[20] researched an investigational PEEK cage with screw integration and found that the device decreased ROM in flexion/extension, lateral bending, and axial torsion compared with an intact spine. The greatest contribution of the integrated screws was in limiting torsional motion and pullout. The authors found that the investigational device was similar to threaded titanium cages, but better resisted anterior displacement.

One author investigated another integrated PEEK ALIF device with a novel fixation system. Yeager et al.[21] researched the Solus PEEK interbody cage with integrated counter-rotating fixation blades (Alphatec Spine, Carlsbad, CA). They found that the integrated device with additional interspinous process clamp significantly reduced lateral bending and axial torsion, whereas a nonintegrated PEEK interbody cage with interspinous process clamp did not.

In previously mentioned study, Chen et al.[4] also investigated the Latero (A-Spine ASIA, Taipei, Taiwan) integrated ALIF device, which consists of a lateral vertebral plate that is bent in the coronal plane to fixate a titanium trapezoid cage. The authors found that Latero had a similar ROM restriction to a nonintegrated ALIF cage with posterior pedicle screw instrumentation. Furthermore, Latero caused superior rigidity in flexion and extension when compared with the SynFix-LR integrated cage. However, Latero was similar to SynFix-LR in bilateral axial rotation and left lateral bending, while being less rigid in right lateral bending. The discrepancy seen in lateral bending is caused by the asymmetric design of the Latero model and the fact that the vertebral plate is inserted on the left side. The authors also noted a decreased spinal stiffness in osteoporotic bone when using Latero, which was especially prevalent in right lateral bending. In addition, the Latero device created minimal annulus stress that was superior to the SynFix-LR device in flexion and extension, and similar to an ALIF cage with posterior instrumentation in all ROM. Furthermore, the Latero device distributed little force to the same-level facet joints in extension, and facet contact force was similar to SynFix-LR in bilateral axial rotation. Notably, the superior endplate of the Latero model was more stressed than all other models in axial rotation, possibly owing to the smaller contact surface of the Latero cage. Additionally, the SynFix-LR device created higher stress on the screw fixation than the Latero device created on the fixation plates in all motions.

Another author investigated a separate integrated titanium ALIF device. Madan et al.[22] studied 29 patients with the Hartshill Horseshoe cage, which is stabilized by inserting screws through holes in the implant. All patients achieved fusion with no implants demonstrating subsidence over an average follow-up of 3.0 years. Furthermore, 23 (85.2%) patients were satisfied with their surgical outcome. One patient did suffer from postoperative sciatica owing to screw impingement.

Femoral ring allografts (FRAs) are commonly used alternatives to synthetic interbody devices. They are vertical rings that incorporate into the fusion mass over time. In an attempt to gain the benefits of an integrated device in the cheaper FRA, Kuzhupilly et al.[23] performed a biomechanical study investigating FRAs (Musculoskeletal Transplant Foundation, Edison, NJ) with and without integrated crossed anterior screws. The authors found that intact spines had stiffer flexion compared with the integrated construct while being statistically similar to the FRAs without screws. However, the integrated FRA was stiffer in extension compared with the screw-less FRA. Lateral bending motion was similar between the integrated FRA, the FRA without screws, and the intact specimens. Conversely, torsion was stiffer in the integrated and nonintegrated FRAs when compared with intact spines.

Lateral Interbody Fusion

The eXtreme lateral interbody fusion (XLIF) technique is among the newest interbody fusion techniques. The XLIF approach allows for abundant disk removal and placement of a large stable interbody implant at the apophyseal ring where the bone is strongest. Furthermore, this approach allows for retention of the anterior longitudinal ligaments and annulus and provides a large fusion surface area. As this is a relatively new technique, integrated interbody devices are limited.

Integrated Lateral Devices (Fig. 18.2)

To date, only two studies have investigated integrated lateral integrated devices. Basra et al.[24] investigated a novel lateral interbody implant consisting of a PEEK spacer with an integrated titanium plate and two hydroxyapatite-coated titanium bone screws. The authors found that stability with the device was increased in flexion/extension, lateral bending, and axial rotation compared with an intact spine. The addition of unilateral pedicle screws and rod did not significantly add to stiffness. However, the addition of bilateral pedicle screws and rods significantly added to stability in flexion/extension. In contrast, the addition of bilateral facet screws

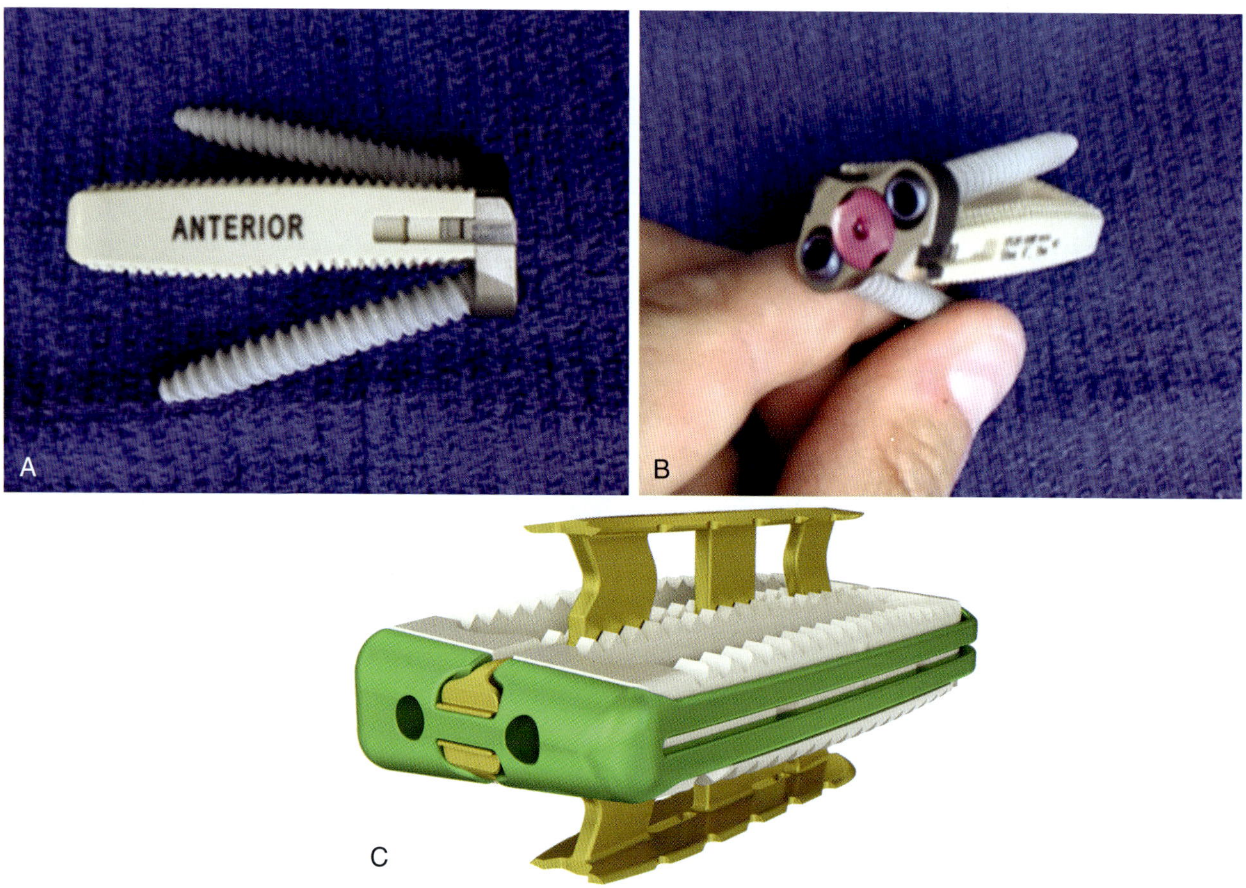

• **Fig. 18.2** A-B. The Globus Intercontinental lateral integrated implant comes in a large variety of lengths, widths, and segmental angulation (lordosis). Two screws are placed into the integrated plate and vertebral body. One screw is placed anterior and one posterior. The screws are locked to the plate with locking screws. This may permit placement of the device at levels where existing pedicle screws have already been placed. Hydroxyapetite screws are available for this implant. **C.** The Aero LL implant from Stryker is a combination PEEK and ring of titanium surrounding the implant. It comes is a variety of lengths, widths, and degrees lordosis. Once impacted in place, two anchors, one rostral and one caudal, are impacted through a groove in the implant into the vertebral body to lock it in place.

to the XLIF device significantly reduced ROM in flexion/extension and axial rotation.

In the aforementioned study by Freeman et al.,[14] the authors also investigated the ROI-A Oblique (LDR Medical) device and found it did not significantly decrease motion compared with intact spinal segments in flexion/extension or lateral bending, and it increased motion in axial torsion owing to incision of the annulus during device placement. However, no significant difference in rigidity was found between the ROI-A Oblique cage and the ROI-A ALIF cage. Similarly to the ROI-A ALIF cage, there was no significant difference in spinal segment rigidity when the integrated plates were deployed on the ROI-A Oblique model. However, the addition of pedicle screws and rods decreased motion significantly in all planes.

TLIF

Integrated transforaminal lumbar interbody fusion (TLIF) cages have not gained as much of an appeal as integrated ALIF or XLIF cages because the insertion point of fixation devices is in the center of the vertebral body where the bone is weakest. In addition, this positioning creates a small lever arm for resisting motion.

Integrated TLIF Devices

Owing to the inherent limitations of integrated TLIF devices, studies are lacking. However, Keiler et al.[25] investigated a prototype steel TLIF cage (DePuy Synthes, West Chester, PA), which can be secured to the adjacent cranial and caudal endplates by two fixation screws. The stand-alone TLIF cage, with and without integrated screw fixation, did not reduce ROM in lateral bending or flexion/extension compared with an intact spine. Furthermore, in axial rotation, the stand-alone TLIF cage resulted in a significant increase in ROM compared to an intact state. However, the placement of integrated screws resulted in significant reduction in lateral bending and flexion/extension compared with the device without screws, but there was no difference in axial rotation.

Conclusion

Numerous integrated interbody cages are available for lumbar spinal surgery. Many of these devices achieve adequate restoration of disk height, segmental lordosis, and restoration of physiologic weight bearing, which are goals for any interbody device. Furthermore, these devices have the benefit of a single approach and negate the need for additional plating and fixation devices. Future devices will continue to improve on the utility of the integrated interbody cages presented herein.

References

1. Schleicher P, Gerlach R, Schär B, et al. Biomechanical comparison of two different concepts for stand alone anterior lumbar interbody fusion. *Eur Spine J.* 2008;17(12):1757–1765. https://doi.org/10.1007/s00586-008-0797-4.
2. Cain CMJ, Schleicher P, Gerlach R, et al. A new stand-alone anterior lumbar interbody fusion device: biomechanical comparison with established fixation techniques. *Spine (Phila Pa 1976).* 2005;30(23):2631–2636.
3. Choi K-C, Ryu K-S, Lee S-H, et al. Biomechanical comparison of anterior lumbar interbody fusion: stand-alone interbody cage versus interbody cage with pedicle screw fixation—a finite element analysis. *BMC Musculoskelet Disord.* 2013;14(1):220. https://doi.org/10.1186/1471-2474-14-220.
4. Chen S-H, Chiang M-C, Lin J-F, et al. Biomechanical comparison of three stand-alone lumbar cages—a three-dimensional finite element analysis. *BMC Musculoskelet Disord.* 2013;14:281. https://doi.org/10.1186/1471-2474-14-281.
5. Siepe CJ, Stosch-Wiechert K, Heider F, et al. Anterior stand-alone fusion revisited: a prospective clinical, X-ray and CT investigation. *Eur Spine J.* 2015;24(4):838–851. https://doi.org/10.1007/s00586-014-3642-y.
6. Cho C-B, Ryu K-S, Park C-K. Anterior lumbar interbody fusion with stand-alone interbody cage in treatment of lumbar intervertebral foraminal stenosis: comparative study of two different types of cages. *J Korean Neurosurg Soc.* 2010;47(5):352–357. https://doi.org/10.3340/jkns.2010.47.5.352.
7. Strube P, Hoff E, Hartwig T, et al. Stand-alone anterior versus anteroposterior lumbar interbody single-level fusion after a mean follow-up of 41 months. *J Spinal Disord Tech.* 2012;25(7):362–369. https://doi.org/10.1097/BSD.0b013e3182263d91.
8. Schimmel JJP, Poeschmann MS, Horsting PP, et al. PEEK cages in lumbar fusion: mid-term clinical outcome and radiologic fusion. *Clin Spine Surg.* 2016;29:E252–E258. https://doi.org/10.1097/BSD.0b013e31826eaf74.
9. Behrbalk E, Uri O, Parks RM, et al. Fusion and subsidence rate of stand alone anterior lumbar interbody fusion using PEEK cage with recombinant human bone morphogenetic protein-2. *Eur Spine J.* 2013;22(12):2869–2875. https://doi.org/10.1007/s00586-013-2948-5.
10. Thaler M, Mayr E, Liebensteiner M, et al. Injury of the right and left inferior epigastric artery during the implantation of a stand-alone ALIF cage through a left retroperitoneal approach: a case report. *Arch Orthop Trauma Surg.* 2010;130(1):31–35. https://doi.org/10.1007/s00402-009-0848-2.
11. Lastfogel JF, Altstadt TJ, Rodgers RB, et al. Sacral fractures following stand-alone L5-S1 anterior lumbar interbody fusion for isthmic spondylolisthesis. *J Neurosurg Spine.* 2010;13(2):288–293. https://doi.org/10.3171/2010.3.SPINE09366.
12. Kwon Y-K, Jang J-H, Lee C-D, et al. Fracture of the L-4 vertebral body after use of a stand-alone interbody fusion device in degenerative spondylolisthesis for anterior L3-4 fixation. *J Neurosurg Spine.* 2014;20(6):653–656. https://doi.org/10.3171/2014.3.SPINE121018.
13. McCarthy MJH, Ng L, Vermeersch G, et al. A radiological comparison of anterior fusion rates in anterior lumbar interbody fusion. *Glob Spine J.* 2012;2(4):195–206. https://doi.org/10.1055/s-0032-1329892.
14. Freeman AL, Camisa WJ, Buttermann GR, et al. Flexibility and fatigue evaluation of oblique as compared with anterior lumbar interbody cages with integrated endplate fixation. *J Neurosurg Spine.* 2016;24(1):54–59. https://doi.org/10.3171/2015.4.SPINE14948.
15. Allain J, Delecrin J, Beaurain J, et al. Stand-alone ALIF with integrated intracorporeal anchoring plates in the treatment of degenerative lumbar disc disease: a prospective study on 65 cases. *Eur Spine J.* 2014;23(10):2136–2143. https://doi.org/10.1007/s00586-014-3364-1.
16. Flouzat-Lachaniette C-H, Ghazanfari A, Bouthors C, et al. Bone union rate with recombinant human bone morphogenic protein-2 versus autologous iliac bone in PEEK cages for anterior lumbar interbody fusion. *Int Orthop.* 2014;38(9):2001–2007. https://doi.org/10.1007/s00264-014-2301-6.
17. Voronov LI, Vastardis G, Zelenakova J, et al. Biomechanical characteristics of an integrated lumbar interbody fusion device. *Int J Spine Surg.* 2014;8. https://doi.org/10.14444/1001.
18. Kornblum MB, Turner AWL, Cornwall GB, et al. Biomechanical evaluation of stand-alone lumbar polyether-ether-ketone interbody cage with integrated screws. *Spine J.* 2013;13(1):77–84. https://doi.org/10.1016/j.spinee.2012.11.013.
19. Drazin D, Hussain M, Harris J, et al. The role of sacral slope in lumbosacral fusion: a biomechanical study. *J Neurosurg Spine.* 2015;23(6):754–762. https://doi.org/10.3171/2015.3.SPINE14557.

20. Beaubien BP, Freeman AL, Turner JL, et al. Evaluation of a lumbar intervertebral spacer with integrated screws as a stand-alone fixation device. *J Spinal Disord Tech*. 2010;23(5):351–358. https://doi.org/10.1097/BSD.0b013e3181b15d00.
21. Yeager MS, Dupre DA, Cook DJ, et al. Anterior lumbar interbody fusion with integrated fixation and adjunctive posterior stabilization: a comparative biomechanical analysis. *Clin Biomech (Bristol, Avon)*. 2015;30(8):769–774. https://doi.org/10.1016/j.clinbiomech.2015.06.015.
22. Madan SS, Harley JM, Boeree NR. Anterior lumbar interbody fusion: does stable anterior fixation matter? *Eur Spine J*. 2003;12(4):386–392. https://doi.org/10.1007/s00586-003-0543-x.
23. Kuzhupilly RR, Lieberman IH, McLain RF, et al. In vitro stability of FRA spacers with integrated crossed screws for anterior lumbar interbody fusion. *Spine (Phila Pa 1976)*. 2002;27(9):923–928.
24. Basra S, Bucklen B, Muzumdar A, et al. A novel lateral lumbar integrated plate-spacer interbody implant: in vitro biomechanical analysis. *Spine J*. 2015;15(2):322–328. https://doi.org/10.1016/j.spinee.2014.09.020.
25. Keiler A, Schmoelz W, Erhart S, et al. Primary stiffness of a modified transforaminal lumbar interbody fusion cage with integrated screw fixation: cadaveric biomechanical study. *Spine (Phila Pa 1976)*. 2014;39(17):E994–E1000. https://doi.org/10.1097/BRS.0000000000000422.

19

Spinous Process Plates for Lumbar Fixation

VINCENT J. ALENTADO AND MICHAEL P. STEINMETZ

Introduction

Lumbar interbody fusion is indicated in the treatment of many degenerative lumbar spinal disorders such as spinal stenosis, spondylolisthesis, trauma, and diskogenic pain of the lumbar spine. Successful outcomes after lumbar interbody fusion are dependent, in large part, on the development of bony fusion. Several operative approaches are commonly used to access the anterior column for interbody fusion, including posterior lumbar interbody fusion (PLIF), transforaminal lumbar interbody fusion (TLIF), anterior lumbar interbody fusion (ALIF), and eXtreme lateral interbody fusion (XLIF).

The interbody cage is often supplemented by posterior internal fixation to increase early postoperative mechanical stiffness and facilitate development of bony fusion. The choice of fixation method is driven by many factors, including presence of instability, bone quality, activity level of the patient, and previous interventions. Bilateral trans-pedicle screw constructs are currently the gold standard for supplemental internal fixation of lumbar interbody fusion. Pedicle screws provide multiplanar stability and have the longest clinical history in supplementing fusion. However, transpedicular fixation is associated with risks. Cerebrospinal fluid leakage (4% of patients), transient neurapraxia (2%), permanent nerve root injury (2%), deep wound infection (4% to 5%), and hardware failure (3% to 12%) are all commonly reported complications after transpedicular fixation.[1,2] Furthermore, some authors have theorized that an increase in adjacent-level intervertebral disk pressures secondary to destabilization from transpedicular fixation may be a leading contributor toward the development of adjacent segment degeneration.[3]

In contrast to the relatively high rates of complications and adverse outcomes after transpedicular fixation, spinous process fixation through plating increases stability at a reduced risk. Furthermore, spinous process plates (SPPs) may be placed with patients in the same lateral decubitus position used for some interbody procedures, avoiding the need for repositioning such as would be required with supplemental transpedicular fixation. Additionally, spinous process plating potentially shortens operative times, decreases blood loss, and reduces fluoroscopic exposure to the operating room team compared with pedicle screw fixation.

Surgical Indications

The main indication for spinous process plating is to provide supplemental fixation following any type of interbody fusion (Fig. 19.1).

Limitations

There are a number of limitations with the use of spinous process plating systems. Foremost is the necessary presence of the spinous processes. This would exclude their use in most revision spine procedures and in many patients who have a traumatic fracture. Owing to the relatively small size of the S1 spinous process, it is often not possible to place these implants at L5-S1. Some implants are designed specifically to accommodate the S1 process, such as the Aspen device (Zimmer Biomet, Denver, CO) featured in the surgical technique section. Spinous process plates' use may be limited in those patients with advanced osteoporosis. In these patients, the plate may fracture or cut through the spinous process during or immediately after implantation. Consideration must also be given to the amount of fixation provided by these implants. In cases where robust fixation is needed (e.g., instability, tumor), these implants may not provide adequate stability. Lastly, it may be difficult and/or biomechanically insufficient to place these devices over multiple levels. The authors have used SPP over two levels, but never more.

Operative Technique

1. Patients are positioned prone in customary fashion on a spine table. Fluoroscopy is typically used during insertion, but not required (Fig. 19.2). The authors prefer a Jackson radiolucent table. Alternatively, patients may be placed in a lateral decubitus position. In this manner the surgeon may sit down and perform surgery looking straight ahead.
2. Following preparing and draping of the lumbar region, an incision is planned. The incision is typically slightly caudal to a typical incision planned for a laminectomy; specifically, it only is required to expose the interspinous space, which is typically slightly caudal to the disk space on lateral imaging. After an approximately 2.5- to 4-cm incision is made, the subcutaneous fat and lumbodorsal fascia are then

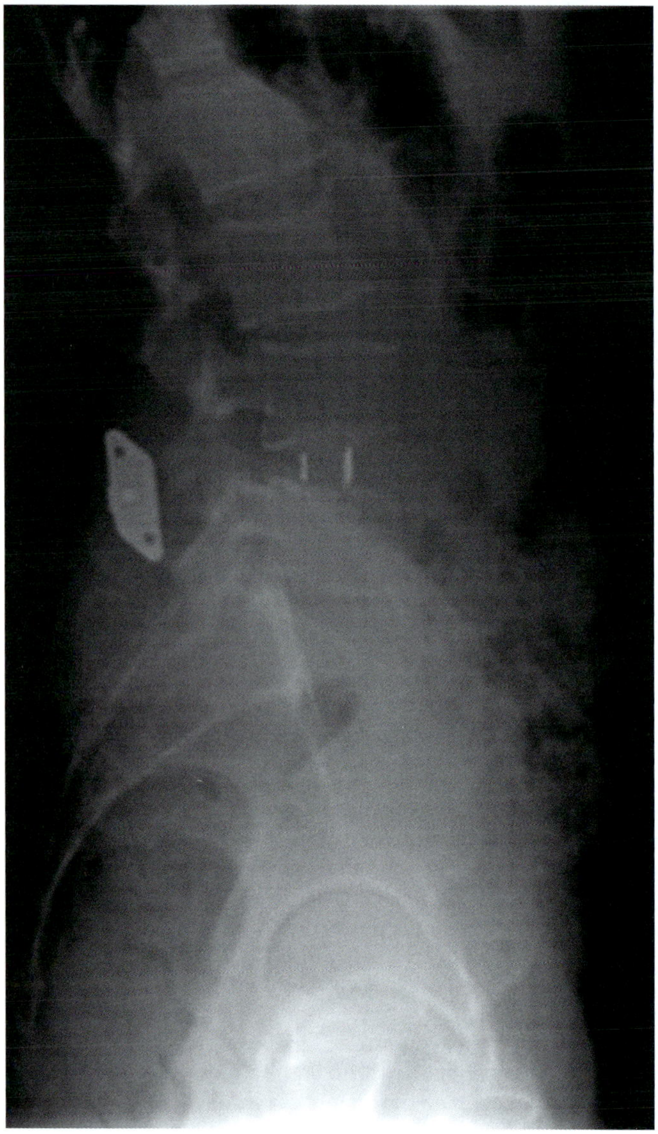

• **Fig. 19.1** Spinous process plates are indicated as supplemental fixation following any type of interbody fusion.

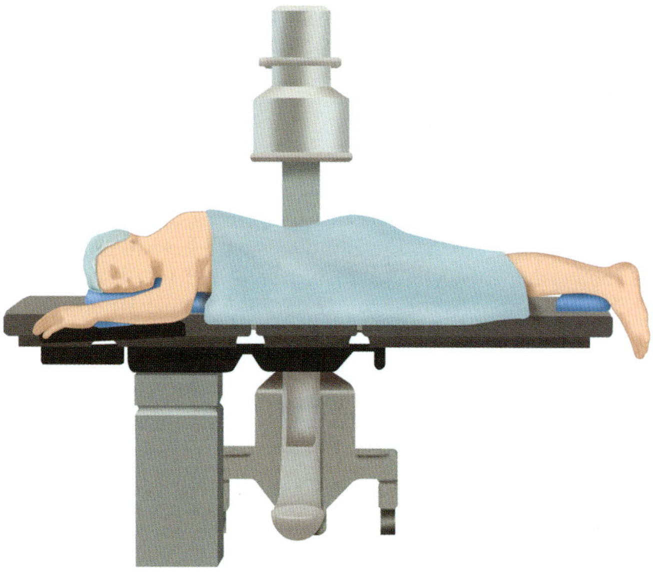

• **Fig. 19.2** The patient is positioned on an appropriate spinal table. Care should be taken not to hyperlordose the patient's spine. (Image courtesy of Zimmer Biomet, Denver, CO.)

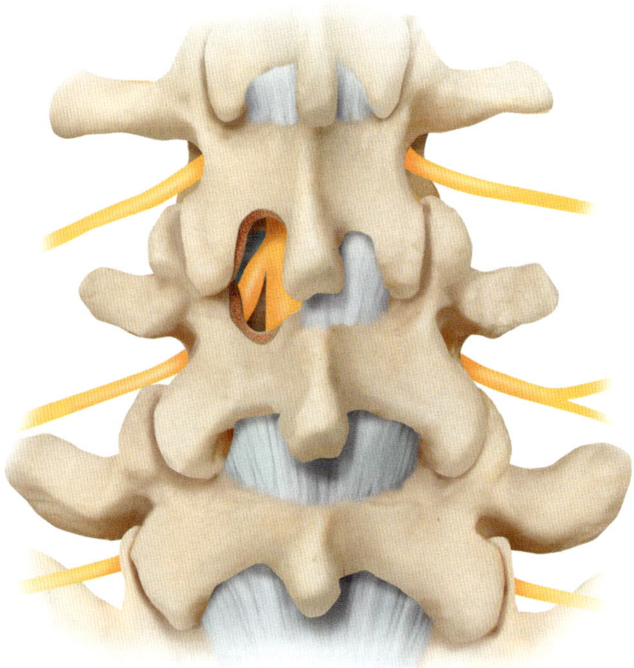

• **Fig. 19.3** Uni- or bilateral hemilaminotomies may be performed to decompress the neural elements. (Image courtesy of Zimmer Biomet.)

divided and retracted. After dividing the fascia, electrocautery is used to perform a subperiosteal dissection so that the bilateral erector spinae muscles can be mobilized off of the cranial and caudal spinous processes to the spinolaminar junction. If desired, for greater visualization or wider decompression, the interspinous ligament at the target level may be removed with rongeurs. The supraspinous ligament can be left in place to facilitate a more anatomic closure, it may be resected completely, or it may be elevated and sutured back in place following placement of the implant. Portions of the spinous processes and/or laminae may also be harvested and placed in the interspinous and/or laminar space for posterior arthrodesis prior to implanting the plate.[4] For decompression, bilateral hemilaminotomies and medial facetectomies may be performed (Fig. 19.3). Care must be taken not to remove too much of the lamina in the midline or facet joint. It is difficult to quantify, but the authors recommend leaving greater than 50% of the lamina and no greater than 50% of the facet joint. This may result in fracture of the spinous process at the laminar junction at the time of implant placement or instability.

3. After adequate decompression or dissection, the SPPs are inserted. The exact placement depends largely on the type and brand of implant used. For this chapter, the technique for placing the Aspen system (Zimmer Biomet) is illustrated (Video 19.1). The interspinous region is first prepared. This preparation depends on the decompression that was performed above. If the interspinous ligament was left in place, a dilator may first be placed into the interspinous space to create a pathway for the implant (Fig. 19.4). Of note, hypertrophic facet joints may prevent adequate placement and overgrown bone may first need to be removed with a rongeur or high-speed drill at this point. It is imperative that the dilator is placed as

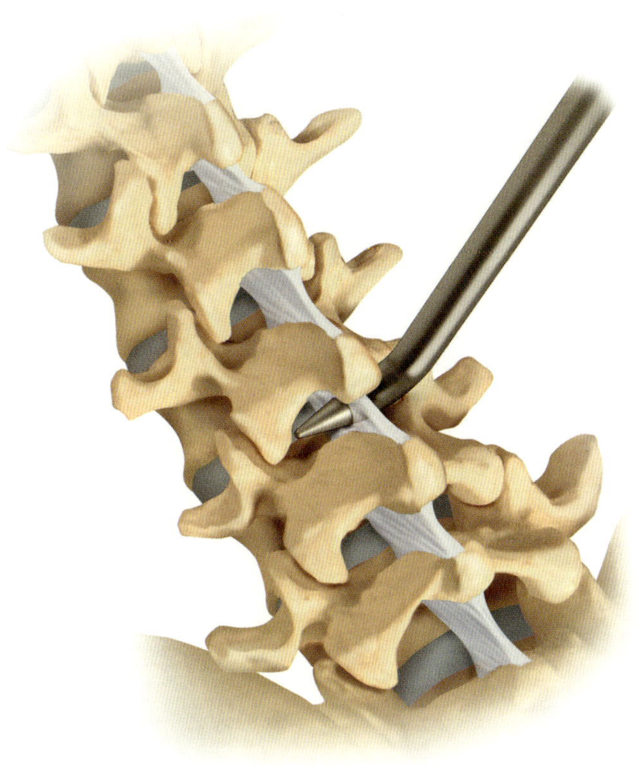

• **Fig. 19.4** A dilator is first placed piercing the interspinous ligament and creating a corridor for the spinous process plating system. Aspen Spinous Process Plating System (Zimmer Biomet). (Image courtesy of Zimmer Biomet.)

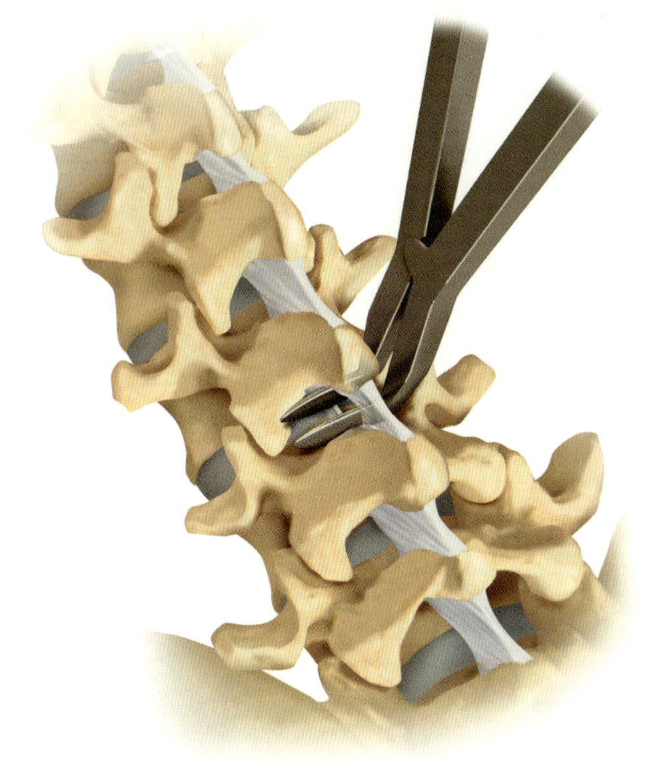

• **Fig. 19.5** A spreader is placed between the spinous processes. The spreader is used to measure the size of the interspinous device. Care must be made not to overdistract the interspace with resultant fracture of the spinous process. (Image courtesy of Zimmer Biomet.)

anterior as possible during this step. This may be ensured with the use of fluoroscopy. Level confirmation may be made during this step as well.

4. A spreader is then placed in order to measure the interspinous space. The spreader is opened, distracting the spinous processes with care not to over distract and fracture the bone (Fig. 19.5). The spreader's ratchet is kept up at this point and when proper distraction is achieved it is dropped down and a measurement may be made. There is risk of fracture of the spinous process. This is especially true in those with osteoporosis. If fractured, the spinous process plate will need to be abandoned. The authors always recommend having a back-up plan for fixation when performing this procedure.
5. If the supraspinous ligament was left in place, a rasp is next placed in the interspinous space (Fig. 19.6A). The rasp is typically one size smaller than the measured distraction on the spreader. The rasp may be rotated cranial and caudal to prepare the interspinous space for fusion (Fig. 19.6B). A larger rasp may then be used if desired. After completion, the corresponding sleeve is placed over the rasp and reinserted in the interspinous space (Fig. 19.7A). After the rasp is removed, the sleeve will serve as a cannula for the plate insertion (Fig. 19.7B).
6. The appropriate size post plate is next chosen. The diameter is based on prior sizing with the spreader and rasp. The length is based on local anatomy. The standard barrel length is typically appropriate; however, if there is significant facet hypertrophy limiting anterior placement, a medium barrel length may be chosen (Fig. 19.8). The chosen plate must engage an appropriate amount of spinous process without extending beyond the bone cranially and caudally; it must be anterior. The Aspen system offers a flared design, which may allow fixation at S1, but also offers anterior placement at all levels. The post plate is placed through the cannula and the cannula then removed (Fig. 19.9). The locking plate is then slid in place over the barrel engaging the opposite side of the spinous process (Fig. 19.10). Once the plate is in place, compression is placed on the cranial and caudal portions of the device, driving the spikes of the plates in to the spinous processes (Fig. 19.11). The spikes should be fully driven in with care not to apply too great a force, which may fracture the bone. Once adequate compression is achieved, the locking screw is finally tightened (Fig. 19.12). The authors utilize fluoroscopy at this point to ensure appropriate placement (Fig. 19.13). Of note, if the supraspinous and intraspinous ligaments were resected during decompression, the above procedure is performed without the need for rasping and the placement of the interspinous cannula. Following sizing, the appropriate implant may be directly placed in the interspinous space.
7. Bone graft may lastly be placed along the decorticated laminae and facet joints. Bone graft may also be placed inside the barrel portion of the Aspen device.
8. If an SPP device has multiple sizes, the smaller-sized plates can be used in smaller patients or on the L5-S1 levels in select patients. In patients requiring SPP fixation to include the S1 level, preoperative radiologic studies can be used to assess whether the S1 spinous process is large enough to accommodate an SPP. Wang et al.[4] anecdotally reported that about 80% of patients had an S1 spinous process that was adequately sized for SPP fixation.

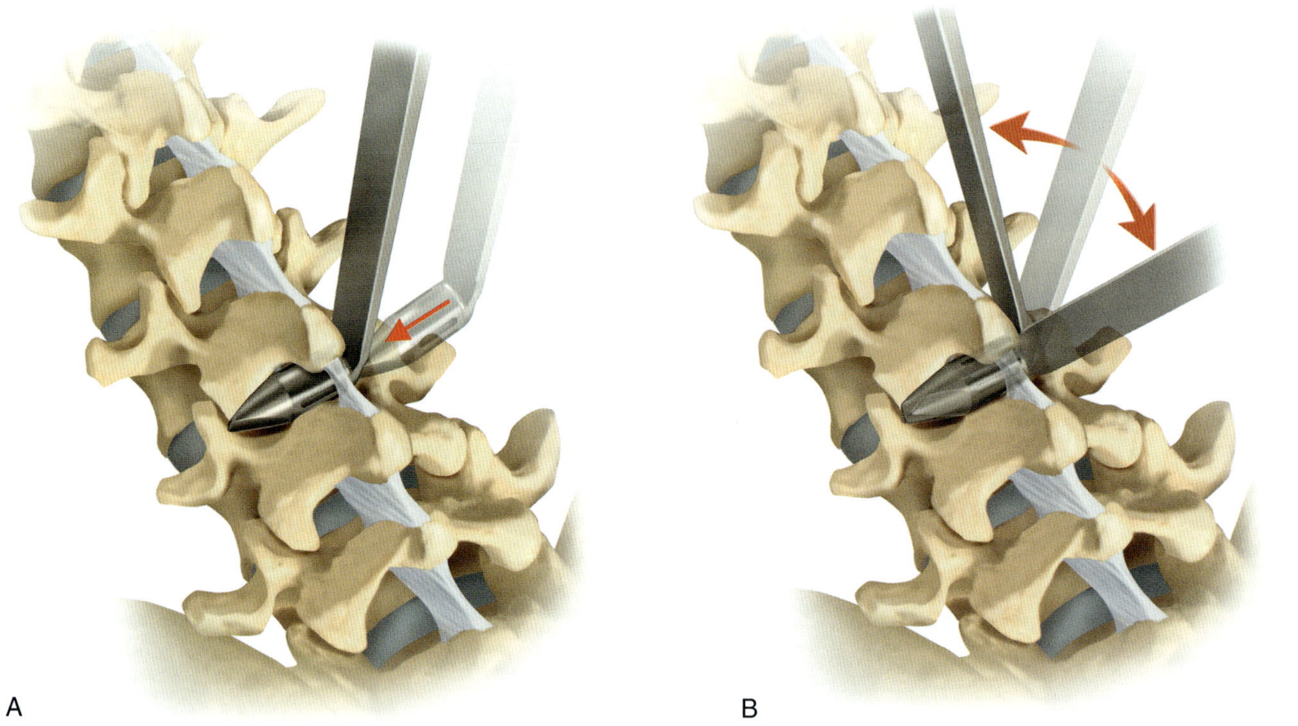

• **Fig. 19.6** A rasp is placed into the interspinous space. **A.** Typically it is one size smaller than the determined size based on the spreaders. **B.** Cranial and caudal rotation prepares the interspinous space for fusion and placement of the device. (Image courtesy of Zimmer Biomet.)

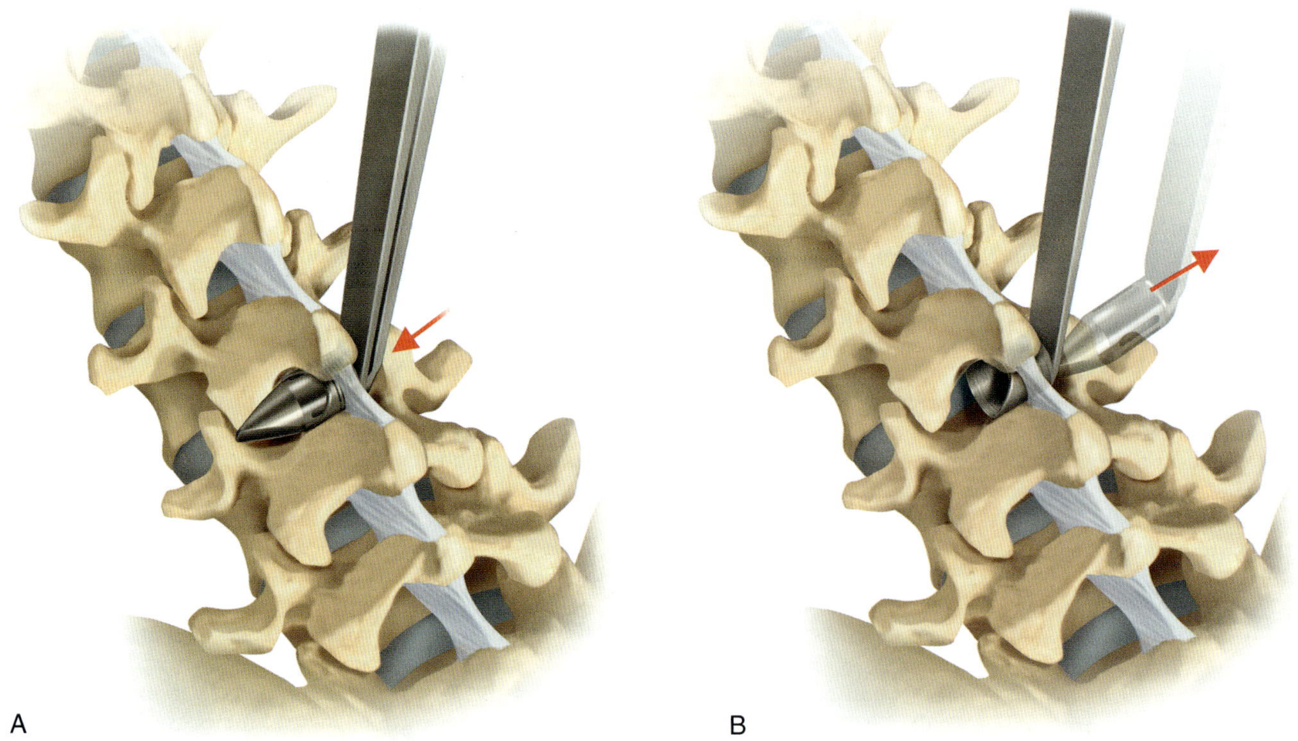

• **Fig. 19.7** **A.** The corresponding sleeve is placed over the rasp and reinserted into the interspinous space. **B.** The rasp is then removed leaving the sleeve in place in the interspinous space. (Image courtesy of Zimmer Biomet.)

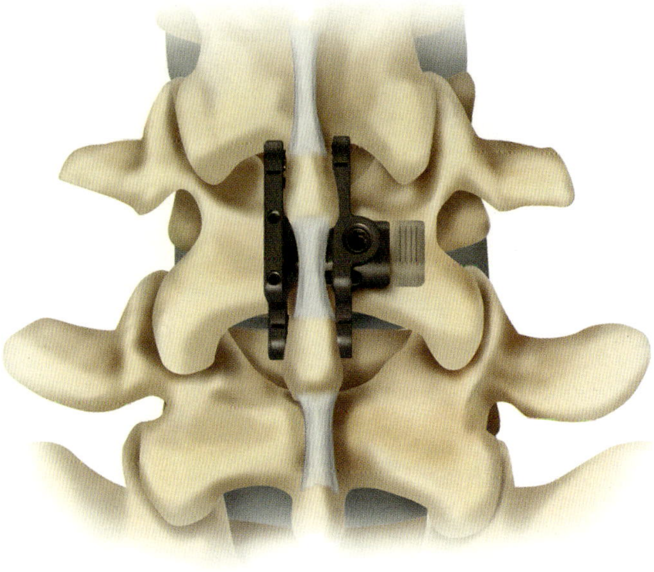

• **Fig. 19.8** **Appropriate size of the chosen device.** The barrel length largely depends on the state of the facet joints. If normal, the standard length is chosen. If hypertrophy, the shorter barrel (medium) is chosen, which is easier to accommodate a narrow interfacet corridor. The length should cover as much of the spinous process bone as possible taking care not to extend beyond the processes. The Aspen design offers a flare that can accommodate maximal caudal spinous process one even at S1. (Image courtesy of Zimmer Biomet.)

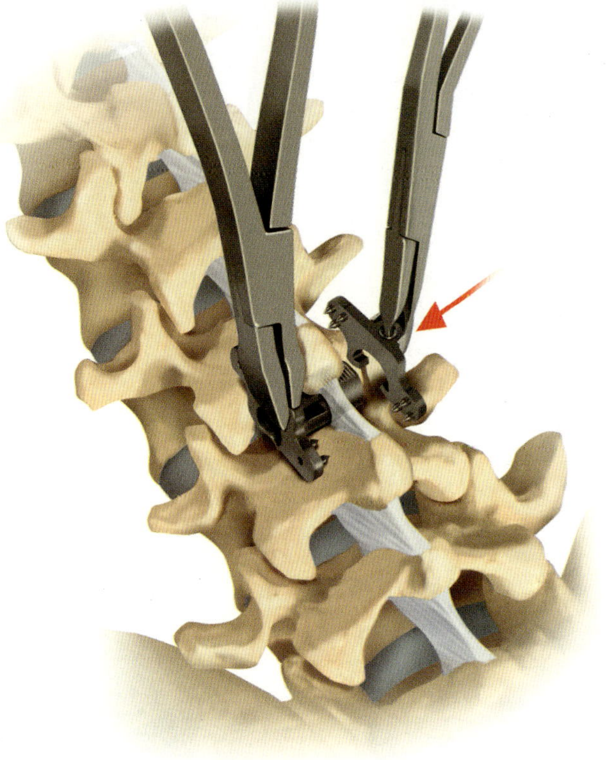

• **Fig. 19.10** The locking plate is placed over the barrel of the post plate. (Image courtesy of Zimmer Biomet.)

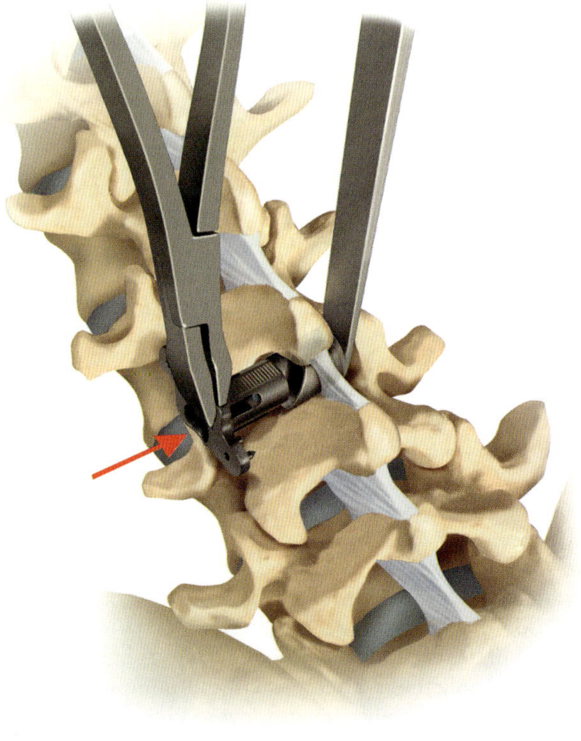

• **Fig. 19.9** The post plate is slid through the cannula and the cannula removed. (Image courtesy of Zimmer Biomet.)

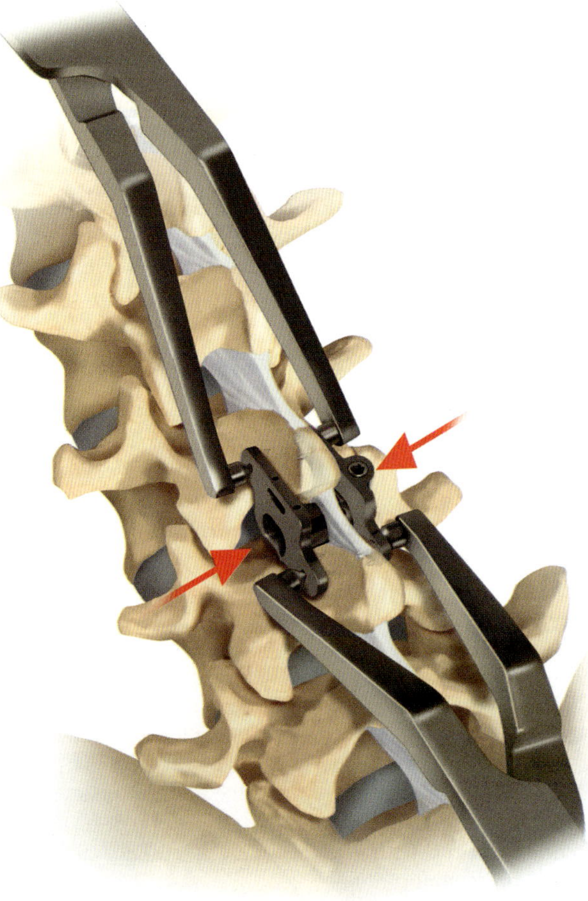

• **Fig. 19.11** Compression is applied across the cranial and caudal portions of the plate. The spikes should fully engage the spinous processes. Overcompression must be avoided. (Image courtesy of Zimmer Biomet.)

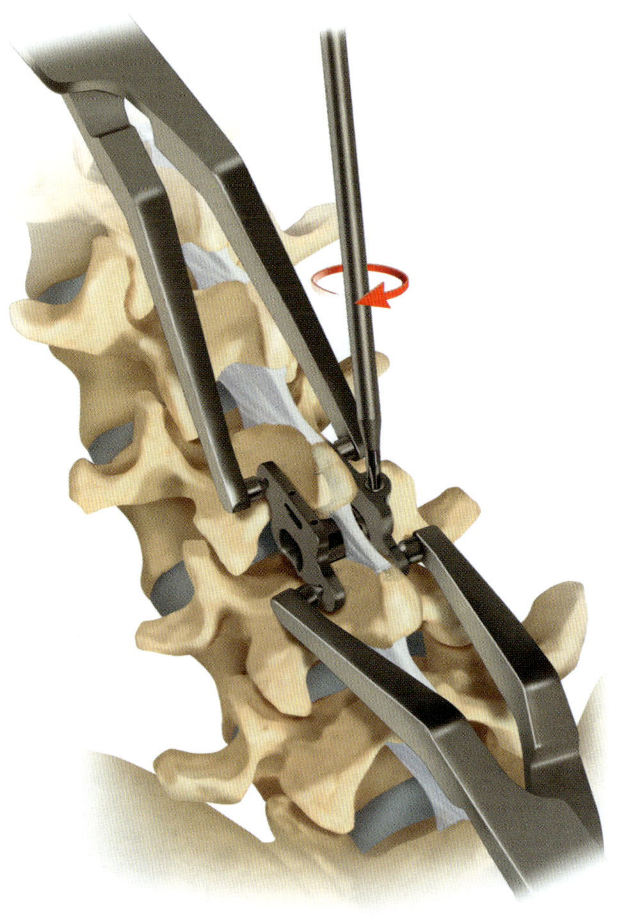

• **Fig. 19.12** Following compression, the locking screw is tightened and locked. (Image courtesy of Zimmer Biomet.)

Closure

The wound is closed in multiple layers. The fascia is closed with 1-0 Vicryl or alternative resorbable suture. This is followed by 2-0 Vicryl in the subcutaneous tissue and dermis. The authors close the skin with 4-0 monocryl in a subcuticular fashion followed by skin glue or Steri-Strips.

Postoperative care

Patients are allowed to mobilize immediately. They typically are discharged from the hospital the following day. Postoperative restrictions are surgeon specific, but typically consist of limited bending and lifting for the first 4 to 6 weeks, followed by physical therapy for core conditioning.

Complications

There are noted complications specifically for spinous process plating. Most may be avoided with meticulous surgical technique. Fracture of the spinous process may occur by overdistraction during sizing, overzealous bone removal of the spinous process or midline lamina, placement of too large of an implant, overcompression of the plates, and lastly dorsal placement of the device. Attention to proper surgical technique as outlined above should mitigate this complication.

Inadequate fixation may result from improper sizing of the implant (i.e., too large or too small), dorsal placement, or inadequate compression. The appropriate barrel size is chosen based on tactile feel during spreading. The plate length is chosen to fully cover the spinous process bone. The plate must be placed anterior; if too posterior, fracture of the spinous process may occur.

Outcomes

Clinical Utility

Utilization of SPPs for spinal pathologies is not new.[5,6] However, new innovations in device design and clinical utility have renewed interest in SPPs. A potential shortcoming of stand-alone interbody cages is that they allow for continuous movement of the facet joints while bony fusion is developing. Facet joint motion can potentially prevent facet arthrodesis and continue to cause postoperative pain for the patient. Thus, surgeons include posterior fixation to stimulate complete fusion. SPPs may be used in patients who have osteoporotic bone that carries a high risk of complications from pedicle screw fixation, such as backing out of screws and fracture of pedicles. In addition, geriatric patients or patients with neoplasms may benefit from the less invasive internal fixation approach provided by SPPs.

Biomechanical studies have shown that SPPs are most effective in reducing flexion-extension range of motion (ROM) because they are at a significant distance from the axis of rotation for this movement. In contrast, these devices provide less rigidity in lateral bending and axial rotation because they lie within or near the axis of rotation for these movements. Compared with interspinous wiring and laminar clamps, SPPs provide more immediate rigidity that is comparable to pedicle screw constructs. Furthermore, there is no risk of dural or neural injury associated with the sublaminar techniques. In addition, SPPs have a low profile and will not violate adjacent facet joints, theoretically lowering rates of hardware-related pain or adjacent segment degeneration.

There are several contraindications for the usage of SPPs. These devices should generally not be used in patients with pars interarticularis defects or any incompetence in the bone between the anterior and posterior spinal columns. In addition, patients with significant translational instability (e.g., medium- to high-grade spondylolisthesis) are not good candidates. From a biomechanical standpoint, it is important to consider that SPPs induce a segmental kyphosis in the normally lordotic lumbar spine. Therefore, the devices could cause an overload of the anterior disk in select patients who do not have adequate anterior spinal column support.

Tomii et al.[7] reported their surgical strategy for treating lumbar spondylolisthesis with instability using a PLIF and SPP. These authors preferred to use the SPP as opposed to pedicle screws in patients who were older than 70 years, based on a previous study that reported people up to age 70 are more active than older patients and thereby had increased chances of developing spondylolisthesis after posterior decompression of the lumbar spine.[8] These authors also favored the SPP in patients younger than 70 years who were found to have osteoporotic bone intraoperatively. They also recommended performing a preoperative CT scan on every patient who was to receive a SPP to rule out pars fracture, because this is a contraindication to utilization of a SPP.

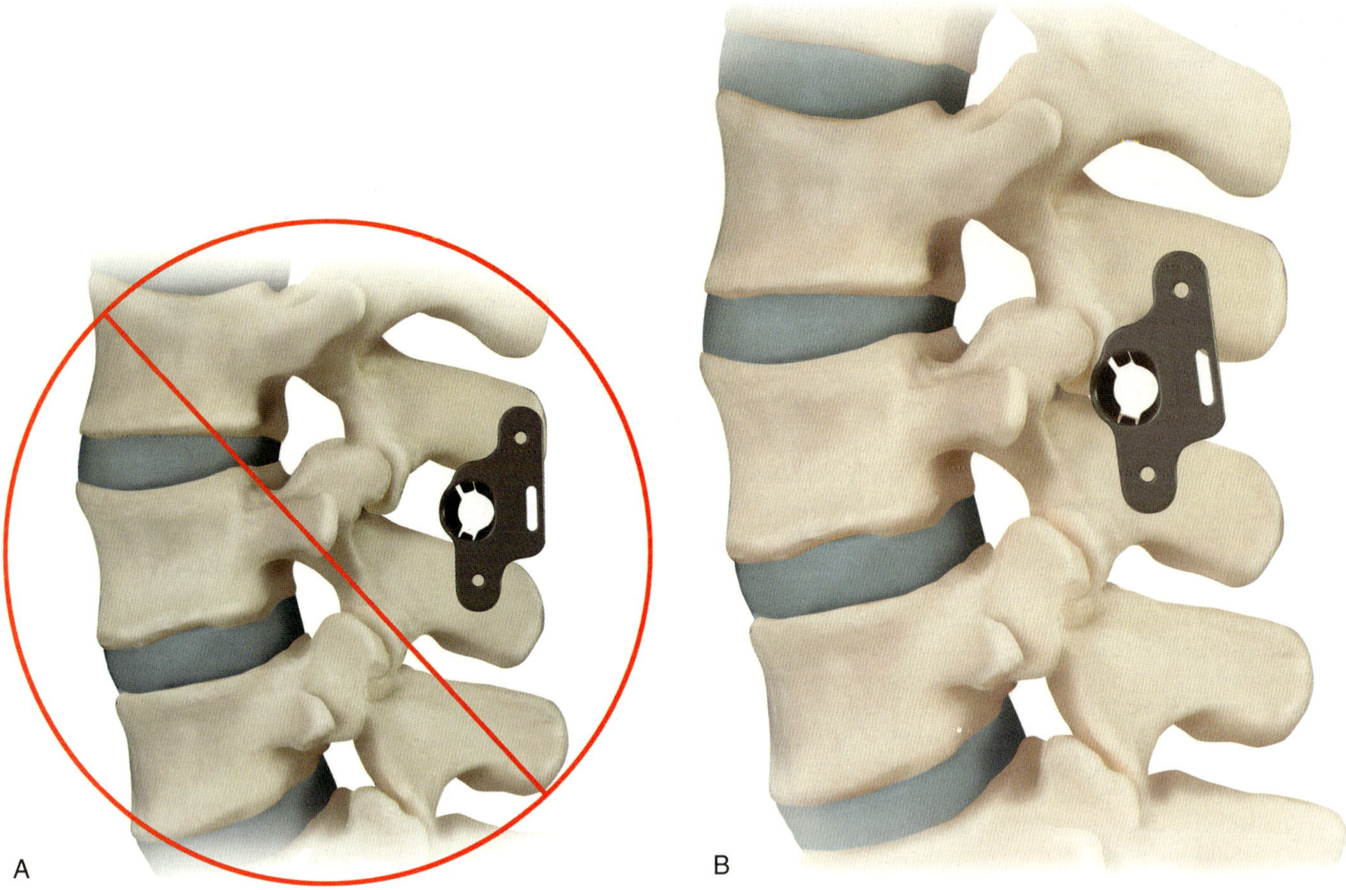

A B

• **Fig. 19.13** Fluoroscopy or other imaging is utilized to confirm appropriate positioning of the implant. The implant must be placed as anterior as possible. **A.** If placed posterior, fracture or dislodgment may occur. **B.** (Image courtesy of Zimmer Biomet.)

Spinous Process Plating Devices

There are multiple SPPs available for spinal surgeons. Most of these devices work in a similar manner and can be used with any interbody fixation technique, as demonstrated by the literature presented below. Owing to the relatively recent renewal of interest in these devices for internal fixation, clinical studies are somewhat sparse.

Spire

The Spire (Medtronic, Dublin, Ireland) SPP is composed of two titanium plates with sharp, opposing spikes connected at their midpoint by a polyaxial stem. The nonparallel, polyaxial design of the stem allows the plates to conform to the anatomy of both sides of each spinous process to maximize bony purchase. The Spire plates are available in two sizes. The standard plate has a length of 45 mm, width of 12 mm, and a thickness of 3 mm. The shorter plate is 35 mm long, with the same width and thickness of the standard plate.

Wang et al.[9] performed a biomechanical analysis of the Spire SPP system used in conjunction with an ALIF cage. They found that, compared with other fixation options, the combined ALIF+SPP construct had the greatest mean limitation of flexion-extension ROM, although this was statistically similar to ALIF with bilateral pedicle screw fixation. These two constructs allowed significantly less flexion-extension ROM compared with ALIF with unilateral pedicle screws and rod, ALIF with posterior translaminar facet screws, and an intact spine. In constructs without an ALIF cage, the Spire SPP again provided the greatest limitation in flexion-extension ROM, but was statistically similar to bilateral pedicle screw and rod fixation. With regard to axial rotation and lateral bending movements, the SPP was similar to unilateral posterior screw and rod fixation. However, fixation with bilateral screws and rods, with or without a supplemental ALIF cage, resulted in the stiffest construct in axial rotation and lateral bending.

Multiple studies have examined clinical outcomes with the Spire SPP system. Wang et al.[4] retrospectively evaluated 32 patients with single-level degenerative disk disease who underwent ALIF. Twenty-one patients received supplemental fixation via the Spire SPP and 11 patients received bilateral pedicle screw fixation. The average follow-up was 5.5 months. The authors found that the median operative time and estimated blood loss was less in those patients who received ALIF+SPP compared with the group who received ALIF with bilateral pedicle screws. In addition, the authors reported that there were no perioperative complications, hardware failure, revision surgery, or cases of pseudarthrosis in patients receiving ALIF+SPP fixation. No clinical outcomes were reported.

Kim et al.[10] retrospectively studied patients receiving PLIF with supplemental internal fixation. Of the 76 patients, 40 received the Spire SPP and 36 had bilateral pedicle screw fixation. Average follow-up was 56.4 months. The authors found that the mean operative time and estimated blood loss were significantly less in patients who had SPP fixation. With regard to quality of life measures, the authors reported that visual analogue scale (VAS) scores significantly improved from 7.2 preoperatively to 1.3 1-year postoperatively in patients receiving supplemental SPP fixation, which was statistically similar to patients receiving bilateral pedicle screws. Furthermore, Korean Oswestry Disability Index (K-ODI) scores were significantly improved 1 year postoperatively in both groups. However, the VAS score on postoperative day 1 was significantly better in the SPP group compared with the pedicle screw group. Postoperative radiographs at 12 months postoperatively indicated that the flexion-extension ROM at the instrumented level was significantly decreased for both SPP and pedicle screw groups compared with preoperatively. Notably, patients with bilateral pedicle screws had more ROM at the superior adjacent segment compared with preoperatively, whereas the SPP group had similar ROM restriction in both cranial and caudal segments compared with preoperatively. In addition, the change in segmental angle of the adjacent segment was significantly increased in the pedicle screw group compared with the SPP group. These findings may explain the higher number of patients with adjacent segment degeneration in the bilateral pedicle screw group (5 patients [12.5%] in SPP group compared with 13 [36.1%] in the pedicle screw group). Overall fusion rates were similar between groups, with the SPP group having a 92.5% fusion rate and the pedicle screw group demonstrating a 91.6% fusion rate. Complications in the SPP group were significant for one patient having sustained back pain that a CT showed to be a fracture of the L4 inferior articular process. Another two patients with SPP fixation had retropulsion of the interbody cage and required reoperation. However, no surgery-related complications were noted, whereas the pedicle screw fixation group had three posterior deep wound infections, two cerebrospinal fluid leaks, and one epidural hematoma.

Aspen

The Aspen (Lanx, Inc., Bloomfield, CO) interspinous anchor is similar to the Spire SPP in that it is secured to the spinous processes by aggressively clamping together two plates with teeth on adjacent spinous processes. The main difference is that during insertion, maximal distraction of the spinous processes is achieved and maintained by the larger-diameter center cylindric post of the Aspen device. This cylinder comes in a variety of diameters to fit interspinous spaces of different sizes. The post serves as a buttress against extension and increases foraminal height. As with all interspinous fusion devices, the aim of the implant is to increase segmental stability with the purpose of improving the fusion rate.

Multiple biomechanical studies have investigated the Aspen SPP with various interbody cages. Both Techy et al.[11] and Kaibara et al.[12] investigated the Aspen SPP with TLIF cages and found that the TLIF+SPP construct resulted in a significant decrease in flexion-extension ROM compared with an intact spine. Although this construct also resulted in the least ROM in flexion-extension, it was statistically similar to TLIF with supplemental bilateral pedicle screw fixation. In addition, both studies determined that TLIF+SPP did not significantly decrease ROM in lateral bending compared with an intact spine, whereas TLIF with unilateral or bilateral pedicle screws increased stiffness in this motion plane. In contrast, the study by Kaibara et al.[12] found that the TLIF+SPP construct created increased stiffness over an intact spine in axial rotation, whereas Techy et al.[11] found no significant difference in axial rotation with this construct compared with an intact spine. However, in both studies TLIF with bilateral pedicle screw fixation was found to result in significantly less ROM in axial rotation compared with TLIF+SPP. In addition to these findings, Kaibara et al.[12] determined that the flexural angle at the L4-5 index level was significantly greater with the SPP compared with an intact spine. Moreover, the SPP created a more extended angle at the L3-4 rostral level, whereas the L5-S1 caudal level was significantly less flexed than normal. The authors also noted that the intervertebral foraminal height at the index level was greatest with the Aspen SPP and that this was significantly higher than both an intact spine and the TLIF with pedicle screw constructs.

Karahalios et al.[13] investigated the Aspen SPP with ALIF in cadaver spines. The authors found that the ALIF+SPP construct increased ROM stiffness over intact spines in flexion-extension, lateral bending, and axial rotation. In addition, the ALIF+SPP construct decreased ROM in flexion-extension and axial rotation compared with ALIF alone. Moreover, the ALIF+SPP construct was stiffer than an ALIF cage with supplemental anterior plating in flexion-extension and lateral bending. Adding the Aspen SPP to the ALIF with anterior plate construct decreased ROM in all planes compared with ALIF with anterior plate only. Compared with ALIF with bilateral pedicle screws, the ALIF+SPP construct provided similar stiffness during flexion, lateral bending, and axial rotation, and was significantly more rigid in extension. The flexural angle at the index level, adjacent rostral level, and adjacent caudal level was statistically greater with the Aspen SPP in place when compared with intact spines. In addition, foraminal height was significantly greater with the SPP compared with intact spines and pedicle screw constructs. Notably, foraminal height did not change in flexion or extension with the ALIF+SPP construct, whereas it decreased with extension in the construct with ALIF and bilateral pedicle screws.

Affix

The Affix (NuVasive, Inc., San Diego, CA) device is a standard spinous process plating device with two 45-mm bilateral plates with teeth. Fogel et al.[14] performed a biomechanical study of the Affix device with XLIF. The authors found that the XLIF+SPP construct led to a significant decrease in ROM in flexion-extension, lateral bending, and axial rotation compared with an intact spine. However, the addition of the SPP decreased ROM only in flexion-extension compared with the stand-alone XLIF cage without additional fixation. In addition, the XLIF+SPP had significantly increased ROM in lateral bending and axial rotation compared with XLIF with unilateral or bilateral pedicle screw placement. Notably, the addition of a lateral plate to the XLIF+SPP construct created a statistically similar decrease in ROM to XLIF with bilateral pedicle screw fixation in all motion planes.

In a separate, but similar, study Fogel et al.[15] tested XLIF with Affix SPP fixation in a degenerative spondylolisthesis biomechanical model. All construct conditions were less stable than their corresponding construct conditions in an intact spine without the spondylolisthesis model. The XLIF+SPP construct created the most rigidity in flexion-extension, but this was similar to XLIF with bilateral pedicle screw fixation. Additionally, the authors noted that under shear loading, supplemental fixation in addition to XLIF reduced shear displacement in all constructs except for those utilizing the SPP, which supports the widely held belief that SPPs should not be utilized in cases of medium- to high-grade spondylolisthesis.

Kornblum et al.[16] performed a biomechanical study of ALIF with the newer Affix II (NuVasive, Inc., San Diego, CA) SPP. The authors found that an un-integrated ALIF cage with SPP fixation resulted in significantly less stiffness in all ROM compared with an integrated ALIF cage with SPP. However, the integrated cage with SPP fixation was more rigid than the integrated cage alone only in flexion-extension ROM, and was similar in lateral bending and axial rotation. Notably, the integrated cage with SPP fixation was similar to an un-integrated cage with bilateral pedicle screws. In addition, the SPP with an integrated ALIF cage also added significantly more stability than an integrated cage with an anterior plate.

Axle

The Axle Interspinous Fusion System (X-Spine Systems, Inc., Miamisburg, OH) is a combined interspinous spacer and SPP. Its design is similar to other SPP, but with a more prominent connecting piece that is constructed as an interspinous spacer. The device comes in multiple sizes ranging from 30 to 46 mm wide and 4 to 15 mm high. Doulgeris et al.[17] performed a biomechanical analysis of cadaveric spines receiving XLIF and the Axle SPP. Incorporation of the Axle system resulted in significantly decreased ROM in flexion-extension and lateral bending compared with intact and XLIF cage-only conditions, but only XLIF with bilateral pedicle screws significantly reduced axial rotation ROM compared with the XLIF cage only. Nevertheless, results of the XLIF with SPP and XLIF with bilateral pedicle screw fixation were statistically similar in all ROM. With regard to neutral and elastic zone stiffness, the authors determined that the cage with SPP increased neutral zone and elastic zone stiffness in all ROM except for axial rotation neutral zone stiffness. However, the addition of the SPP did not increase neutral zone stiffness compared with the cage alone in lateral bending or axial rotation. Additionally, the XLIF with bilateral pedicle screws construct had a significantly stiffer neutral zone and trended toward significantly stiffer elastic zone ($P = .06$) in lateral bending compared with XLIF+SPP.

Gonzalez-Blohm et al.[18] also investigated the Axle system but with PLIF. These authors found that the PLIF+SPP construct significantly reduced ROM in all motions compared with intact segments. Furthermore, they noted that flexion-extension and axial rotation movements were similar compared with PLIF with bilateral pedicle screws. However, PLIF with bilateral pedicle screws was significantly more rigid in lateral bending compared with the PLIF+SPP construct. With regard to neutral and elastic zone stiffness, the PLIF+SPP and PLIF with bilateral pedicle screw constructs had similar stiffness for neutral and elastic zones in flexion, extension, and axial rotation, but the PLIF and bilateral pedicle screw construct resulted in more neutral and elastic zone stiffness in lateral bending.

Other Devices

Several authors have presented their experience with various additional SPP devices. Yeager et al.[19] studied an ALIF cage with the BridgePoint SPP (Alphatec Spine, Carlsbad, CA). With an integrated ALIF cage and the SPP, all ROM were stiffer than with an intact spine. However, an unintegrated ALIF cage and the SPP did not provide additional rigidity over an intact spine in lateral bending or axial torsion ROM. Additionally, the authors found that the integrated ALIF cage and SPP were similar to an ALIF cage with bilateral pedicle screw in all ROM, whereas a nonintegrated ALIF cage with SPP had more ROM than an ALIF cage with bilateral pedicle screws in lateral bending and axial torsion.

Yu et al.[20] studied a novel titanium alloy SPP, the Interspinous Fastener (Shandong Wego Orthopedic Device Co., Ltd, Weihai, China), for potential use with PLIF. The PLIF+SPP construct was significantly stiffer than an intact spine in all ROM and was similar to PLIF with bilateral pedicle screws in all ROM.

Tomii et al.[7] performed a retrospective study of 15 patients with lumbar spinal stenosis secondary to degenerative spondylolisthesis with instability that were treated with PLIF and the S-plate (Kisco DIR, Osaka, Japan) SPP. The authors found that every patient had improvement in their symptoms postoperatively. Mean Japanese Orthopaedic Association scores increased from a mean of 12.1 preoperatively to 19.4 at discharge, and to 21.9 at final follow-up of 1.5 to 4 years. The authors also noted that the mean intervertebral height increased from 65.4 mm preoperatively to 73.7 mm on postoperative day 1 and 61.4 mm at final follow-up. However, there were no cases of recurrent symptomatic foraminal stenosis owing to subsidence of the intervertebral space. Furthermore, there were no perioperative complications or cases of pseudarthrosis in any patient.

Lopez et al.[21] recently reported a systematic review of the literature pertaining to lumbar spinous process fixation and fusion. They reviewed 293 articles, with only 15 remaining after applying exclusionary criteria. No class I or II data have been published to date. Methodologically flawed and class III studies have demonstrated that interspineous fusion devices reduce instability at one year. No statistical comparison of complications rates to other processes of fixation have been presented. The authors noted that these interspinous devices are commonly used and heavily marketed; however, data on their efficacy and safety are very limited.

Conclusions

Spinous process plates can be successfully utilized as supplemental fixation to lumbar interbody fusion techniques in the correct clinical scenario. Biomechanical studies demonstrate the substantial rigidity of these constructs in flexion-extension ROM, and the potential for increased rigidity in all motion planes with the correct SPP and interbody fusion technique. Furthermore, the few available clinical studies in the literature demonstrate good quality of life outcomes, high fusion rates, and low morbidity rates with these devices for supplemental fixation. Future studies will continue to expand on the role and outcomes of these devices in spinal surgery.

References

1. Esses SI, Sachs BL, Dreyzin V. Complications associated with the technique of pedicle screw fixation. A selected survey of ABS members. *Spine (Phila Pa 1976)*. 1993;18(15):2231–2238; discussion 2238–2239.
2. Jutte PC, Castelein RM. Complications of pedicle screws in lumbar and lumbosacral fusions in 105 consecutive primary operations. *Eur Spine J*. 2002;11(6):594–598. https://doi.org/10.1007/s00586-002-0469-8.
3. Cunningham BW, Kotani Y, McNulty PS, et al. The effect of spinal destabilization and instrumentation on lumbar intradiscal pressure: an in vitro biomechanical analysis. *Spine (Phila Pa 1976)*. 1997;22(22):2655–2663.

4. Wang JC, Haid RW, Miller JS, et al. Comparison of CD HORIZON SPIRE spinous process plate stabilization and pedicle screw fixation after anterior lumbar interbody fusion. Invited submission from the Joint Section Meeting On Disorders of the Spine and Peripheral Nerves, March 2005. *J Neurosurg Spine*. 2006;4(2):132–136. https://doi.org/10.3171/spi.2006.4.2.132.
5. Cobey MC. The value of the Wilson plate in spinal fusion. *Clin Orthop*. 1971;76:138–140.
6. Böstman O, Myllynen P, Riska EB. Posterior spinal fusion using internal fixation with the Daab plate. *Acta Orthop Scand*. 1984;55(3):310–314. https://doi.org/10.3109/17453678408992363.
7. Tomii M, Itoh Y, Numazawa S, et al. Spinous process plate (S-plate) fixation after posterior interbody fusion for lumbar canal stenosis due to spondylolisthesis. *Neurosurg Rev*. 2013;36(1):139–143. https://doi.org/10.1007/s10143-012-0402-5.
8. Shenkin HA, Hash CJ. Spondylolisthesis after multiple bilateral laminectomies and facetectomies for lumbar spondylosis. Follow-up review. *J Neurosurg*. 1979;50(1):45–47. https://doi.org/10.3171/jns.1979.50.1.0045.
9. Wang JC, Spenciner D, Robinson JC. SPIRE spinous process stabilization plate: biomechanical evaluation of a novel technology. Invited submission from the Joint Section Meeting on Disorders of the Spine and Peripheral Nerves, March 2005. *J Neurosurg Spine*. 2006;4(2):160–164. https://doi.org/10.3171/spi.2006.4.2.160.
10. Kim HJ, Bak KH, Chun HJ, et al. Posterior interspinous fusion device for one-level fusion in degenerative lumbar spine disease: comparison with pedicle screw fixation—preliminary report of at least one year follow up. *J Korean Neurosurg Soc*. 2012;52(4):359–364. https://doi.org/10.3340/jkns.2012.52.4.359.
11. Techy F, Mageswaran P, Colbrunn RW, et al. Properties of an interspinous fixation device (ISD) in lumbar fusion constructs: a biomechanical study. *Spine J*. 2013;13(5):572–579. https://doi.org/10.1016/j.spinee.2013.01.042.
12. Kaibara T, Karahalios DG, Porter RW, et al. Biomechanics of a lumbar interspinous anchor with transforaminal lumbar interbody fixation. *World Neurosurg*. 2010;73(5):572–577. https://doi.org/10.1016/j.wneu.2010.02.025.
13. Karahalios DG, Kaibara T, Porter RW, et al. Biomechanics of a lumbar interspinous anchor with anterior lumbar interbody fusion. *J Neurosurg Spine*. 2010;12(4):372–380. https://doi.org/10.3171/2009.10.SPINE09305.
14. Fogel GR, Parikh RD, Ryu SI, et al. Biomechanics of lateral lumbar interbody fusion constructs with lateral and posterior plate fixation: laboratory investigation. *J Neurosurg Spine*. 2014;20(3):291–297. https://doi.org/10.3171/2013.11.SPINE13617.
15. Fogel GR, Turner AWL, Dooley ZA, et al. Biomechanical stability of lateral interbody implants and supplemental fixation in a cadaveric degenerative spondylolisthesis model. *Spine (Phila Pa 1976)*. 2014;39(19):E1138–E1146. https://doi.org/10.1097/BRS.0000000000000485.
16. Kornblum MB, Turner AWL, Cornwall GB, et al. Biomechanical evaluation of stand-alone lumbar polyether-ether-ketone interbody cage with integrated screws. *Spine J*. 2013;13(1):77–84. https://doi.org/10.1016/j.spinee.2012.11.013.
17. Doulgeris JJ, Aghayev K, Gonzalez-Blohm SA, et al. Biomechanical comparison of an interspinous fusion device and bilateral pedicle screw system as additional fixation for lateral lumbar interbody fusion. *Clin Biomech (Bristol, Avon)*. 2015;30(2):205–210. https://doi.org/10.1016/j.clinbiomech.2014.10.003.
18. Gonzalez-Blohm SA, Doulgeris JJ, Aghayev K, et al. Biomechanical analysis of an interspinous fusion device as a stand-alone and as supplemental fixation to posterior expandable interbody cages in the lumbar spine. *J Neurosurg Spine*. 2014;20(2):209–219. https://doi.org/10.3171/2013.10.SPINE13612.
19. Yeager MS, Dupre DA, Cook DJ, et al. Anterior lumbar interbody fusion with integrated fixation and adjunctive posterior stabilization: a comparative biomechanical analysis. *Clin Biomech (Bristol, Avon)*. 2015;30(8):769–774. https://doi.org/10.1016/j.clinbiomech.2015.06.015.
20. Yu X, Zhu L, Su Q. Lumbar spine stability after combined application of interspinous fastener and modified posterior lumbar interbody fusion: a biomechanical study. *Arch Orthop Trauma Surg*. 2014;134(5):623–629. https://doi.org/10.1007/s00402-014-1977-9.
21. Lopez AJ, Scheer JK, Dahdaleh NS, et al. Lumbar spinous precess fixation and fusion: a systematic review and critical analysis of an emerging spinal technology. *Clin Spine Surg*. 2017;30(9):E1279–E1288.

20

Instrumentation for Stability After Lumbar Interbody Fusion

PIERCE D. NUNLEY AND KELLY A. FRANK

Introduction

Posterior fixation (PF) after lumbar interbody fusion (LIF) is a standard practice in spine surgery. As stand-alone LIF devices and techniques continue to advance, there is debate around the necessity of PF. Data and literature substantiating fusion outcomes is lacking for stand-alone devices, and therefore the US Food and Drug Administration (FDA) has yet to approve stand-alone LIF as equivalent to LIF with PF.

As a surgeon, one of the first tenets of surgery is to accomplish the desired goal with the highest benefit-to-risk ratio. Stated another way, the surgeon wants to execute the surgical procedure that has the best opportunity to provide the greatest benefit to the patient while minimizing risks. In LIF, solid fusion allows the patient the best opportunity for relief and positive clinical outcomes. However PF, although understood to facilitate a solid fusion, is a greater surgical risk.

Requirements to achieve a fusion can be categorized into two groups. The first is to provide the *biological environment* that will be conducive to allow a fusion to occur (e.g., preparing bony surfaces and endplates until they are bleeding, maximizing graft and host interface by removing as much disk as possible and appropriately preparing the endplates).[1] The second is to provide *stability* that will allow the fusion to occur postoperatively. There is very little to debate regarding the first principle, but the second principle is the focus for this chapter.

There are many ways to perform PF of the lumbar spine, and new techniques and implants are evolving. This chapter will discuss the history and rationale for the use of PF and the three most common techniques used today: facet screws (FS), pedicle screws (PS), and interspinous process (ISP) devices.

Facet Screws

History

In 1944, King[2] was first to publish on vertebral screw fixation. These screws were placed parallel to the inferior border of the lamina and perpendicular to the lumbar vertebrae facets joints. Recovery time was long, required bed rest, and the rate of pseudoarthrosis was extremely high— 55.1% in a study of 49 patients.[3–5]

Difficulties in the surgical technique and poor results continued until 1959 when Boucher reported a new material and method of screw insertion that improved fixation. The screws were placed through the inferior facet and into the inferior pedicle. He utilized stainless steel, machined screws that were 1.5 to 2 inches in length.[2] In 1964, Pennel[6] used a similar fixation technique to that of Boucher. These screws would be considered 'unilateral' or transfacet screws as they were directed from each ipsilateral facet (Fig. 20.1).

In the 1980s, Magerl[7] developed the technique of 'translaminar' facet screw fixation, a variation of the transfacet method. These screws started on the contralateral side of the spinous process, traversed through the ipsilateral lamina, and then crossed the joint and exited laterally at the posterolateral inferior aspect of the pedicle. In 1989, Jacobs[8] reported 91% solid arthrodesis with 93% clinical success in 88 consecutive patients with a prospective average follow up of 16 months using Magerl's technique.

Although translaminar and transfacet fixation are both less costly than pedicle screws, transfacet fixation is believed to have greater incidence of incomplete fusion.[9–11]

Translaminar fixation has remained the more popular technique, although it does not come without complications. It requires a larger surgical area, has been associated with a 10% incidence of laminar wall violation and improper screw position, and higher neurologic complications.[10,12]

In recent years, there have been some novel ideas for facet fixation to include the facet gun that was last marketed by US Spine (Javelin MIS Locking Facet System, Amedica/US Spine, Salt Lake City, UT). Not all ideas or techniques are successful as this product is no longer available and no papers could be found to report on outcomes. It remains to be seen if other devices or techniques will prove to be safe and efficacious.

Several companies have developed specific screws to be utilized in transfacet and translaminar facet fixation; however, the most frequently used screw to date is a simple 4.5 mm titanium cortical bone screw found in all orthopedic trauma sets. These screws are extremely inexpensive in comparison to pedicle screws. From an industry point of view, it is unlikely that there will be significant marketing for this technique. However, when clinical results have been excellent[13] and cost-effectiveness is vitally important, we may likely see a resurgence of this technique in the future (Fig. 20.2).

Indications

The clinical indications for facet screws are broad in nature, but the most common indication from the surgeon's perspective is posterior fixation with or without interbody support on patients with an intact lamina (no previous laminectomy or pars intra-articularis defect).

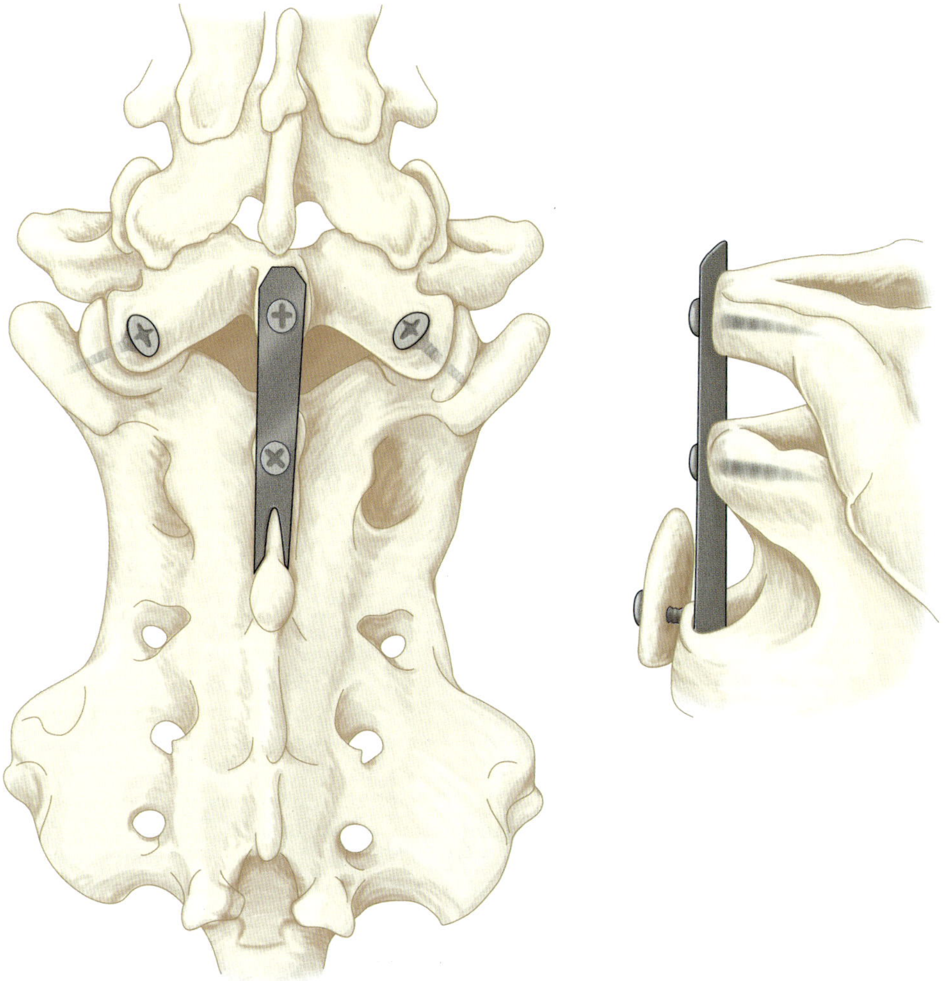

• **Fig. 20.1** Metal screws placed through the lateral articulations as first described by King. When the spinous processes were well developed, a tibial graft was fastened with small screws. (Reproduced with permission from King, D: Internal fixation for lumbosacral fusion. *J Bone Joint Surg* 1948;30-A:560–565.)

Technique

The technique for placing facet or Magerl screws is straightforward, but requires a keen sense of three-dimensional vertebral anatomy. The typical screw is 4.5 mm titanium or stainless steel with cortical threads. A few screws have been developed specifically for this purpose, but no data have been reviewed by this author that demonstrate superiority over basic screws.

Surgically, a midline incision is made to expose the lamina of the superior vertebrae in the segment to be fused (e.g., L4 for and L4-5 fusion). This dissection allows for clear visual identification of the entire lamina. Further dissection should be done to reveal the caudal edge of the inferior vertebral transverse process at the attachment to the pedicle (e.g., L5 transverse process for an L4-5 fusion). The trajectory is a line that is coplanar with the lamina where the starting point is from the contralateral side of the spinous process at the junction of the lamina aiming toward the intersection of the caudal junction of the transverse process of the caudal vertebrae at its attachment to the pedicle.

In order for the midline incision to remain small with minimally invasive exposure, a separate stab wound has to be made cranial and laterally on each side that will be collinear with the facet screw.

A 3.0-mm drill bit is advanced through the stab wound and docked on the lamina and advanced in this trajectory and exits the cortical bone of the inferior lateral pedicle at the junction of transverse process. A 4.5-mm tap is then advanced just beyond the joint. The purpose of this is so that the screw will engage the caudal vertebrae immediately, so there is no distraction of the facet joint before the screw engages distally. The screw is then inserted, with typical screw lengths between 44 and 54 mm. The second screw is placed on the contralateral side using the same technique. Decortication of the lamina and facet joints is accomplished with a high-speed bone dissector and graft is placed to facilitate a posterior fusion.

Limitations

Obviously the patient must have intact pars intra-articularis and lamina to perform the technique.

Biomechanically the technique is not as robust as pedicle screw fixation; however, with anterior column support (e.g., anterior lumbar interbody fusion, lateral lumbar interbody fusion, posterior lumbar interbody fusion, or transforaminal lumbar interbody fusion), the fixation is essentially clinically equivalent.

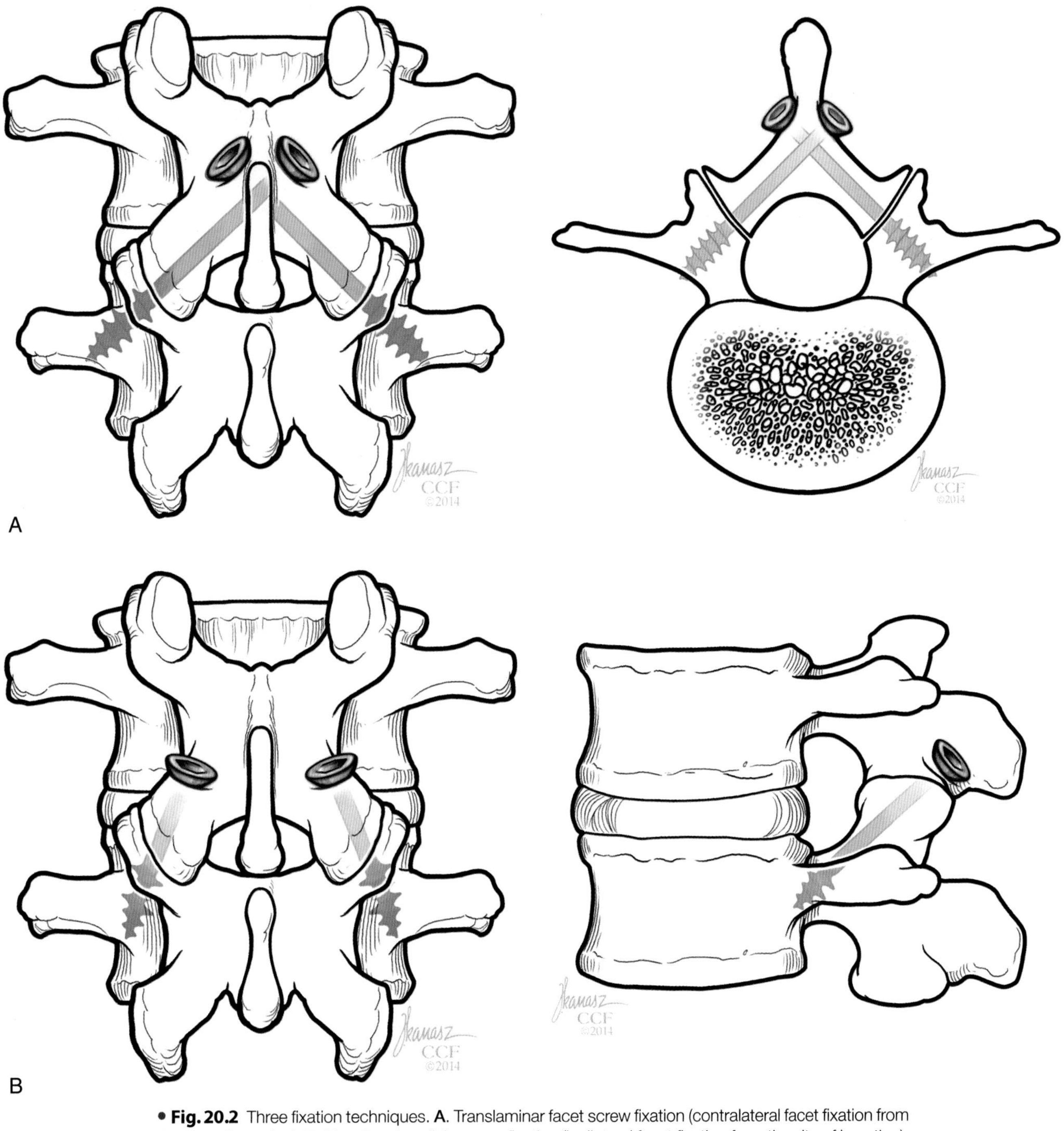

• **Fig. 20.2** Three fixation techniques. **A**. Translaminar facet screw fixation (contralateral facet fixation from the site of insertion). **B**. Transfacet pedicle screw fixation (ipsilateral facet fixation from the site of insertion).

Facet screw technique requires a keen understanding of the 3D anatomy of the spine, whether unilateral or translaminar. The technique currently requires open exposure, but may be successfully and reliably performed percutaneously in the future with the use of navigation and/or robotics.

Tips and Tricks

In the past, there have been guide devices available to assist with facet screw implantation, but their availability at this time is unknown. Ideally, the drill bits and taps are calibrated to a sleeve that passes through the soft tissue to provide protection of the paraspinous processes during instrumentation. If such a system is not available, this technique can be done with the instrumentation from most large fragment trauma sets.

Always start with the most cranial screw first and stay as cranial as possible to allow for ample room for the second screw. If the first screw is placed in the middle, then there will not be enough room for the caudal screw.

There are no reliable and repeatable fluoroscopic landmarks to place these screws with 2D fluoroscopy. This technique requires understanding 3D anatomy, specifically the

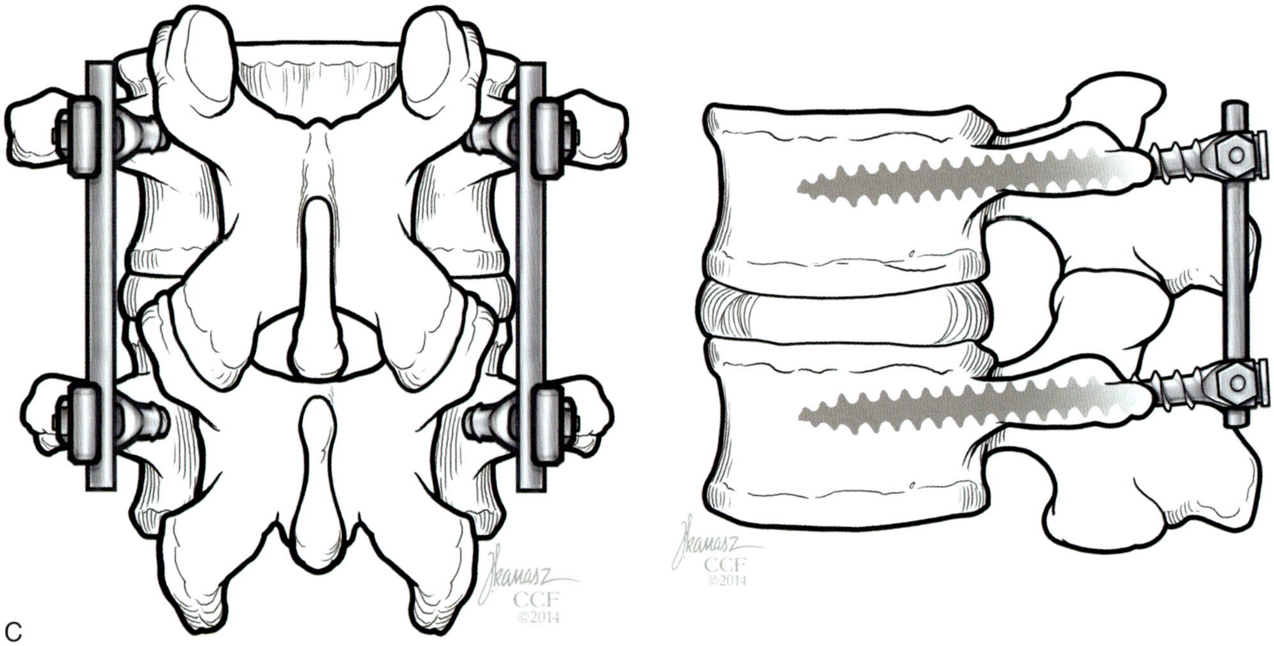

Fig. 20.2, cont'd C. Traditional pedicle screw fixation. (Reprinted with permission, Cleveland Clinic Center for Medical Art & Photography © 2014. All Rights Reserved.) *World Spinal Column Journal* 2014;5(2):97.

start point and exit point with the ability to drill in that specific trajectory.

A patient may have a previous one-side hemilaminotomy, and the cranial screw needs to be placed on the side of the previous decompression.

Complications

Many complications can occur using facet screw fixation. Intraoperative complications include screw misdirection that could lead to dural tear, nerve compression, and/or nerve injury. Lamina and facet fractures may also occur if screws are not placed in the correct trajectory. Postoperative complications are rare, but would include loosening or failure of the hardware, typically in the presence of a pseudoarthrosis. If the screws fracture, it is almost always at the facet joint. Reoperation for pseudoarthrosis can be accomplished with pedicle screws. It is important to note that the caudal segment may have a screw pass through the pedicle so that the facet screw will need to be removed before placing the caudal pedicle screw. Careful examination of the preoperative x-rays and computed tomography scan will help with planning.

Pedicle Screws

History

Harrington and Tullous[14] reported in 1969 on what most people credit as the first "true" pedicle screw. The screws were inserted into pedicles with modified Harrington instrumentation and were wired to Harrington distraction rods.

In 1970, Roy-Camille et al.[15,16] reported the use of posterior plates and sagittal screws through the pedicle and articular processes. Although the trajectory was not the same as standard pedicle screw fixation today, this was a similar concept that showed significant success. Louis and Maresca[17] reported success with a modified technique and instrumentation. The report on 455 cases with 31.6 months of average follow-up indicated solid arthrodesis was achieved in 97.4% of posterior only cases and 100% of the combined approach cases.

Roy-Camille then presented the pedicle screw technique in 1984 at the Academy of Orthopaedic Surgeons meeting in San Francisco.[18] Steffee et al.[19] was very interested in this technique and, in 1986, he published on a variable screw placement plate that could be used from the thoracic spine to the sacrum (Fig. 20.3).

Pedicle screw fixation became the gold standard by the mid-1990s[10] and, in 1993 and 1996, the North American Spine Society endorsed the use of pedicle screws by experienced surgeons.[20]

Despite this, the 1990s were marred by unfortunate events for physicians, manufacturers, and medical societies supporting the pedicle screw. In August of 1993 the FDA sent a letter to six companies instructing them not to 'advertise or promote' the use of pedicle screws in the spine. As a class III device, the screws were approved as bone screws, but not specifically for the spine. By December of 1993, the infamous 20/20 episode aired and sparked litigation that continued throughout the United States. Acromed settled for $100 million in 1997, just before the FDA reclassified the devices from class III to class II in July 1998. The reclassification resulted in the dismissal of the majority of the remaining litigation cases.[21]

Minimally Invasive Surgery (MIS) Pedicle Screws

Magerl[7] was first to introduce MIS, the percutaneous placement of screws in 1977. The technique was cumbersome, and utilized an external spinal skeletal fixation (ESSF) system. Over time, this particular technique did not achieve good results primarily owing to wound issues from the external nature and was no longer used, but the concept of MIS screw placement remained (Fig. 20.4).[22]

Foley et al.[23] were the first to publish a clinical series of a percutaneous technique in fusion of degenerative lumbar pathologies

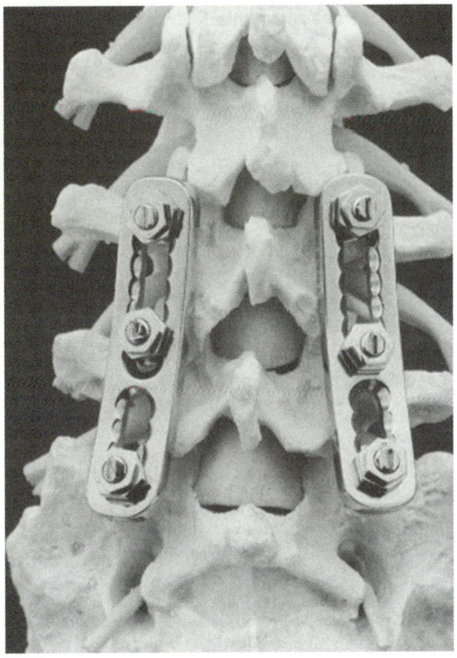

• **Fig. 20.3** The variable screw placement (Steffee) system. (Courtesy of DePuy Synthes.)

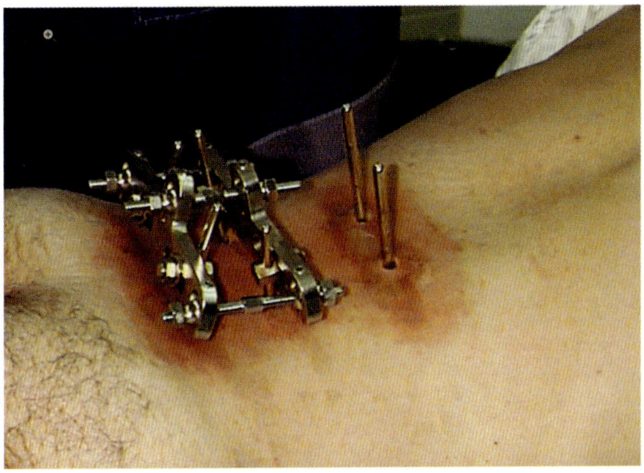

• **Fig. 20.4** Minimally invasive surgery (MIS) screw placement. (Courtesy Pierce D. Nunley, MD, 1996, Switzerland.)

(Sextant; Medtronic, Minneapolis, MN, USA). A major step toward percutaneous screw placement, the Sextant system used fluoroscopic imaging to assist in the trajectory. The multiaxial screw was modified and placed percutaneously using an extension sleeve/tower. The engineering of Foley's design was significant as it used the mechanics of the radius of an arc to deliver the rod percutaneously. Unfortunately, this required a separate incision to be made in order to pass the rod, and anatomic variations further made this a challenge. This original system could only be used with two screws, but a two-level system was subsequently developed (Fig. 20.5).[23,24]

The results with the early percutaneous pedicle screws showed good stability and fusion and the technology advanced to be used with multiple pathologies (trauma, tumors, deformity, and degenerative disease.[25,26] More recent studies have confirmed these results.

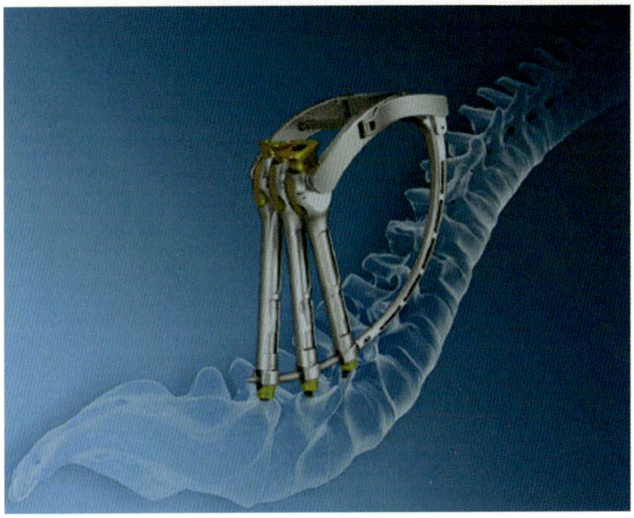

• **Fig. 20.5** Two-level rod insertion system, CD Horizon Sextant II. (Courtesy of Medtronic Inc., Minneapolis, MN, USA.)

In 2012, Kruger et al. published a report on 51 prospective patients using Sextant II Rod insertion system. A total of 204 screws were used; 197 were correctly placed, with all fractures showing fusion after 6 weeks. "However, the authors reported that the multiaxial pedicle screws were not able to conserve the slight correction obtained perioperatively via positioning and longitudinal traction."[27]

In 2014, Wang et al.[28] reported a retrospective review of 100 patients with kyphosis using the Sextant system. They concluded that Sextant was superior to conventional open posterior short segment four screw system.

Design Evolution of Minimally Invasive Surgery (MIS) Pedicle Screws

The evolution of minimally invasive systems flourished as designers and manufactures raced to develop better ways to place pedicle screws percutaneously.

The MIS pedicle screws required cannulation for the majority of the early systems. The technique first involved targeting the pedicle via C-arm guidance and then inserting a large gauge biopsy-style needle through the pedicle and into the vertebral body. The needle stylet is removed and a guidewire placed into the vertebral body and the needle removed. This would then allow taping, if indicated, and screw guidance through the pedicle into the vertebral body. There were biomechanical concerns as cannulation affected the overall strength of the screws, particularly in the smaller diameters. Guidewire diameter and screw designs were altered by many manufactures to account for these challenges.

Subsequent generations of MIS systems can be categorized as either rigid tower (Sextant II, Medtronic, Minneapolis, MN and Expedium, Depuy, Raynham, MA) or flexible tower systems (Serengeti, K2M, Leesburg, VA). Many manufactures had different designs of detachable towers that would be placed over conventional screws and then removed after the screws and rod were secure (Fig. 20.5).

The concept of a flexible tower/retractor was developed that had certain advantages over the rigid tower designs. Notably, it was easier to pass rods for certain spinal deformities, including hyperlordosis, rotatory scoliosis, and spondylolisthesis.

More recent generations of the rigid tower systems incorporate the 'tower' into tabs that are manufactured with the screws and

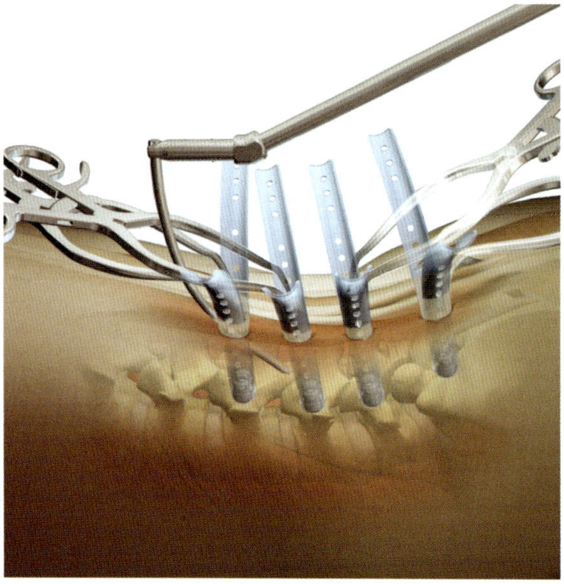

• **Fig. 20.6** Flexible retractor system for minimally invasive surgery pedicle screw placement. (Courtesy of K2M, Inc., Leesburg, VA, USA.)

then 'break away' after the screw is placed and rod secured. Many of these systems have built-in screw reduction tabs that allow for easier placement and seating of the rod and reduction of spinal deformities (Figs. 20.6 and 20.7). There are potential advantages of these systems, but at the time of publication no data on these new systems can be reported.

As with all systems, there are advantages and disadvantages and today spine surgeons have many options from which to choose (Figs. 20.6–20.9).

Indications

Pedicle screws are utilized in posterior fixation of the spine with or without interbody support.

Technique

There are a variety of techniques for placing MIS pedicle screws. Flouroscopy is most commonly used, but navigation with the aid of 3D intraoperative imaging has recently gained in popularity. Currently, multiple companies are developing robots to assist in the placement of these screws as another option. However, navigation and robotics are beyond the scope of this chapter and proprietary to the specific hardware, software, and implants for each system.

Flouroscopy can be used either with one or two machines, and there are two basic techniques. The first technique uses pure anteroposterior and lateral images to aim from 'outside to inside' starting at the posterior lateral aspect of the pedicle to the anterior medial pedicle at its attachment to the vertebral body. The typical starting point is at the junction of the transverse process and the inferior articulating facet.

A styletted large-bore needle is advanced across the pedicle. The stylet is removed and the guide pin is placed into the vertebral body. Cannulated screws are placed by either tapping first or advancing the screw directly without tapping. The second flouroscopic technique is often called the "down the barrel" technique and the C-arm is rotated 15 to 30 degrees laterally to "look" straight down the pedicle. The needle and subsequent screw are advanced in a "bullseye" view down the pedicle. Some techniques allow for solid screws to be inserted under flouroscopy after the needle is removed. Rods are then placed and any desired reduction maneuvers are performed prior to tightening the construct to the manufacturer's specifications.

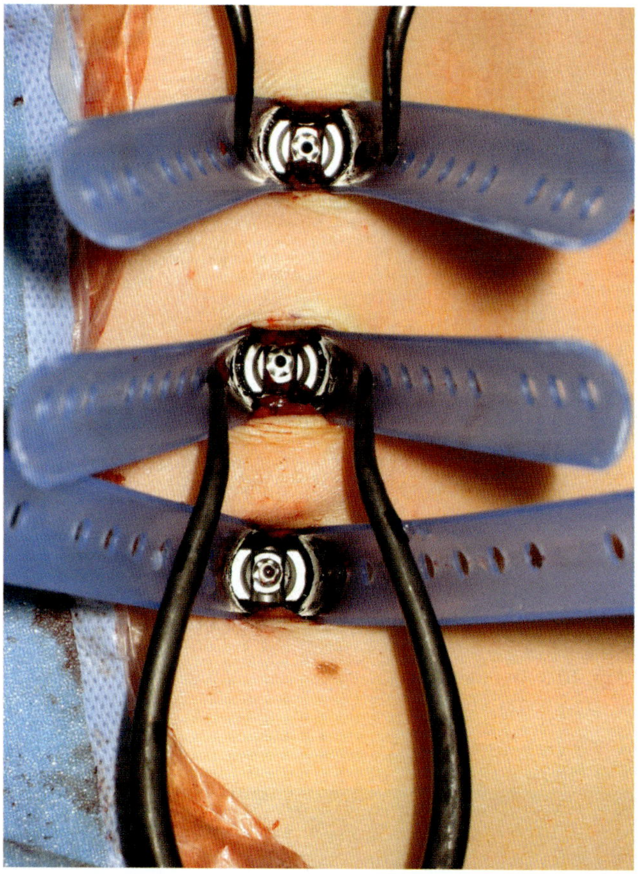

• **Fig. 20.7** Surgeon's view of tulips using a flexible minimally invasive surgery retractor. (Courtesy of K2M, Inc., VA, USA.)

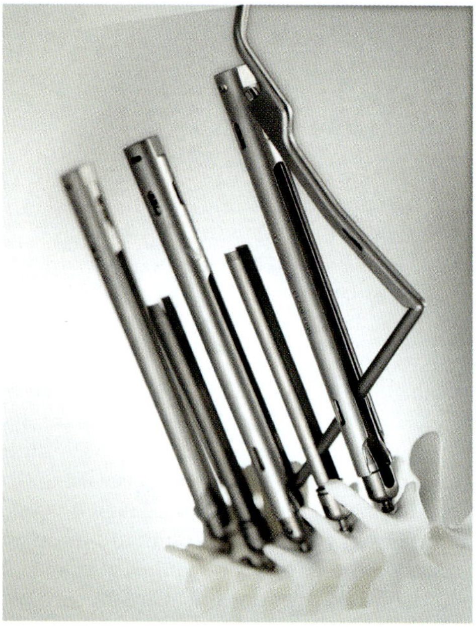

• **Fig. 20.8** Rod placement with rigid tower design. (Courtesy of DePuy Synthes.)

Grafting is then performed either by a formal posterolateral decortication and grafting or, alternatively, by percutaneously decorticating the facet joint complexes and leaving the fragments of the decortication with or without supplemental grafting to facilitate a posterior fusion.

Tips and Tricks

If available, use two C-arms for biplanar fluoroscopy. Pay close attention to entry points for screws and be consistent. Altering the entry points can make connecting the rod very difficult. Place wires on both sides before placing screws, because a screw will block the lateral image on the contralateral side. At the S1 level, it can be difficult to clearly identify the medial board of the pedicle. Canting the C-arm cranial and caudal under live fluoroscopy will often help identify landmarks in these difficult cases. Intraoperative triggered electromyography can be a helpful tool, particularly for questionable screws, since the medial pedicle cannot be visualized or probed.

Limitations

There are many potential limitations to MIS pedicle screw fixation. The first is that the technique requires either fluoroscopy or navigation. There is a growing awareness of the dangers of radiation exposure and MIS techniques with fluoroscopy expose the surgeon and staff with increased radiation. Depending on the imaging modality used with navigation there is a chance to decrease radiation exposure to the team and, possibly, the patient.

MIS screw fixation requires a keen understanding of the three-dimensional anatomy of the spine, particularly when there are abnormalities regarding size and trajectory of specific pedicles and difficulty viewing critical anatomic landmarks (e.g., medial border of the pedicle frequently challenging at S1).

Complex spine and multiple level cases require consistency with screw placement in order to be able to place the rods without excessive bends or stress on the screws. This is more difficult in the MIS case where the surgeon does not "see" the lineup of screws as they are placed.

Accessing the transverse processes for decortication and placement of bone graft (if desired by the surgeon) can be challenging with most systems as the 'towers' are in the way. This can be accomplished by a secondary tube or even using a flat retractor, such as a small Hibbs, to provide soft tissue retraction.

A "requirement" for a midline exposure for a formal decompression would require a separate midline incision. However, in most cases the decompression can be performed first by indirect decompression created by the combination of the anterior and posterior fixation and second via a unilateral transforaminal decompression utilizing the same wound as the pedicle screw fixation.

Cortical Bone Trajectory

It is worth mentioning an emerging technique for placing posterior screws that has been most often referred to as cortical bone trajectory screws.[29] In 2009, Santoni et al.[30] first reported in *Spine* a 30% increase in pullout failure load compared with traditional pedicle screws. They theorized that in osteoporotic bone these screws and trajectory may be incrementally more beneficial, as osteoporosis affects cortical bone to a lesser extent than cancellous bone. Multiple studies in recent years have been published,

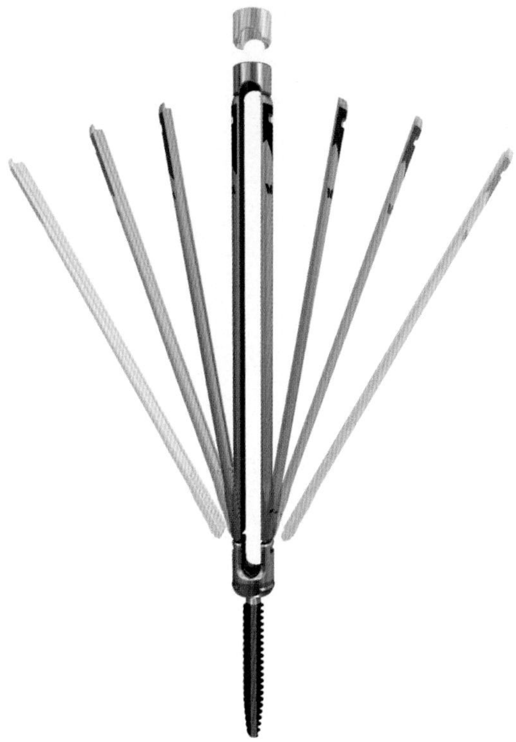

• **Fig. 20.9** Low profile rigid built-in tower with reduction threads built into breakaway tabs. (Courtesy of K2M, Inc., Leesburg, VA, USA.)

most notably by Matsukawa, Radcliff, and Calvert and their colleagues.[31–33] The analysis in these papers concluded that cortical bone trajectory tends to have greater insertional torque and pull-out strength. However, it remains to be seen if this technique will stand the test of time as the clinical papers released to date are all small number cohorts.

Indications are the same as for pedicle screw fixation; however, for midline wounds this technique requires significantly less soft tissue dissection and is considered by some to be an MIS technique.

The technique for placing these screws varies significantly and will not be a focus of this chapter. The author encourages the interested reader to attend a hands-on course to learn this very useful technique.

Limitations include learning and working in a different anatomic trajectory than traditionally trained and the learning curve needs to become proficient. It is also difficult to connect this screw to adjacent segment traditional pedicle screw trajectory constructs, which can be challenging in revision surgeries.

MIS Spinal Deformity

The advancement of devices and instrumentation has led to nearly an unlimited number of levels that can be instrumented in the spine. Several systems now allow for multilevel instrumentation and fixation to correct spinal deformity. The use of rigid or flexible towers, as described previously, has changed the landscape of MIS spinal deformity surgery and challenges the traditional open surgical technique (Fig. 20.10). A large number of ongoing studies are comparing surgical techniques for spinal deformity, including traditional open, hybrid, and MIS techniques. In 2015, the International Spine Study Group presented that MIS techniques improved patients' spinal deformity,

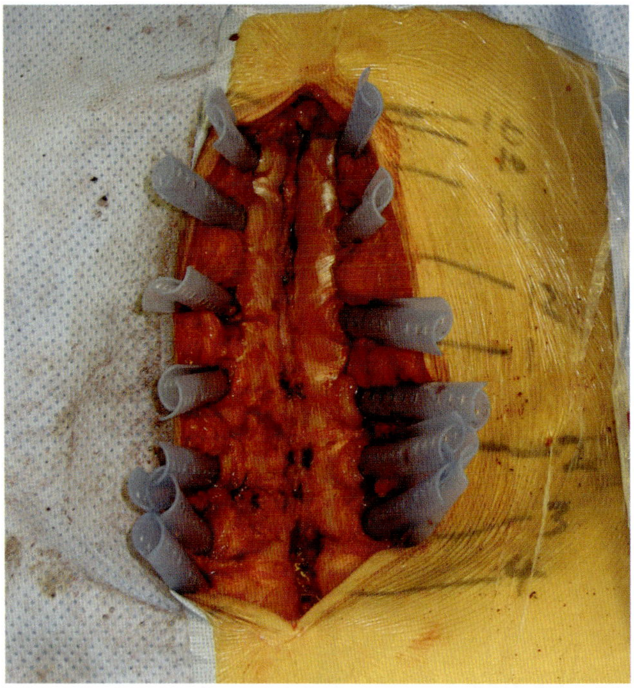

• **Fig. 20.10** Multilevel scoliosis case with flexible retractor design. (Courtesy of Pierce Nunley, Shreveport, LA, 2008.)

although substantial deformity did not improve. They also found that MIS surgery had significantly lower estimated blood loss and shorter intensive care unit stay.[34,35] In the coming years it seems highly probable the majority of deformity surgery will be able to be performed partially or entirely using MIS techniques (Fig. 20.10).

Interspinous Process Device

History

Knowles filed the first patent in 1952, approved in 1954, for an interspinous process device (ISP).[36] The only publication on this device was a letter to the editor, Whiteside in 2003 that stated the device was no longer used after frequent rotation or loosening (Fig. 20.11).[37]

The Wallis system, 1986, by Abbott Spine (Park, IL) was the next generation of ISP: it has gone through multiple enhancements since its creation.[38,39] Minns' reported on a soft preformed implant in 1996, but the device did not progress past biomechanical cadaver testing.[40]

The 1990s were a period for the design of several new ISPs, beginning with Paradigm's Coflex (formerly Interspinous U) in 1994.[41] Medtronic's XTOP was approved by the FDA in 2005, and launched to market in 2008.[42] Although still available outside the United States (OUS), Medtronic discontinued sales of XSTOP in the United States in 2015.

DIAM, by Medtronic, has been Conformite Europene (CE) marked in Europe since 2006, and was approved for an Investigational Device Exemption (IDE) study in the United States the same year. However, in 2016 the FDA rejected approval of DIAM in the United States.[42,43]

Although the first ISPs designed were Wallis, Coflex, DIAM, and XSTOP, only Coflex remains available in the United States. The current landscape includes other devices such as Aspen (ZimmerBiomet, Warsaw, IN) (Fig. 20.12), Interbridge (ZimmerBiomet), Stabilink (Southern Spine, Macon, GA), and Bridgepoint (Alphatec Spine, Carlsbad, CA).[42]

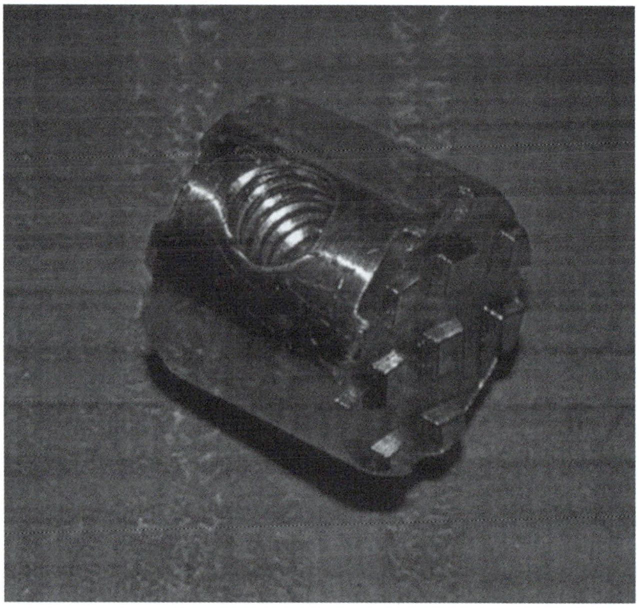

• **Fig. 20.11** Knowles device. (From Whitesides TE. The effect of an interspinous implant on intervertebral disk pressures. *Spine* 2003;28(16):1906–1907; author reply 7–8.)

Many of these interspinous process devices have been used in nonfusion techniques. Nonfusion techniques are not the focus of this chapter.

Technique

These devices are placed through a midline approach after exposure of the lamina. Some allow or require the removal of the supraspinous ligament, whereas others leave the ligament intact as a checkrein. The device is trialed and inserted per the manufacture's guidelines. Most devices require bilateral exposure, but some allow for only unilateral exposure. In order to create an environment for fusion, there must be an appropriate biologic placed in or around the device in the interspinous space.

Because there is a great deal of variability in the constructs available on the market, the reader is referred to the specific device to be appropriately trained by expert users and the manufacturer.

Not enough is known about these devices to discuss their limitations; however, used as fixation and fusion devices, the future is unknown for these devices as a supplemental fixation after interbody fixation. Although promising, we need more quality research to prove the safety and efficacy of these devices.

Biomechanical Testing

Biomechanical testing of pedicle screws began in 1986, with pedicle screws and fixed plate implants.[44,45] Load sharing or load transfer across the implant was established within the surgeon community as important for fusion success.[45] The bone-implant interface, bone density, screw pullout, and proper fit in the pedicle have been shown to be important for the biomechanical success of pedicle screw fixation.[46–49] Additional biomechanics studies compare pedicle and facet screws with equivalent or improved stabilization with pedicle screws.[19,50]

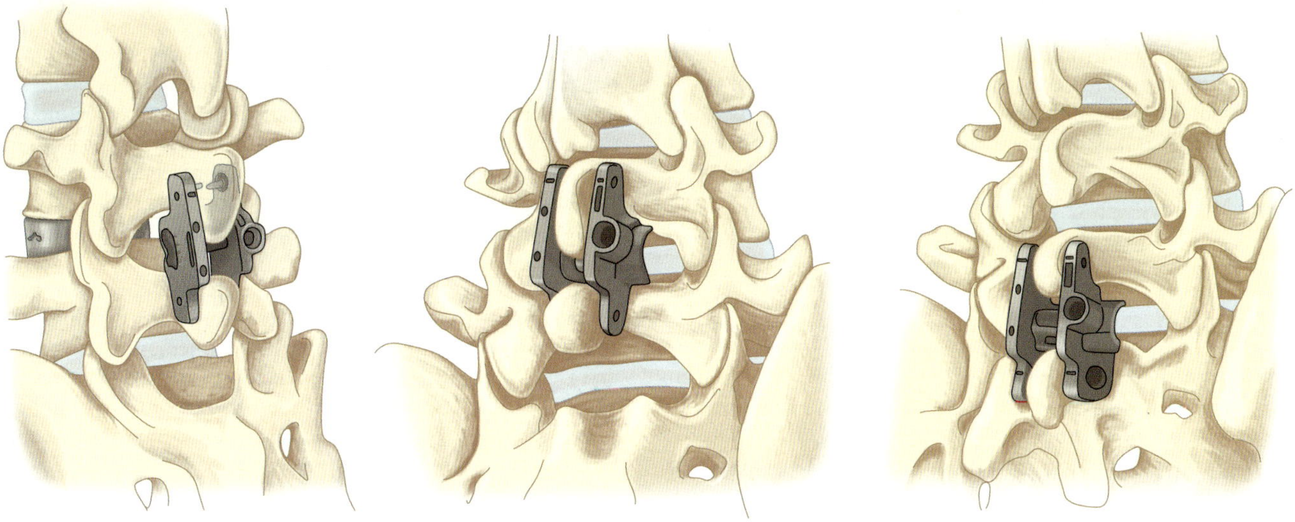

• **Fig. 20.12** Aspen system. (Courtesy of ZimmerBiomet, Warsaw, IN.)

Facet Screw Biomechanics

The anatomy of facets during extension causes the superior facet of the lower vertebra to block the inferior facet of the upper vertebra. This blocking restricts any further extension, creating spinal stability during extension.[51,52] Biomechanically, facet screws, when used to immobilize the facet joints, should stabilize the spine to allow for fusion.[52] Multiple biomechanics studies have shown that translaminar fixation provides adequate stability after interbody fusion.[12,53,54]

Biomechanical testing indicates that both facet screws and pedicle screws provide adequate stability to achieve solid fusion.[12,50,53,54] Multiple studies have looked at the results of surgeries with pedicle screws versus facet screws.[13,15,54]

In 2016, Liu et al.[55] studied TLIF at two levels and compared unilateral pedicle screws (UPS), hybrid with unilateral pedicle screws plus contralateral translaminar facet screws (UPSFS), and bilateral pedicle screws (BPS). The surgery was significantly shorter for UPS and UPSFS compared with BPS. However, clinical outcomes were not significantly different between groups (Visual Analogue Scale, Japanese Orthopedic Association (JOA), Oswestry Disability Index). There was no significant difference in fusion rates or complication rates, although fusion did increase from UPS (81.8%) to UPSFS (89.3%) to BPS (94.1%). Screw rod failure was significantly higher in the UPSFS group.[55]

Interspinous Process Device Biomechanics

Wang et al.[56,57] presented to the Joint Section in 2005 and later published in 2006 their results of the SPIRE device. They performed anterior column support and then compared pedicle screw, translaminar facet screw, and ISP fixation. No statistically significant differences were found in this in vitro biomechanical testing environment, leading them to conclude that SPIRE was biomechanically appropriate for posterior fixation.

Techy et al.[58] performed a biomechanical study in a TLIF model with posterior instrumentation. They concluded that ISP fixation was equal to pedicle screws in flexion and extension; however, ISP provided minimal stability in axial rotation and lateral bending as compared with pedicle screws. They did also note that an ISP with unilateral pedicle screws was the same as bilateral pedicle screws.

Fogel et al.[59] reported on a cadaveric study of 10 specimens in 2014 where they showed that pedicle screw fixation and ISP were significantly superior to either a lateral interbody or lateral interbody with lateral plate in all ranges of motion. However, in flexion/extension and rotation, pedicle screws were significantly better than the ISP. They concluded that the relative values were so close that ISP may offer an alternative to pedicle screw placement in the clinical setting.

Finally, Godzik et al.[60] reported on the use of the SPIRE in 2016 using a protocol of ISP versus supplementing with unilateral pedicle screws or unilateral or bilateral facet screws. Although ISP alone was significantly better than intact in flexion and extension as well as axial rotation, significant improvements were seen in biomechanics when additional posterior fixation was performed.

The conclusion from currently available biomechanical data is that ISP (not simple spacers [e.g., X-Stop, Coflex]) do significantly increase the biomechanical stability in the spine, particularly in flexion and extension and when there is interbody fixation. The clinical question is whether this is sufficient fixation so as not to adversely affect the clinical outcome. Further studies will be required to determine the future of ISP as a supplement to interbody fixation.

Future Trends

MIS

Minimally invasive spine surgery is the fastest growing market segment in spine surgery. New techniques and improvements in established techniques will allow for continued growth. It is important that these techniques and instrumentation are carefully studied and reported to provide safety and efficacy that our patients deserve. It is likely that in the near future, the majority of spine surgeries performed will incorporate at least some elements of minimally invasive surgery.

Image Guidance and Robotics

Although not the focus of this chapter, it should be mentioned that the increased development of navigation systems and robotics will likely, once again change how these systems are placed and will likely be an integral part of spinal instrumentation. The current challenges are the cost of the systems and increased time in the operating room. However, with the growing concerns of radiation exposure it is likely that we will continue to see a growth of this technology. It is likely that there will be a point when the cost is reasonable and the technology advances to the point where a surgeon will be more likely to ask the question "why not" rather than "why" would I use navigation and robotics to place spinal hardware.

Conclusion

In summary, there is a long history of posterior spinal instrumentation with many choices available for today's spine surgeon. Although stand-alone interbody likely has a place in selected patients, it remains controversial in identifying exactly which are appropriate patients. It is clear from the biomechanics data that posterior fixation increases the stability of the spine. The ultimate question is "how much stability is needed" and "when do we need more stability?"

Circumferential fusion has a distant history of being a morbid technique owing to outdated techniques and implants. With modern techniques and implants, supplemental instrumentation can be placed after interbody fusion with relatively low increased risk to the majority of our patients. Biomechanical and clinical studies have repeatedly shown that fusion rates and outcomes are as good and generally better when a circumferential construct is utilized.

As can be ascertained from the content of this chapter, there are no 'right or wrong' answers necessarily for which construct is best for posterior supplemental instrumentation, but the general trend is that MIS posterior fixation is better when indicated and potentially there could be a resurgence of translaminar facet screws as navigation systems become more commonplace and the health care system continues to look for less expensive ways to achieve the same clinical results.

References

1. Rihn JA, Gandhi SD, Sheehan P, et al. Disc space preparation in transforaminal lumbar interbody fusion: a comparison of minimally invasive and open approaches. *Clin Orthop Relat Res.* 2014;472(6):1800–1805.
2. Boucher HH. A method of spinal fusion. *J Bone Joint Surg Br.* 1959;41-B(2):248–259.
3. King D. Internal fixation for lumbosacral fusion. *Am J Surg.* 1944;66:357–361.
4. King D. Internal fixation for lumbosacral fusion. *J Bone Joint Surg Am.* 1948;30A(3):560–565.
5. Thompson WA, Ralston EL. Pseudarthrosis following spine fusion. *J Bone Joint Surg Am.* 1949;31A(2):400–405.
6. Pennel GF, McDonald GA, Dale GG. A method of spinal fusion using internal fixation. *Clin Orthop Rel Res.* 1964;35:86–94.
7. Magerl FP. Stabilization of the lower thoracic and lumbar spine with external skeletal fixation. *Clin Orthop Relat Res.* 1984;(189): 125–141.
8. Jacobs RR, Montesano PX, Jackson RP. Enhancement of lumbar spine fusion by use of translaminar facet joint screws. *Spine (Phila Pa 1976).* 1989;14(1):12–15.
9. Agarwala A, Bucklen B, Muzumdar A, et al. Do facet screws provide the required stability in lumbar fixation? A biomechanical comparison of the Boucher technique and pedicular fixation in primary and circumferential fusions. *Clin Biomech (Bristol, Avon).* 2012;27(1):64–70.
10. Ferrara LA, Secor JL, Jin BH, et al. A biomechanical comparison of facet screw fixation and pedicle screw fixation: effects of short-term and long-term repetitive cycling. *Spine (Phila Pa 1976).* 2003;28(12):1226–1234.
11. Best NM, Sasso RC. Efficacy of translaminar facet screw fixation in circumferential interbody fusions as compared to pedicle screw fixation. *J Spinal Disord Tech.* 2006;19(2):98–103.
12. Shim CS, Lee SH, Jung B, et al. Fluoroscopically assisted percutaneous translaminar facet screw fixation following anterior lumbar interbody fusion: technical report. *Spine. (Phila Pa 1976).* 2005;30:838–843.
13. Buttermann GR, Thorson TM, Mullin WJ. Outcomes of posterior facet versus pedicle screw fixation of circumferential fusion: a cohort study. *Eur Spine J.* 2014;23(2):347–355.
14. Harrington PR, Tullos HS. Reduction of severe spondylolisthesis in children. *South Med J.* 1969;62(1):1–7.
15. Roy-Camille R, Saillant G, Mazel C. Internal fixation of the lumbar spine with pedicle screw plating. *Clin Orthop Relat Res.* 1986;203: 7–17.
16. Roy-Camille R, Saillant G, Berteaux D, et al. Osteosynthesis of thoraco-lumbar spine fractures with metal plates screwed through the vertebral pedicles. *Reconstr Surg Traumatol.* 1976;15:2–16.
17. Louis R, Maresca C. Stabilisation chirurgicale avec Reduction des pondylolyses et des spondylolisthesis. *Int Orthop (S.I.C.O.T.).* 1977;1:215.
18. Roy-Camille R, Saillant G, Lapresle P, et al. A secret in spine surgery: The pedicle. Proceedings of the 51st annual meeting of the American Academy of Orthopaedic Surgeons, 1984.
19. Steffee AD, Biscup RS, Sitkowski DJ. Segmental spine plates with pedicle screw fixation. A new internal fixation device for disorders of the lumbar and thoracolumbar spine. *Clin Orthop Relat Res.* 1986;203:45–53.
20. Gaines RW. The use of pedicle-screw internal fixation for the operative treatment of spinal disorders. *J Bone Joint Surg Am.* 2000;82-A(10):1458–1476.
21. In the United States District Court for the Eastern District of Pennsylvania in Re: Orthopedic Bone Screw Products Liability Litigation. *Daniel Fanning et al and Margaret Schmerling, et al. v. AcroMed Corporation* (C.A. No. 97–381 1997). https://www.paed.uscourts.gov/documents/opinions/97D1164P.pdf.
22. Soini JR, Seitsalo SK. The external fixation test of the lumbar spine. 30 complications in 25 of 100 consecutive patients. *Acta Orthop Scand.* 1993;64:147–149.
23. Foley KT, Gupta SK, Justis JR, et al. Percutaneous pedicle screw fixation of the lumbar spine. *Neurosurg Focus.* 2001;10(4):E10.
24. Foley KT, Gupta SK. Percutaneous pedicle screw fixation of the lumbar spine: preliminary clinical results. *J Neurosurg.* 2002;97(suppl 1):7–12.
25. Mobbs RJ, Sivabalan P, Li J. Technique, challenges and indications for percutaneous pedicle screw fixation. *J Clin Neurosci.* 2011;18(6):741–749.
26. Phan K, Rao PJ, Mobbs RJ. Percutaneous versus open pedicle screw fixation for treatment of thoracolumbar fractures: systematic review and meta-analysis of comparative studies. *Clin Neurol Neurosurg.* 2015;135:85–92.

27. Krüger A, Rammler K, Ziring E, et al. Percutaneous minimally invasive instrumentation for traumatic thoracic and lumbar fractures: a prospective analysis. *Acta Orthop Belg.* 2012;78:376–381.
28. Wang H, Zhou Y, Li C, et al. Comparison of open versus percutaneous pedicle screw fixation using the Sextant system in the treatment of traumatic thoracolumbar fractures. *Clin Spine Surg.* 2017;30(3):E239–E246.
29. Phan K, Hogan J, Maharaj M, et al. Cortical bone trajectory for lumbar pedicle screw placement: a review of published reports. *Orthop Surg.* 2015;7(3):121–213.
30. Santoni BG, Hynes RA, McGilvray KC, et al. Cortical bone trajectory for lumbar pedicle screws. *Spine J.* 2009;9(5):366–373.
31. Matsukawa K, Yato Y, Imabayashi H, et al. Biomechanical evaluation of lumbar pedicle screws in spondylolytic vertebrae: comparison of fixation strength between the traditional trajectory and a cortical bone trajectory. *J Neurosurg Spine.* 2016;24(6):910–915.
32. Radcliff K, Klocke N, Harris J, et al., eds. *Can Cortical Screws Provide the Same Resistance to Catastrophic Hardware Failure as Traditional Pedicle Screws Following Simulated Fatigue: a Biomechanical Investigation.* Miami, FL: Presented at: Society for Minimally Invasive Spine Surgery Global Forum; 2014.
33. Calvert GC, Lawrence BD, Abtahi AM, et al. Cortical screws used to rescue failed lumbar pedicle screw construct: a biomechanical analysis. *J Neurosurg Spine.* 2015;22(2):166–172.
34. International Spine Surgery Group, Mundis Jr GM, Turner JD, et al. In: *A Critical Analysis of Sagittal Plane Deformity Correction With Minimally Invasive Adult Spinal Deformity Surgery: a Two-Year Follow-Up Study.* Chicago, IL: Presented at: North American Spine Society, 30th Annual Meeting; 2015.
35. International Spine Surgery Group, Chou D, Wang M, Blaskiewicz D, et al. In: *The Impact of Minimally Invasive Spinal Deformity Surgery on Icu and Hospital Stay.* Chicago, IL: Presented at: North American Spine Society, 30th Annual Meeting; 2015.
36. Knowles F. Apparatus for treatment of the spinal column. US patent 2677369 A. 1952. https://www.google.com/patents/US2677369#backward-citations.
37. Whitesides TE. The effect of an interspinous implant on intervertebral disc pressures. *Spine (Phila Pa 1976).* 2003;28(16):1906–1907; author reply 1907–1908.
38. Senegas J, Etchevers JP, Vital JM, et al. [Recalibration of the lumbar canal, an alternative to laminectomy in the treatment of lumbar canal stenosis]. *Rev Chir Orthop Reparatrice Appar Mot.* 1988;74(1):15–22. [in French].
39. Sénégas J. Mechanical supplementation by non-rigid fixation in degenerative intervertebral lumbar segments: the Wallis system. *Eur Spine J.* 2002;11(suppl 2):S164–S169.
40. Minns RJ, Walsh WK. Preliminary design and experimental studies of a novel soft implant for correcting sagittal plane instability in the lumbar spine. *Spine (Phila Pa 1976).* 1997;22(16):1819–1825; discussion 1826–1827.
41. Richter A, Schütz C, Hauck M, et al. Does an interspinous device (Coflex) improve the outcome of decompressive surgery in lumbar spinal stenosis? One-year follow up of a prospective case control study of 60 patients. *Eur Spine J.* 2010;19(2):283–289.
42. Gazzeri R, Galarza M, Alfieri A. Controversies about interspinous process devices in the treatment of degenerative lumbar spine diseases: past, present, and future. *Biomed Res Int.* 2014;2014:975052.
43. Caserta S, La Maida GA, Misaggi B, et al. Elastic stabilization alone or combined with rigid fusion in spinal surgery: a biomechanical study and clinical experience based on 82 cases. *Eur Spine J.* 2002;11(suppl 2):S192–S197.
44. Gaines RW, Carson WL, Satterlee CC, et al. Improving quality of spinal internal fixation —evolution toward "ideal immobilization"—a biomechanical study. *Orthop Trans.* 1987;11:86–87.
45. Gaines RW, Carson WL, Satterlee CC, et al. Experimental evaluation of seven different spinal fracture internal fixation devices using nonfailure stability testing. The load-sharing and unstable-mechanism concepts. *Spine (Phila Pa 1976).* 1991;16(8):902–909.
46. Bennett GJ, Serhan HA, Sorini PM, et al. An experimental study of lumbar destabilization. Restabilization and bone density. *Spine (Phila Pa 1976).* 1997;22(13):1448–1453.
47. Coe JD, Warden KE, Herzig MA, et al. Influence of bone mineral density on the fixation of thoracolumbar implants. A comparative study of transpedicular screws, laminar hooks, and spinous process wires. *Spine (Phila Pa 1976).* 1990;15(9):902–907.
48. Law M, Tencer AF, Anderson PA. Caudo-cephalad loading of pedicle screws: mechanisms of loosening and methods of augmentation. *Spine (Phila Pa 1976).* 1993;18(16):2438–2443.
49. McLain RF, Fry MF, Moseley TA, et al. Lumbar pedicle screw salvage: pullout testing of three different pedicle screw designs. *J Spinal Disord.* 1995;8(1):62–68.
50. Chin KR, Reis MT, Reyes PM, et al. Stability of transforaminal lumbar interbody fusion in the setting of retained facets and posterior fixation using transfacet or standard pedicle screws. *Spine J.* 2015;15(5):1077–1082.
51. Kim SM, Lim TJ, Paterno J, et al. A biomechanical comparison of supplementary posterior translaminar facet and transfacetopedicular screw fixation after anterior lumbar interbody fusion. *J Neurosurg Spine.* 2004;1(1):101–107.
52. Oxland TR, Lund T. Biomechanics of stand-alone cages and cages in combination with posterior fixation: a literature review. *Eur Spine J.* 2000;9(suppl 1):S95–S101.
53. Deguchi M, Cheng BC, Sato K, et al. Biomechanical evaluation of translaminar facet joint fixation. A comparative study of poly-L-lactide pins, screws, and pedicle fixation. *Spine (Phila Pa 1976).* 1998;23(12):1307–1312; discussion 1313.
54. Kandziora F, Schleicher P, Scholz M, et al. Biomechanical testing of the lumbar facet interference screw. *Spine (Phila Pa 1976).* 2005;30(2):E34–E39.
55. Liu F, Cao Y, Feng Z, et al. Comparison of three different posterior fixation techniques in transforaminal lumbar interbody fusion for two-level lumbar degenerative diseases: at a mean follow up time of 46 months. *Clin Neurol Neurosurg.* 2016;141:1–6.
56. Wang JC, Spenciner D, Robinson JC. SPIRE spinous process stabilization plate: biomechanical evaluation of a novel technology. Invited submission from the Joint Section Meeting on Disorders of the Spine and Peripheral Nerves, March 2005. *J Neurosurg Spine.* 2006;4(2):160–164.
57. Wang JC, Haid RW, Miller JS, et al. Comparison of CD HORIZON SPIRE spinous process plate stabilization and pedicle screw fixation after anterior lumbar interbody fusion. Invited submission from the Joint Section Meeting On Disorders of the Spine and Peripheral Nerves, March 2005. *J Neurosurg Spine.* 2006;4(2):132–136.
58. Techy F, Mageswaran P, Colbrunn RW, et al. Properties of an interspinous fixation device (ISD) in lumbar fusion constructs: a biomechanical study. *Spine J.* 2013;13(5):572–579.
59. Fogel GR, Parikh RD, Ryu SI, Turner AW. Biomechanics of lateral lumbar interbody fusion constructs with lateral and posterior plate fixation: laboratory investigation. *J Neurosurg Spine.* 2014;20(3):291–297.
60. Godzik J, Kalb S, Martinez-Del-Campo E, Newcomb AG, Singh V, Walker CT, et al. Biomechanical Evaluation of the CD HORIZON Spire Z Spinal System With Pedicle and Facet Fixation. *Spine (Phila Pa 1976).* 2016;41(15):E902–E907.

21 Revision Interbody Fusion

JACOB R. JOSEPH AND PAUL PARK

Introduction

Revision lumbar surgery is a technically challenging operation that requires careful planning and patient selection. In the case of previous interbody fusion, there are particular considerations the surgeon needs to address when planning a revision operation, such as the approach taken at the index surgery. Compared with posterolateral fusions, interbody fusions may be more challenging, as a more complicated dissection involving the thecal sac and nerves may be required owing to cage migration or the need to remove the cage from within the disk space. Indications for revision of interbody fusion include, but are not limited to excessive graft subsidence, pseudoarthrosis, graft extrusion, and infection. Factors that need to be taken into account include type of interbody cage used, spinal levels involved, presence or absence of bony fusion, and presence or absence of posterior supplementation. In this chapter, we review the various interbody fusion techniques, potential complications requiring revision, and treatment options.

Interbody Fusion Techniques

Posterior Lumbar Interbody Fusion and Transforaminal Lumbar Interbody Fusion

Posterior lumbar interbody fusion (PLIF) and transforaminal lumbar interbody fusion (TLIF) are widely accepted procedures for achieving interbody arthrodesis. They use either a direct posterior (PLIF) or a posterolateral (TLIF) approach to enter the disk space. TLIF most commonly involves a unilateral approach via the foramen with insertion of a single oblique or banana-shaped cage. Some surgeons utilize a bilateral approach with placement of two cages obliquely. PLIF traditionally involves a wide laminectomy and at least partial facetectomies with orthogonal placement of a cage on each side of the vertebral disk spaces. Because of the posterolateral approach used in TLIF, less dural sac and exiting nerve root retraction is necessary than in PLIF. These procedures can be performed with a traditional open or minimally invasive approach.

Graft extrusion after PLIF or TLIF has been widely reported in the literature, with an incidence ranging from 0.35% to 6% (Fig. 21.1). Bakhsheshian et al.[1] reported their series of 513 patients undergoing minimally invasive TLIF and found 5 cases of graft extrusion. Of these 5 cases, 2 patients were asymptomatic and did not require surgery. Three patients had evidence of neurologic decline and underwent revision surgery. Similarly, Zhao et al.[2] reported their series of 512 patients undergoing mini-open TLIF, with 6 patients having graft extrusion. They reported that small cages, rectangular cage shape, and multi-level procedures increased the risk of cage extrusion. Furthermore, the presence of linear endplates as opposed to concave presented a higher likelihood of extrusion. Other studies have reported similar risk factors.[3]

Currently no direct comparative studies are investigating the rates of graft extrusion in open TLIF versus minimally invasive TLIF. Several studies have examined the relationship between unilateral versus bilateral pedicle screw fixation in TLIF. Although the data are not yet conclusive, it does appear that there may be a higher rate of cage migration in patients with unilateral pedicle screw fixation, suggesting that bilateral screws provide greater stability to the graft.[4]

Lateral Lumbar Interbody Fusion

Lateral lumbar interbody fusion (LLIF) is a technique that was first described in 2006 by Ozgur et al., although variations of this technique have existed prior to that report.[5] This procedure classically involves a retroperitoneal transpsoas approach to access the disk space orthogonally. It has been an increasingly popular technique that offers the advantages of a less-invasive approach with minimal blood loss, as well as providing an alternative means of achieving a more robust diskectomy with placement of a larger cage than with PLIF or TLIF. LLIF has been utilized both in a stand-alone fashion, as well as with posterior pedicle screw fixation or lateral plate fixation.

Overall reported rates of graft extrusion in LLIF have been low (Fig. 21.2), although there are several case reports in the literature. However, larger case series describe graft subsidence to be a bigger complication of LLIF. Le et al.[6] reported a 14.3% rate of radiographic subsidence and a 2.1% rate of clinical subsidence in a group of 140 LLIF patients, and noted that increasing construct length was associated with higher subsidence rates. Many cases of reported subsidence did require revision surgery, although the nature of the surgery has been inconsistently reported. In addition, the definition of subsidence has varied among authors. Several studies report associated vertebral body fractures. Owing to the heterogeneity of subsidence, some studies advocate conservative management, whereas other authors advocate for either placement of posterior instrumentation in cases with stand-alone cages, or supplementation with vertebroplasty/kyphoplasty in cases of vertebral body fracture.[7]

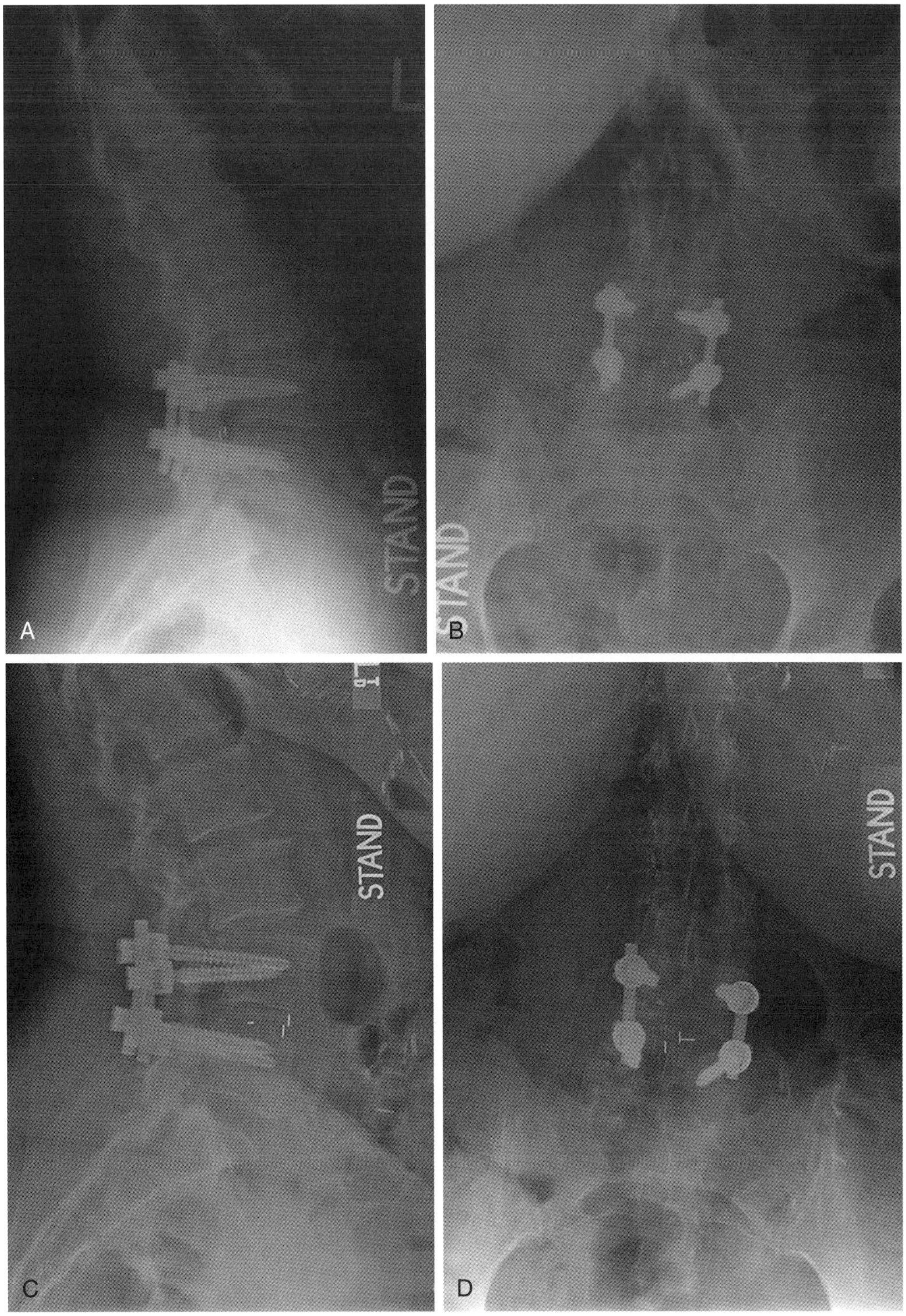

• **Fig. 21.1** A 51-year-old woman with a history of left L4-5 transforaminal lumbar interbody fusion (TLIF) at an outside institution presented for another opinion owing to severe back and leg pain. **A, B.** Lateral and anteroposterior x-rays show retropulsion of interbody cage. Patient underwent revision surgery with removal of existing cage and placement of a cage of greater height further anteriorly via the same left-sided TLIF approach. **C, D.** X-rays 1 year after revision surgery showing fusion.

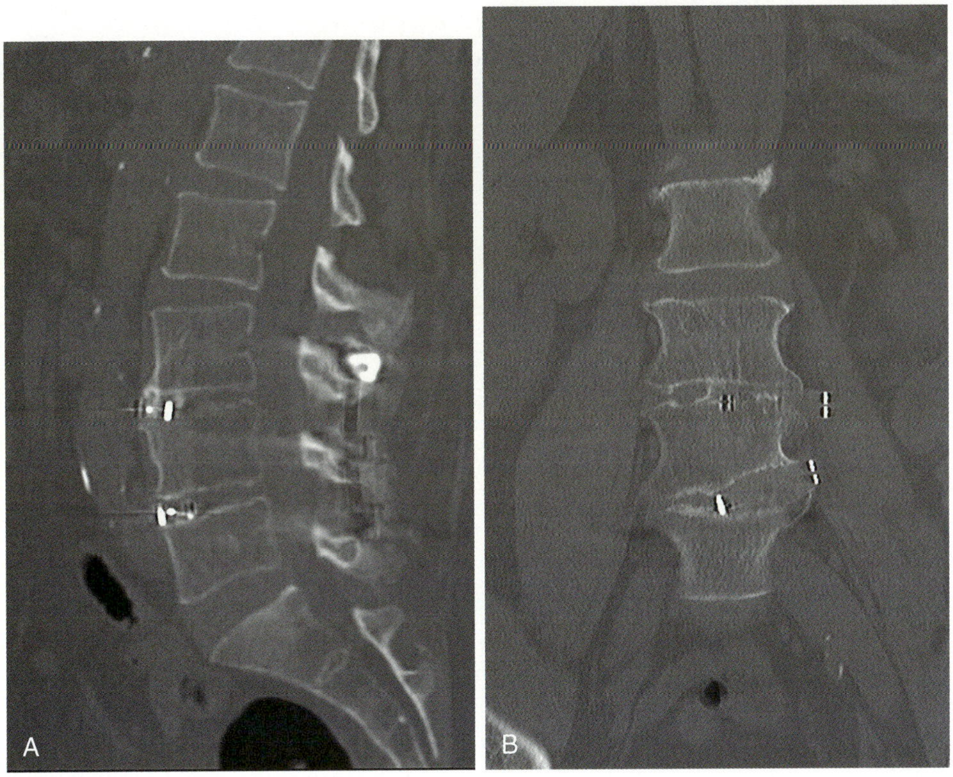

• **Fig. 21.2** A 61-year-old woman with a history of L3-4 and L4-5 lateral lumbar interbody fusion and posterior instrumented fusion at an outside institution 6 years previously. **A.** Sagittal reformatted computed tomography (CT) scan showing anterior placement of cages. **B.** Coronal reformatted CT showing lateral migration of both cages.

Anterior Lumbar Interbody Fusion

Anterior lumbar interbody fusion (ALIF) is a technique that provides direct access to the anterior spine. It is typically performed by a vascular or general surgeon using either a transperitoneal or, more commonly, a retroperitoneal approach to expose the anterior disk space. With this approach, a robust diskectomy can be performed and a large interbody cage placed. ALIF can be performed as a stand-alone, with integral fixation, anterior plate fixation, or with posterior supplemental fixation. Although graft extrusion and implant migration have been described, they are relatively rare with the use of modern techniques.[8] However, subsidence has been reported commonly, particularly in stand-alone ALIF (Fig. 21.3).

Axial Lumbar Interbody Fusion

Axial lumbar interbody fusion (AxiaLIF) is a minimally invasive percutaneous technique that can achieve fusion at L5-S1, or from L4-S1. This technique utilizes a small paracoccygeal incision that gives access to the presacral area with serial dilation, allowing for diskectomy, placement of interbody graft to promote fusion, and placement of a threaded rod to serve as the interbody fixation device.[9,10] Although AxiaLIF has reported good fusion rates, there is a risk of rectal or bowel injuries. There is a reported revision rate of 8.8% owing to pseudoarthrosis at 3-year follow-up.[11] Revision techniques, including anterior and posterior approaches with or without removal of the AxiaLIF implant, have been described.

Surgical Indications

Many cases of pseudoarthrosis or graft extrusion can be managed with nonoperative treatment. In asymptomatic patients, serial imaging may be the appropriate management. However, cases of progressive migration or development of deformity will likely warrant operative intervention, even with a lack of symptoms.

For those cases of simple graft symptomatic subsidence or pseudoarthrosis in which surgery is needed, a posterior approach can frequently be utilized. These would be cases in which alignment correction or increased foraminal height are not needed. Particularly in instances where only stand-alone ALIF or LLIF cages were utilized, supplementation with posterior pedicle screws and posterolateral fusion can be efficacious to provide additional stability to the involved segments, eventually leading to adequate bony fusion. This approach provides the advantage of being relatively simple to perform using a straightforward standard technique. Posterior approaches are also indicated in posterior graft extrusions, both to remove the mal-positioned graft and to perform a redo interbody fusion with additional pedicular fixation.

Anterior approaches to the lumbar spine can be helpful in multiple instances of interbody failure. They can be particularly helpful in revision of anterior graft extrusions. Whereas TLIF cages are more likely to retropulse, they can extrude anteriorly as well. Similarly, ALIF and LLIF grafts can also extrude anteriorly. In cases of LLIF, this may become more common with release of the anterior longitudinal ligament. In the case of graft extrusion anteriorly, computed tomography (CT) angiography and consultation with a vascular surgeon should be strongly considered to evaluate

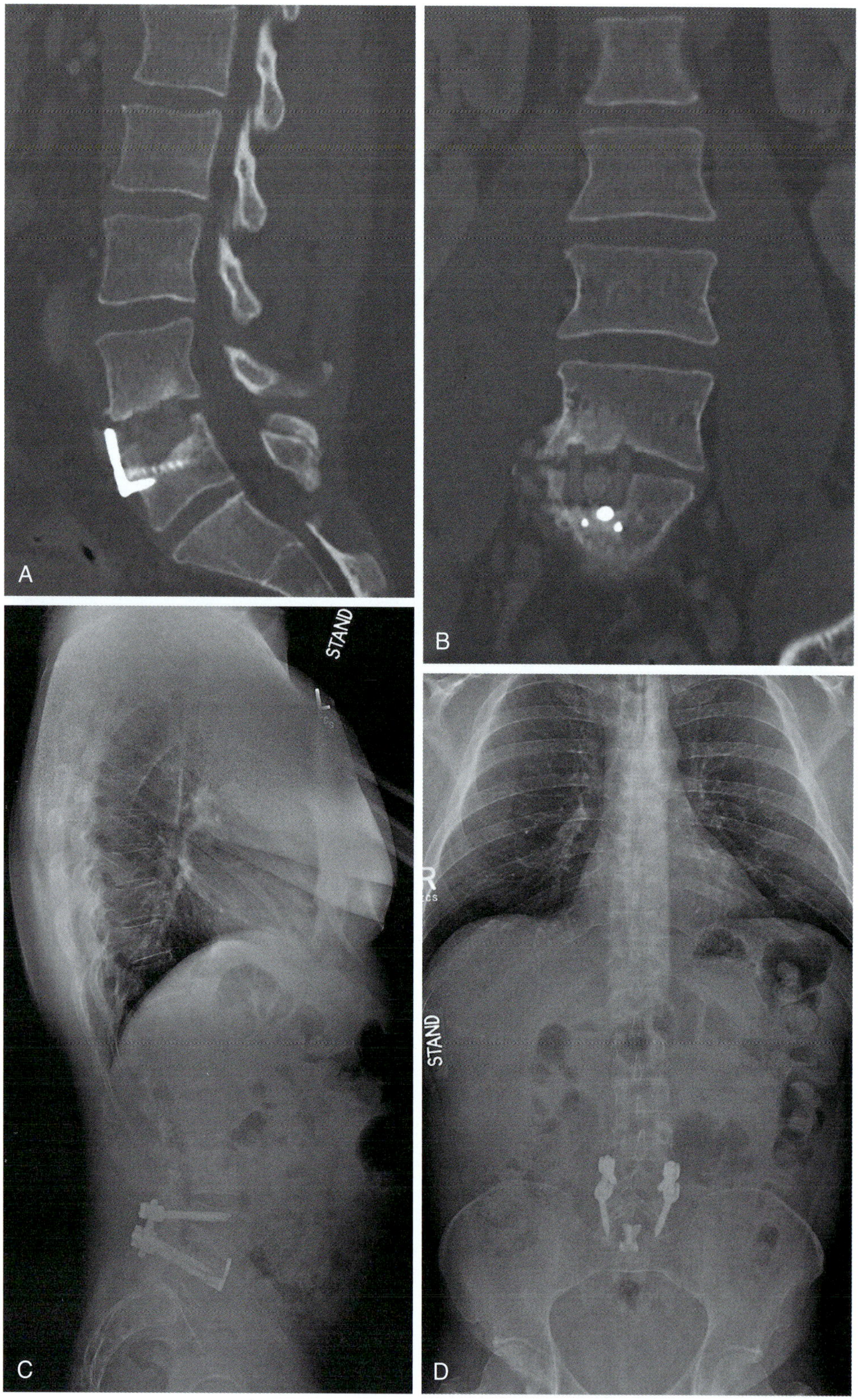

• **Fig. 21.3** A 37-year-old man presented with low back and leg pain after undergoing L4-5 anterior lumbar interbody fusion with anterior plate at an outside institution. ALIF was complicated by retrograde ejaculation. **A, B.** Sagittal and coronal reformatted computed tomography images show eccentric placement of cage, significant subsidence, and minimal bone formation. Patient underwent foraminotomy and L4-5 posterior instrumented fusion. **C, D.** X-rays 1 year after revision surgery.

proximity to the great vessels. However, the morbidity with this approach should also be considered against the risk of nonoperative intervention, as anteriorly migrated grafts may rarely cause significant morbidity such as pseudoarthrosis or delay injury to the great vessels on their own.[12,13] The retroperitoneal transpsoas approach has also been described in revision of interbody cages. In cases of lateral extrusion of LLIF cages, a repeat lateral surgery can be performed to access the cage.

Endoscopic approaches to the spine are relatively new, but are being performed for lumbar diskectomy, foraminotomy, and interbody fusions. In conjunction with this increasing popularity, endoscopic approaches are being investigated for their utility in revision surgery. McGrath et al.[14] described a case in which a patient with a previous TLIF had cage retropulsion causing symptomatic nerve compression. The patient was also noted to have a solid bony interbody fusion. The authors elected to perform an endoscopic interlaminar partial resection of the interbody cage, resulting in decompression of the lateral recess and complete resolution of symptoms.[14] In the setting of a solid fusion, this procedure allowed for avoidance of a more extensive procedure requiring removal of the interbody cage.

Surgical Technique

Posterior Approaches

Posterior approaches for supplemental fusion can be utilized for cases in which subsidence or pseudoarthrosis resulted after standalone anterior or lateral interbody fusions. In addition, posterior approaches are useful in cases in which there has been cage migration posteriorly, usually after PLIF/TLIF.

Step 1: Standard positioning on a Jackson frame or equivalent, followed by standard preparing and draping.

Step 2: If the index case was an anterior approach, a midline incision is made followed by a standard subperiosteal dissection. After adequate lateral exposure, pedicle screws are inserted in the targeted segments followed by rod placement and the traditional steps for posterolateral fusion. In the case of prior posterior surgery, incision incorporating the existing midline scar is made. Careful dissection and release of scar tissue is performed until the bony defect is fully exposed. The initial dissection and exposure of the normal bony anatomy (i.e., adjacent normal spinous process and lamina) is helpful to determine the approximate location of the bony defect.

Step 3: Once the bony defect has been exposed, attention is turned to releasing the often extensive scar tissue within the spinal canal. The use of a curette to develop a plane between scar tissue and dura is essential. Use of a microscope can also be helpful during this dissection and may minimize inadvertent durotomy.

Step 4: Further bone removal cranially will allow identification of the dural margin and assist in developing the plane between dura and scar. Careful development of this plane caudally will eventually result in exposure of the traversing nerve root as it crosses the targeted disk space. Mobilization of the traversing nerve root is typically a challenge owing to the scar tissue. Again, use of a curette—specifically, a down-going curette—is helpful to release the scar. Initial ventral dissection cranial to the disk space where there is less scar tissue is recommended. Once a ventral plane is established, careful dissection caudally is more easily accomplished. In the case of a posterior extruded cage, the same technique is applied and is generally successful. Integrity of the dura should be noted. Although rare, if the cage is intradural, then some authors advocate a transdural approach for removal of the cage.[15]

Step 5: Typically, once the surrounding scar has been adequately released, a posteriorly migrated cage can be mobilized and removed relatively easily. If the cage is not mobile, such as when a cage is predominantly within the disk space, an osteotome can be used to loosen the cage. Care must be taken to minimize endplate damage, and use of fluoroscopy is highly recommended.

Step 6: Once the cage is removed, the disk space should be prepared again, with extra care taken to preserve what is left of the endplates. Ideally, the new cage will be positioned in a different region of the disk space. Use of an expandable cage is recommended, as positioning is more easily accomplished with a shorter-height implant that can subsequently be expanded to contact the endplates. Adequate bone graft placement is essential and is typically added prior to cage insertion.

Step 7: An alternative option is to place a cage from the contralateral side if the index operation was a TLIF.

Step 8: If any lucency is noted around the pedicle screws on preoperative imaging, the screws should be replaced with larger diameter screws. Even without evidence of lucency on imaging, the pedicle screws should be assessed intraoperatively with replacement if screw purchase is poor. If adequate fixation is unable to be achieved, then consider extension of the construct to the adjacent segments.

Step 9: A traditional posterolateral fusion should be undertaken with decortication of the remaining bony elements followed by sufficient bone graft placement. Note that the use of biologics, such as recombinant human bone morphogenetic protein-2 (rhBMP2), can be considered, given the need to achieve fusion. The rationale and potential risks of rhBMP2 should be discussed with the patient.

Step 10: The incision should be closed in anatomic layers.

Anterior Approaches

Anterior approaches can be useful in cases of pseudoarthrosis after PLIF/TLIF. This approach also provides access to any cage that is anteriorly migrated, including those placed via a PLIF/TLIF, LLIF, or ALIF procedure. The anterior approach has the advantage of providing the widest view of the disk space, thus allowing for removal of a mal-positioned cage and residual disk as well as allow placement of a larger cage to help promote fusion. In revision of AxiaLIF, it may be possible to place a new cage adjacent to the AxiaLIF rod. If the AxiaLIF needs to be removed, options include anterior sacral resection or presacral device retrieval (utilizing the same working corridor as for implantation). In revision of PLIF/TLIF, removal of the cage and replacement with a larger cage may be the best option.

In cases requiring anterior exposure for anteriorly extruded interbody grafts, an access surgeon, using either a transperitoneal or retroperitoneal approach, should be utilized. Fluoroscopy should be used to ensure that the access corridor would be ideal for cage removal and replacement. The extruded graft should be visualized directly, and the great vessels must be dissected and retracted off, again with the assistance of a vascular surgeon. Next, removal of scar and any remaining disk material with preparation of the endplates should be completed, followed by a standard ALIF. In cases of revision surgery, it may be prudent to use integrated screws or an anterior plate followed by posterior fixation, if not already present.

Lateral Approaches

Lateral approaches for revision interbody fusion are typically used for laterally migrated cages, but can also be used for retrieval of PLIF/TLIF cages. In laterally migrated cages, if the patient was symptomatic from lumbar plexus compression or irritation, special care is warranted in transpsoas exposure of the cage. As with all lateral spine exposure, EMG monitoring is indicated to ensure safety of the lumbar plexus. Once the cage is identified and exposed, it may be necessary to reimpact the cage into the disk space prior to its careful extraction. Reimpaction has been described when there is concern that lateral cage migration is impacting the lumbar plexus directly, and direct removal could result in further nerve injury.[16] Once the cage is removed, care must be taken to remove granulation tissue and residual disk material without further injuring the endplates, which need to be adequately prepared for regrafting. In addition, special attention should be paid to ensure that the contralateral annulus is completely released, as incomplete release has been previously theorized to contribute to lateral migration.[17] Several previous reports advocate placement of a lateral plate as well, to prevent further migration. In addition, if the cage was originally stand-alone, consideration should be given to posterior fixation as well.

Lateral approaches have also been described in retrieval of migrated PLIF/TLIF cages. Moisi et al.[18] described their technique to retrieve fractured, migrated, or subsided cages. They recommend positioning the retractor onto the lateral disk space per the standard approach, with use of an osteotome to dissect superiorly and inferiorly to the implanted cage. Once the cage is loosened, a hook or pituitary can be used to remove the cage. Finally, the remaining disk material should be removed with preparation of the endplates so that a standard LLIF cage can be inserted. Importantly, the authors note limitations with this approach if the existing cage has migrated too far anteriorly or posteriorly.

Postoperative Care

Postoperatively, the patient should be admitted to the general care ward. Depending on the circumstances of surgery, such as excessive blood loss, intensive care admission may be warranted. Regular neurologic checks should be performed to identify any potential neurologic decline. Pain should be controlled with a combination of opioids and muscle relaxants, although they should be weaned as soon as possible. Bracing is left to the discretion of the surgeon. Early mobilization with physical and occupational therapy can be helpful.

Complications/Side-Effects

Potential complications are similar to that of the index spinal procedure and are dependent on the approach used, spinal level, and extent of the necessary surgery. Major approach-related complications associated with ALIF include injury (1) to vascular structures; (2) to retroperitoneal structures, such as the ureters; and (3) to the superior hypogastric plexus, which can lead to retrograde ejaculation in males. Previous case series have reported high morbidity and mortality with retrieval of interbody cages from an anterior approach.[19] Most of these complications are related to injury to the vascular structures or the viscera. Prior to surgery, the anesthesiologist should be made aware of the potential for massive blood loss during the procedure. During cage removal, particular care must be taken in cases where rhBMP2 was used in the graft, as it may induce vessel fibrosis and scarring.[20] In lateral approaches, the lumbar plexus is at particular risk, as described above.

Outcomes in a Nutshell

There are no high-quality studies that have investigated revision of interbody fusion cages. However, based on reported small series as well as institutional experience, most patients tolerate revision of interbody cages well, with low overall morbidity.

Conclusion

Given the increasing popularity of lumbar interbody fusion procedures, knowledge of revision strategies for interbody fusion failure is critical. Hardware failure, cage migration, and/or subsidence are the most common indications for revision surgery. Treatment options include conservative management in asymptomatic cases. However, in symptomatic cases, a variety of approaches are available to retrieve fractured or migrated cages and/or perform redo fusion. The revision strategy must be tailored to the individual patient with pertinent anatomy and pathology in mind.

References

1. Bakhsheshian J, Khanna R, Choy W, et al. Incidence of graft extrusion following minimally invasive transforaminal lumbar interbody fusion. *J Clin Neurosci*. 2016;24:88–93.
2. Zhao FD, Yang W, Shan Z, et al. Cage migration after transforaminal lumbar interbody fusion and factors related to it. *Orthop Surg*. 2012;4:227–232.
3. Aoki Y, Yamagata M, Nakajima F, et al. Examining risk factors for posterior migration of fusion cages following transforaminal lumbar interbody fusion: a possible limitation of unilateral pedicle screw fixation. *J Neurosurg Spine*. 2010;13:381–387.
4. Yuan C, Chen K, Zhang H, et al. Unilateral versus bilateral pedicle screw fixation in lumbar interbody fusion: a meta-analysis of complication and fusion rate. *Clin Neurol Neurosurg*. 2014;117: 28–32.
5. Ozgur BM, Aryan HE, Pimenta L, et al. Extreme Lateral Interbody Fusion (XLIF): a novel surgical technique for anterior lumbar interbody fusion. *Spine J*. 2006;6:435–443.
6. Le TV, Baaj AA, Dakwar E, et al. Subsidence of polyetheretherketone intervertebral cages in minimally invasive lateral retroperitoneal transpsoas lumbar interbody fusion. *Spine (Phila Pa 1976)*. 2012;37:1268–1273.
7. Graham RB, Wong AP, Liu JC. Minimally invasive lateral transpsoas approach to the lumbar spine: pitfalls and complication avoidance. *Neurosurg Clin N Am*. 2014;25:219–231.
8. Mobbs RJ, Loganathan A, Yeung V, et al. Indications for anterior lumbar interbody fusion. *Orthop Surg*. 2013;5:153–163.
9. Louwerens JK, Groot D, van Duijvenbode DC, et al. Alternative surgical strategy for AxiaLIF pseudarthrosis: a series of three case reports. *Evid Based Spine Care J*. 2013;4:143–148.
10. Aryan HE, Newman CB, Gold JJ, et al. Percutaneous axial lumbar interbody fusion (AxiaLIF) of the L5-S1 segment: initial clinical and radiographic experience. *Minim Invasive Neurosurg*. 2008;51: 225–230.
11. Lindley EM, McCullough MA, Burger EL, et al. Complications of axial lumbar interbody fusion. *J Neurosurg Spine*. 2011;15:273–279.
12. Pawar UM, Kundnani V, Nene A. Major vessel injury with cage migration: surgical complication in a case of spondylodiscitis. *Spine (Phila Pa 1976)*. 2010;35:E663–E666.
13. Villavicencio AT, Nelson EL, Rajpal S, et al. Case series of anterior intervertebral graft extrusions in transforaminal lumbar interbody fusion surgeries. *World Neurosurg*. 2016;85:130–135.
14. McGrath Jr LB, Madhavan K, Chieng LO, et al. Early experience with endoscopic revision of lumbar spinal fusions. *Neurosurg Focus*. 2016;40:E10.
15. Zaidi HA, Shah A, Kakarla UK. Transdural retrieval of a retropulsed lumbar interbody cage: technical case report. *Asian J Neurosurg*. 2016;11:71.

16. Daffner SD, Wang JC. Migrated XLIF cage: case report and discussion of surgical technique. *Orthopedics*. 2010;33(518):2010.
17. Towers WS, Kurtom KH. Stand-alone LLIF lateral cage migration: a case report. *Cureus*. 2015;7:e347.
18. Moisi M, Page J, Paulson D, et al. Technical note: lateral approach to the lumbar spine for the removal of interbody cages. *Cureus*. 2015;7:e268.
19. Nguyen HV, Akbarnia BA, van Dam BE, et al. Anterior exposure of the spine for removal of lumbar interbody devices and implants. *Spine (Phila Pa 1976)*. 2453;31:2449–2453.
20. Rodgers SD, Marascalchi BJ, Grobelny BT, et al. Revision surgery after interbody fusion with rhBMP-2: a cautionary tale for spine surgeons. *J Neurosurg Spine*. 2013;18:582–587.

22

Interbody Fusion Strategies in Thoracic and Sacral Overlap Diseases

TIMOTHY T. ROBERTS, COLIN HAINES, AND JASON W. SAVAGE

Introduction

The thoracolumbar junction is subject to unique biomechanical forces owing to its existence as a transition zone. The thoracic spine is relatively rigid, largely in part to the costovertebral joints as well as coronally oriented facet joints.[1] In contrast, the lumbar spine is more flexible because there are no rib articulations and more sagittally oriented facet joints.[2] Importantly, this relationship may change with aging, as mild to moderate disk degeneration typically increases segmental lumbar motion. However, severe disk degeneration is often accompanied by subchondral sclerosis, ankylosis, and osteophyte formation, which limit lumbar mobility, thus reducing the motion difference of the thoracolumbar spine.[3] In addition, segmental lordosis decreases as the spine progresses toward the apex of kyphosis, underscoring its importance with regard to sagittal balance.

The lumbosacral junction is also subject to "overlap" disease. Historically, lumbosacral fusion has been associated with a high rate of pseudarthrosis. The advent of interbody fusion and the use of pelvic fixation, with either iliac screw fixation or sacral alar iliac screws (S2AI), has improved the rate of arthrodesis across the lumbosacral (LS) junction.[4]

Indications: Thoracolumbar Overlap Disease

Fusion

Bony fusion of this region is often required to maximize patient outcomes. The thoracolumbar junction is subject to higher biomechanical stresses that may lead to increased nonunion at region of the spine.[5] As such, many surgeons support interbody devices to augment fusion rates.

Spondylolisthesis, although more common in the lumbar spine, is a common indication for instrumented fusion. Although the authors' are unaware of any reports of interbody fusion rates at thoracolumbar junction owing to this pathology, lumbar interbody fusion rates have been shown to be equivalent or better than posterolateral fusion[6,7] in the lumbar spine. By extrapolation, one may consider this technique to achieve similarly high bony fusion.

Tumor/Infection

Both tumor and infection may involve variable destruction of vertebral bodies and endplates. Malignancies, of which metastases are the most common, typically involve the vertebral bodies and spare the disk. Therefore, vertebral body cage constructs are more commonly needed than interbody cages. However, there may be isolated instances in which interbody cages are helpful if there is disk destruction with relative sparing of the body and endplates.

Spondylodiscitis is often amenable to interbody devices owing to anatomic involvement of this disease. Most commonly, the vertebral body becomes seeded via arterial spread and the disk subsequently is infected through local extension. Because of this, there is often significant disk space collapse, sclerotic endplate changes, and infected body, but with variable degrees of body destruction.[8] If debridement of the collapsed disk space is all that is surgically needed, then an interbody device may be ideal both to restore vertebral body height and to assist in fusion.

Deformity

Adult spinal deformity is often treated with decompression and thoracolumbar fusion to address neurologic symptoms and provide postural correction. An understanding of relevant radiographic parameters and goals of deformity correction surgery are critical in minimizing complications and maximizing patient outcomes. Sagittal imbalance is the key driver of pain and disability in the adult patient with deformity. Regional alignment, global balance, and spinopelvic parameters are key measurements that must be taken into account when evaluating adjacent segment disease (ASD). In general, the accepted goals of deformity surgery are sagittal vertical axis less than 5 cm, pelvic tilt (PT) less than 15 degrees, and pelvic incidence minus lumbar lordosis plus or minus 10 degrees (Fig. 22.1). It is important to note that these goals likely change in the aging population, and over correction often leads to postoperative complications, most notably instrumentation failure and proximal junction kyphosis/failure.

Sagittal balance has major implications on patient reported outcomes and thus patients with a kyphotic deformity at the T12-L1 level may benefit from interbody support to maximize lordosis or make a correction at that level. Importantly, the type of technique may have implications on focal alignment. Whereas threaded interbodies have been shown to be kyphogenic, vertically oriented cages typically result in lordosis, albeit often under 5 degrees of change.[9] More promising, direct lateral interbody fusion has been shown to result in 9 degrees of lordosis creation.[10]

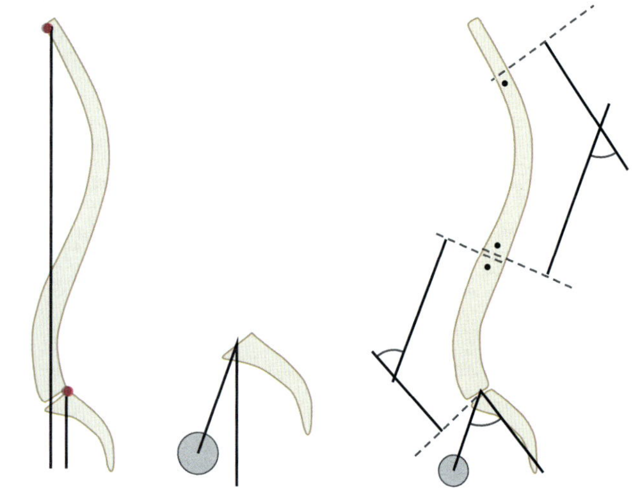

• **Fig. 22.1** Realignment objectives in the sagittal plane. Alignment parameters change with age and are likely different in the elderly population. (From Schwab F, Patel A, Ungar B, et al. Adult spinal deformity-postoperative standing imbalance: how much can you tolerate? An overview of key parameters in assessing alignment and planning corrective surgery. *Spine* 2010;35(25):2224–2231.)

Proximal junctional kyphosis (Fig. 22.2), a known complication of multilevel instrumented constructs, may be amenable to interbody instrumentation to help restore lordosis and provide anterior column support. Importantly, the integrity of the associated endplates must be assessed if a bony proximal junctional kyphosis is suspected. If damaged, interbody cages have a high rate of subsidence. Lateral interbody fusion is also often useful to address nonunion at the site of a previous pedicle subtraction osteotomy (Fig. 22.3).

Fracture

Certain thoracic injuries may be conducive to transforaminal interbody fusion. In a series of lower thoracic and thoracolumbar fracture dislocations, lordosis and high fusion rates were achieved.[11] Without adequate endplate and vertebral body structural integrity, implant subsidence is common. Therefore, using interbody instrumentation to maintain disk space height as a primary endpoint has variable efficacy, even in the setting of pedicle screw instrumentation. However, interbody placement to assist in fracture healing may be beneficial.

Disk Herniation

Surgical management of thoracic and thoracolumbar disk herniations varies based on location. Laterally based herniations may be addressed with unilateral transpedicular decompressions, whereas more centrally based disks often need more extensile approaches, such as costotransversectomy, lateral extracavitary, or thoracotomy. More recently, a minimally invasive lateral approach for thoracic and thoracolumbar disk herniations has recently been described.[12] Regardless of the approach, fusion is often indicated if enough bone was resected to cause instability. Because of the disk void after fragment removal, interbody fusion may be an ideal choice.

The type of interbody instrumentation is best dictated by the surgical approach used. From a posterior approach, both unilateral and bilateral transforaminal implants have been described.[13] Lateral cage placement is ideal with either a formal thoracotomy or minimally invasive lateral approach.[12] Regardless of the choice, an interbody instrument may be a good option to assist in disk height restoration and increase the fusion surface area.

Limitations

Accessing the anterior column or disk space at the thoracolumbar junction is often challenging owing to its unique anatomy and the presence of the spinal cord or conus medullaris. Unlike in the lumbar spine, the thecal sac cannot be retracted at the thoracolumbar (TL) junction. The traditional way to access the disk space at the TL junction is via a thoracotomy. Owing to the associated risks and morbidity with that approach, less invasive procedures have been developed. The direct lateral approach to the TL junction is a facile way to access the disk space and implant an interbody device for deformity correction and/or fusion. This can be done through a traditional retroperitoneal approach, or via a minimally invasive lateral approach (e.g., direct lateral anterior lumbar interbody fusion, eXtreme lumbar interbody fusion). A more traditional transforaminal decompression and interbody fusion is another option at the TL junction. For the purposes of this chapter, we describe the direct lateral approach.

SURGICAL TECHNIQUE

Step 1: Following standard single lumen intubation, the patient is carefully placed in the lateral decubitus position on a radiolucent table. Our preference is to use a sand bag and tape to hold the patient in place during surgery. It is critical to have a perfect anteroposterior (AP) and lateral x-ray of the disk space. The operative table should be adjusted so that the disk space is orthogonal to the floor.

Step 2: The incision is then marked out using intraoperative fluoroscopy. An oblique 2- to 3-cm incision is then made over the disk space and the muscle fibers are sharply incised overlying the corresponding rib. For level 1 diskectomy and fusion, rib resection is typically not required. The chest cavity is then entered and the lung is swept anteriorly with the surgeon's finger. At T12-L1 it is often necessary to cross the diaphragm, which should be done at the junction of the chest wall to allow for repair. A specialized retractor system with light source and neuromonitoring is then placed centered over the disk space. This is confirmed using AP and lateral intraoperative fluoroscopy.

Step 3: The disk and endplate cartilage is then removed using a combination of curettes, endplate shavers, and pituitary rongeurs. Trial-sized cages are then inserted into the disk space. Care should be taken not to over distract the disk, as this may increase the risk of subsidence. Once the disk space is satisfactorily prepared, the contralateral annulus is released using a Cobb elevator. This will allow for symmetric distraction, and assist in deformity correction if desired.

Step 4: The interbody cage is then filled with the bone graft substitute and/or biologic of choice and inserted into the disk space. Proper positioning of the implant is confirmed using AP and lateral fluoroscopy.

Step 5: Posterior pedicle screw fixation is then placed. The authors do not perform stand-alone direct lateral interbody fusions at the TL junction.

Step 6: The wound is then closed in layers using absorbable suture. If necessary, the insertion of the diaphragm is repaired to the chest wall. A chest tube is often placed if the pleural space was entered during the exposure.

Postoperative Care

Postoperative care of patients undergoing fusion across the thoracolumbar junction depends largely on the nature of the preoperative

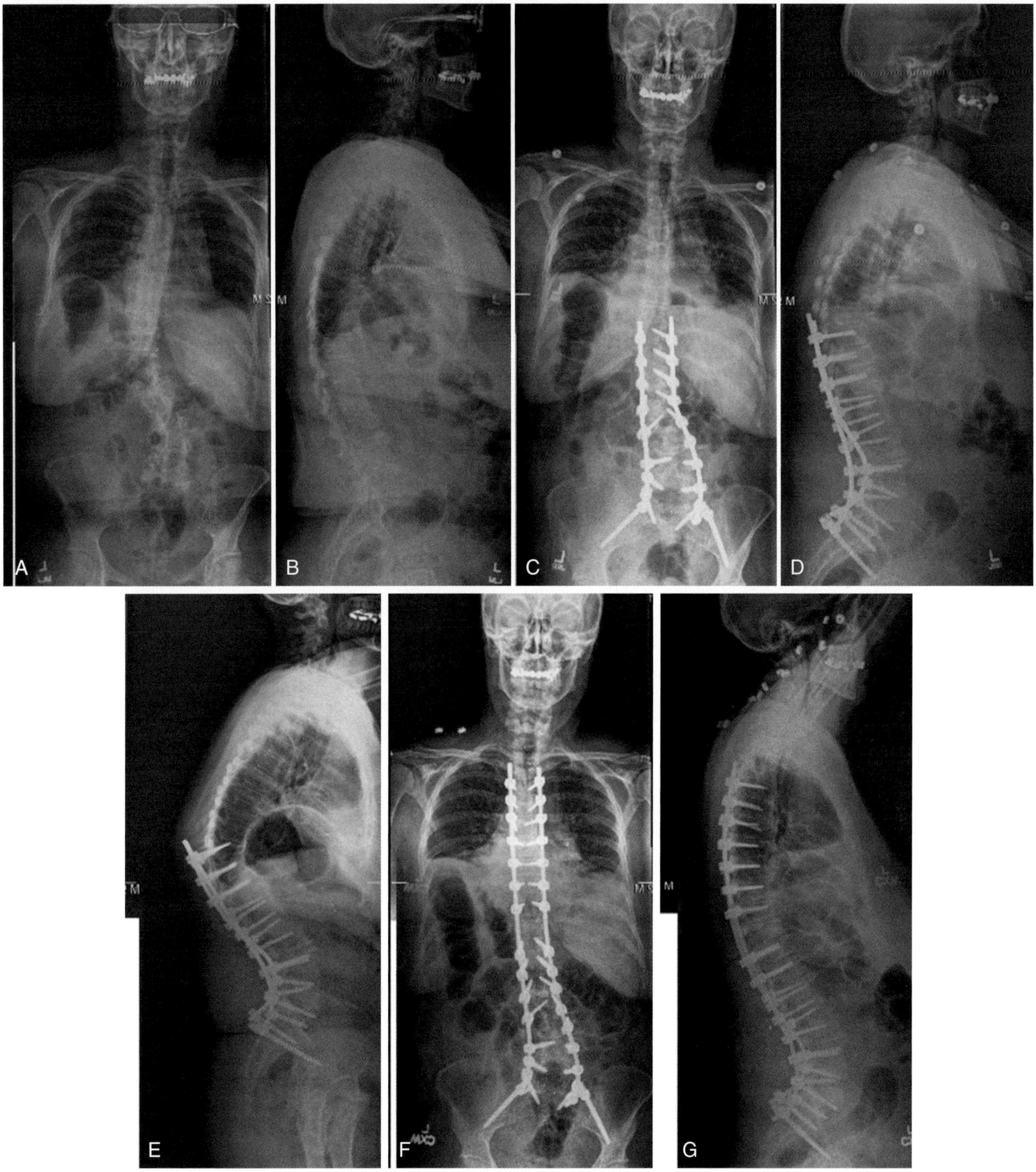

• **Fig. 22.2** A 63-year-old female patient with severe back and leg pain underwent a multilevel lumbar decompression with posterior column osteotomies and T10-ileum to address her stenosis and adult spinal deformity. She developed acute proximal junctional failure that required an extension of the fusion to T4.

pathology, the surgical approach, the extent and morbidity of the procedure, and the incidence of intraoperative complications.

For anterior and lateral procedures requiring deflation of the ipsilateral lung, chest tubes are commonly left postoperatively to reduce the incidence of persistent pneumothoraxes, potentially obstructive serous and/or bloody fluid collections, and potentially to reduce strain on the healing diaphragm and parenchymal tissues.

Patients are mobilized with therapy services as soon as possible. It is rare that we use an orthosis in this patient population.

Complications

Potential for intraoperative complications at the thoracolumbar junction is high, owing to the complex and vulnerable anatomy of

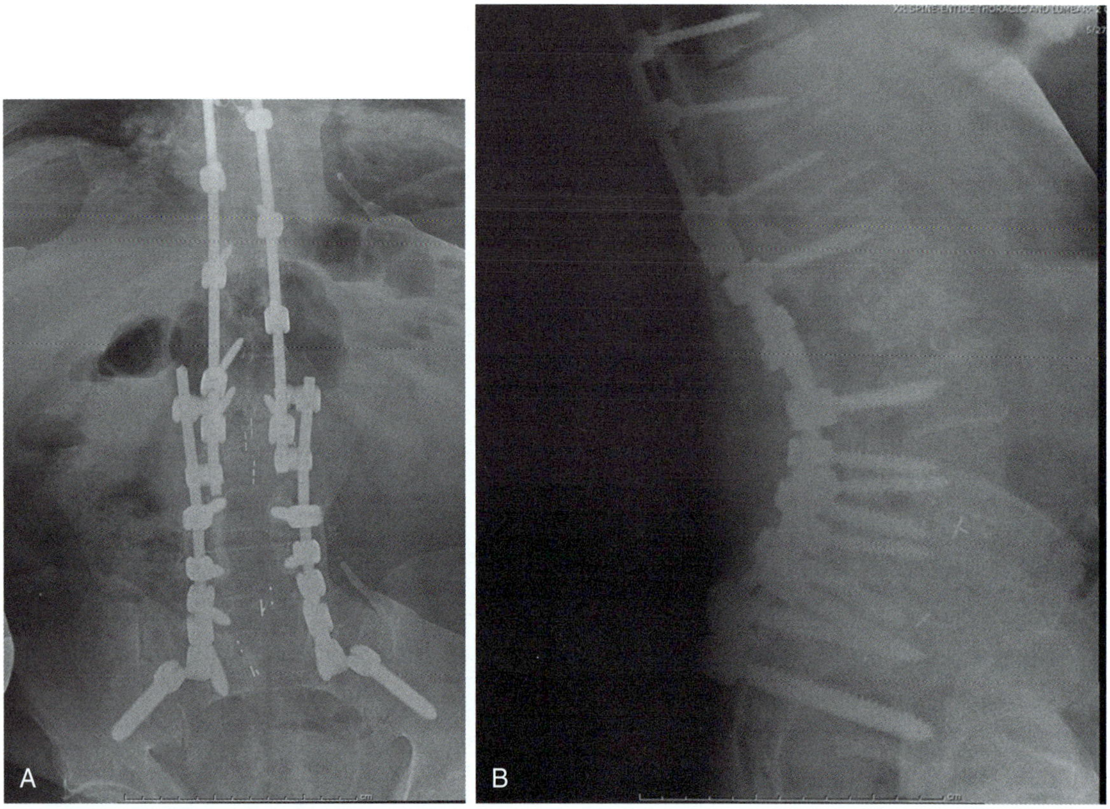

• **Fig. 22.3** A 67-year-old male patient underwent a L2 pedicle subtraction osteotomy for sagittal plane imbalance. He developed a nonunion at the osteotomy site and required a revision L1-2 and L2-3 direct lateral interbody fusion.

the abdominal-thoracic junction. The aorta lies just anterior and to the left of midline at the T12-L1 level, while the azygos vein lies to its right, along with the splanchnic nerves and thoracic duct. The inferior vena cava lies more anteriorly at this level, penetrating the diaphragm as high as at the T8 level and descending relatively anterolateral to these accessory veins and lymphatic structures. Much of this delicate and unforgiving anatomy may be unfamiliar to the orthopedic or neurologic surgeon who should employ added caution, vigilance, and patience during these procedures.

The thoracic duct is a thin-walled vesicular structure that returns lymphatic fluid from the abdominal viscera and lower extremities into the main circulation. The thoracic duct originates from the confluence of the lymphatic lumbar and intestinal trunks, known as the *cisterna chyli*, which is located midline at the mid-to-low lumbar spine. The thoracic duct ascends alongside the aorta as it pierces the diaphragm (T12 level), then ascends immediately anterior to the vertebral bodies and discoligamentous complexes on the right side of the body. Here it is especially vulnerable to transection or indirect tearing via overly aggressive diskectomy or distraction techniques. The thoracic duct terminates at the junction of the left internal jugular vein and the subclavian vein (approximately the T5 level).[14] Injury to the thoracic duct can result in lymphatic spillage—up to 4 liters daily—resulting in a life-threatening chylothorax, which requires drainage and typically operative repair or ligation.[15]

Surgeons accessing the thoracolumbar region must possess an intimate understanding of the anatomy of the diaphragm and its traversing structures. The diaphragmatic crura are a sling of tendons that ascend from the level of the L1 body and travel up and around the aorta and esophagus, which typically pierce the diaphragm at the T12 and T10 levels, respectively.[16] The crura have left and right tendons that are contiguous with the anterior longitudinal ligament. During anterior and lateral approaches, the crura may need to be mobilized for access to the T12-L1 vertebral bodies and adjacent disk spaces. This is typically performed by leaving a tendinous cuff of about 1 cm from the vertebral body. Repair of the diaphragmatic crura during closure must be meticulous, robust, and anatomic. Failure to repair both the diaphragm, as well as the abdominal musculature fascia superficially, can result in a postoperative diaphragmatic or incisional abdominal hernia, respectively.[14]

Complications associated with lateral approaches depend in part on the laterality of the approach. Left-sided approaches are often preferred in the upper lumbar spine as they avoid the liver and the mobilization of the vena cava. Vena cava lacerations or perforations are notoriously morbid, owing to their relatively thin-walled structures and extremely high current. Right-sided approaches, however, may be necessary for certain pathology such as accessing the convexity of a dextroscoliotic thoracolumbar curve. If extension above the thoracolumbar junction is anticipated, some authors advocate for a right-sided approach, given its avoidance of the artery of Adamkiewicz.[17]

For extension into the lumbar spine, psoas muscle retraction and/or mobilization may be necessary. The complications associated with psoas violation or aggressive retraction are well documented, and often include L4 root injuries, psoas and/or quadriceps weakness, and thigh numbness.[18] Complications are less likely to occur at the cranial regions of the psoas' origin (L1-3) than in the thicker, caudal regions (L3-5); however, they can occur throughout.[19] At the thoracolumbar junction and the superior lumbar spine, the psoas may be elevated subperiosteally, as opposed to using a trans-psoas approach; this may reduce chance of injury to the lumbar roots.[16]

The mid-to-lower thoracic spine is considered a watershed area of the spinal cord and thus may be vulnerable to ischemia in the event of excessive manipulation, misplaced implants or instruments, or overly aggressive reduction maneuvers. Injury to the artery of Adamkiewicz, the largest anterior segmental medullary artery that supplies the inferior third of the spinal cord, is reported with anterior or lateral approaches at the thoracolumbar junction.[14] Classically, the artery arises from a left posterior intercostal artery at a level between the 9th to 12th thoracic vertebra; however, in up to 25% to 30% of people, it arises on the right side. It can also originate as low as L2 and branch from the aorta proper or from other lumbar vessels.[20] Injury to the artery of Adamkiewicz classically results in anterior spinal artery syndrome, marked by distal and disproportionate motor versus sensory loss, coupled with urinary and fecal incontinence.

Other intraoperative complications associated with accessing the thoracolumbar junction include injury to the sympathetic plexus, which can occur when exposing and/or ligating the intercostal vessels.[14] Conus medullaris syndrome has also been reported with this approach, as has hepatic ischemia resulting from aggressive deformity correction and resultant tethering of the vascular celiac trunk by the diaphragmatic crura.[21]

Pulmonary complications are relatively common in the postoperative setting, especially following procedures in which ipsilateral lung deflation is performed. Such complications include lung contusions, pulmonary effusions, atelectasis, persistent pneumothoraces, and pneumonia.[14, 22] Failure to perform a meticulous closure or intraoperative pleural injury can result in a postoperative pneumothorax. Postoperative chest tubes are often used to decrease related morbidities. Intraoperative vascular injury and failure to achieve adequate hemostasis—especially when ligation of segmental vessels is required—are associated with postoperative hemothoraces, requiring chest-tube decompression and often surgical reexploration.[17]

Outcomes

Surgical outcomes of fusions performed at the thoracolumbar junction depend largely on the inciting pathology, patient comorbidities, and the nature and extent of the procedure. Overall, the thoracolumbar junction is a region vulnerable to both implant failure and bony nonunion, owing, in part, to its kyphotic inflection and the lever-arm generated by the rigid thoracic spine.

In a notable retrospective analysis of 96 patients with adult idiopathic scoliosis patients undergoing primary instrumented fusion demonstrated a 17% overall pseudoarthrosis rate, almost 60% of which occurred between T9 and L1. Additional risk factors identified for thoracolumbar pseudarthrosis include advanced age (>55 years), longer fusion constructions (12 or more vertebral levels), and preoperative thoracolumbar kyphotic curves of 20 or greater degrees.[5] The same study team also identified osteoarthritis of the hip as well as use of the thoracoabdominal approach (versus the paramedian approach) as additional pseudarthrosis risk factors.[23]

Despite the elevated risk of nonunion, several case series have demonstrated that effective kyphotic deformity correction can be achieved using thoracolumbar osteotomies and instrumentation junctional fusions. One study demonstrated an average 46-degree improvement in overall sagittal alignment, as well as improvements in lumbar lordosis and sagittal imbalance, utilizing posterior-only approaches.[24] In patients with ankylosing spondylitis (AS), the thoracolumbar junction (especially T11-12 and T12-L1) is the single most common region for focal kyphotic deformity and *pre*interventional pseudarthrosis in an otherwise autofused spine. Historically, these patients with complex and rigid deformity have required combined anterior or extensive anterior alone procedures to correct their imbalance; however, improved instrumentation and osteotomy techniques are allowing surgeons to achieve excellent outcomes using posterior approaches alone. In a series of 30 consecutive adult patients with AS, Chang et al.[25] reported an average of 38-degrees of junctional kyphosis correction without radiographic evidence of postoperative pseudarthrosis at an average of 4.7 years.

For shorter segmental fusions, including single- or double-level procedures, lateral interbody fusion has been demonstrated to be an effective and safe technique. A retrospective analysis of 22 lateral interbody fusions (14 patients) performed at the thoracolumbar junction (T11-12 and T12-L1) demonstrated bony union in all but one patient who died soon thereafter from metastatic cancer. The majority of such cases were augmented with posterior instrumented fixation. Albeit a retrospective and clinically disparate series, there were relatively few complications, allowing the authors to conclude that lateral interbody techniques can be effective in the thoracolumbar junction.[22]

The thoracolumbar junction is disproportionately vulnerable to posttraumatic kyphotic deformity The case detailed in Fig. 22.4 demonstrates the occurrence and treatment of such sequelae. Several studies have explored the potential use of minimally invasive surgical (MIS) transforaminal interbody fusion techniques between T10 and L2 with somewhat mixed results. In a series of 15 patients with posttraumatic junctional deformities undergoing single-level MIS-TLIF procedures in an attempt to correct an average of 19.1 degrees of focal kyphosis, there was no significant improvement in kyphosis at an average follow-up of 26 months.[24] Despite this less than ideal outcome, the authors reported no significant complications and union was achieved in 13 of 15 patients.

Lumbosacral Overlap Disease

The problems that arise at the TL junction are similar to those seen at the LS area. Fusion to the sacrum should be avoided unless absolutely necessary. Fusion of the LS junction is often reserved for instability at L5-S1 (isthmic or degenerative spondylolisthesis, severe foraminal stenosis requiring complete facetectomy for neural decompression) or in the setting of adjacent segment disease with significant sagittal plane imbalance. Iatrogenic flatback syndrome is a common cause of failure at L5-S1, necessitating revision fusion at the LS junction or extension down to the sacrum below a previous fusion construct. Many of these complications are illustrated in the case seen in Fig. 22.5, including postlaminectomy syndrome, pseudoarthrosis, removal of failed instrumentation with severe iatrogenic flatback and sagittal imbalance (Fig. 22.5A and B).

The nonunion rate at L5-S1 is relatively high, especially in the setting of a long fusion construct. The addition of an interbody fusion at L5-S1, the use of iliac fixation, and the advent of biologics have increased the fusion rate at this biomechanically challenging area of the spine. The use of a third or fourth rod across an osteotomy site and/or across junctional pathologies (thoracolumbar or lumbosacral) may also decrease the rate of rod failure/breakage and improve fusion rates at high risk areas. Our preference is to place iliac fixation in all deformity constructs that extend up to or past L2. We typically also place an interbody cage at L5-S1 (Fig. 22.5C), unless there is advanced spondylosis with disk space collapse and osteophyte formation at that level, and always use a third rod across a three-column osteotomy site.

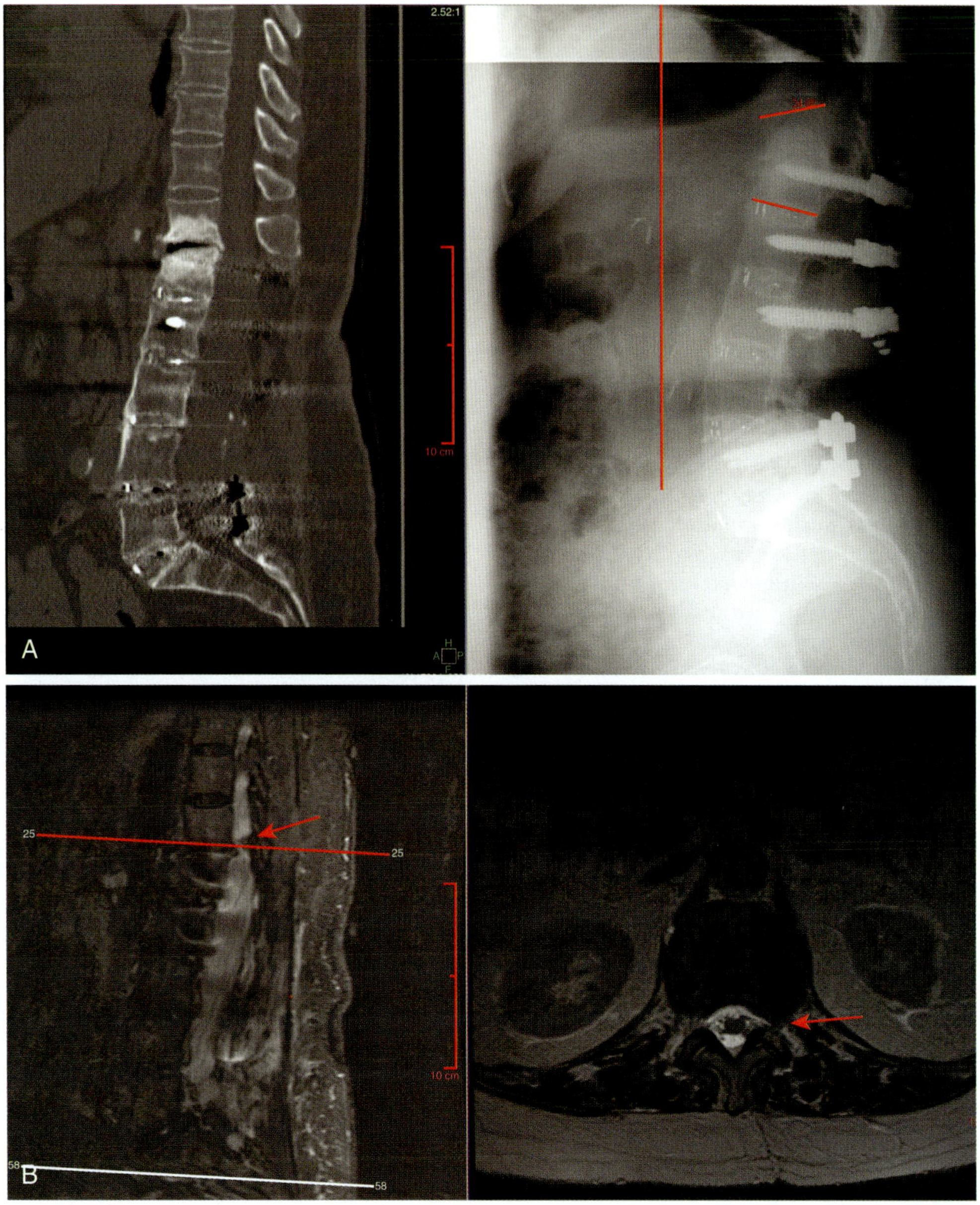

• **Fig. 22.4** A. 76-year-old female patient status post (s/p) multiple L1-S1 posterior lumbar interbody fusion procedures, the most recent of which, L1-4, was performed 2 years prior. Standing lumbar radiographs *(right)* demonstrate 25 degrees junctional kyphosis *(red lines)*. Computed tomography sagittal midline reconstruction *(left)* demonstrates marked disk degeneration, endplate and vertebral body sclerosis, and a vacuum effect within the disk space when supine, indicating mechanical instability. B. Magnetic resonance imaging sequences of the same patient preoperative. Sagittal short tau inversion recovery (STIR) images *(left)* and axial T2-weighted images demonstrate marked left-sided lateral recess and foraminal stenosis, with osteophyte formation, disk bulging, and ligamentous hypertrophy and infolding *(red arrows)*.

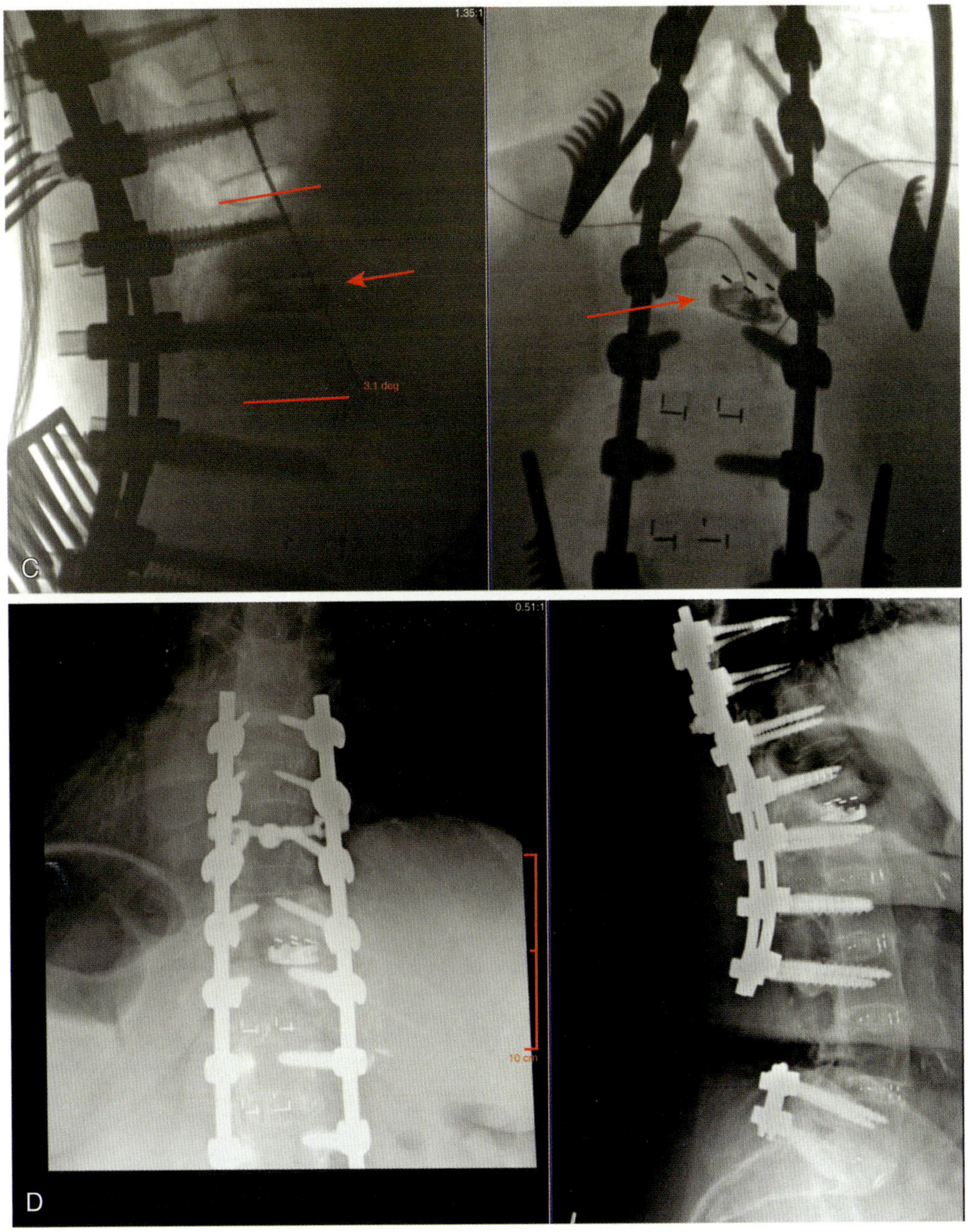

Fig. 22.4,cont'd C. Intraoperative fluoroscopic imaging, lateral *(left)* and posteroanterior (PA) *(right)* demonstrating deployment of an interbody cage *(red arrows)* at the T12-L1 interbody space. An expandable "bullet" or "straight line" cage (Elevate expandable cage by Medtronic, Minneapolis, MN) was chosen for its small size to allow it to maneuver relatively safely around the conus medullaris without excessive manipulation. It was then expanded in situ to restore the junction to approximately neutral sagittal alignment (3.1 degrees of lordosis as measured). **D**. A 3 months postoperative images of T10-L3 posterior lumbar fusion with interbody cage at thoracolumbar junction. Junctional and global sagittal balance was restored and patient was pain-free.

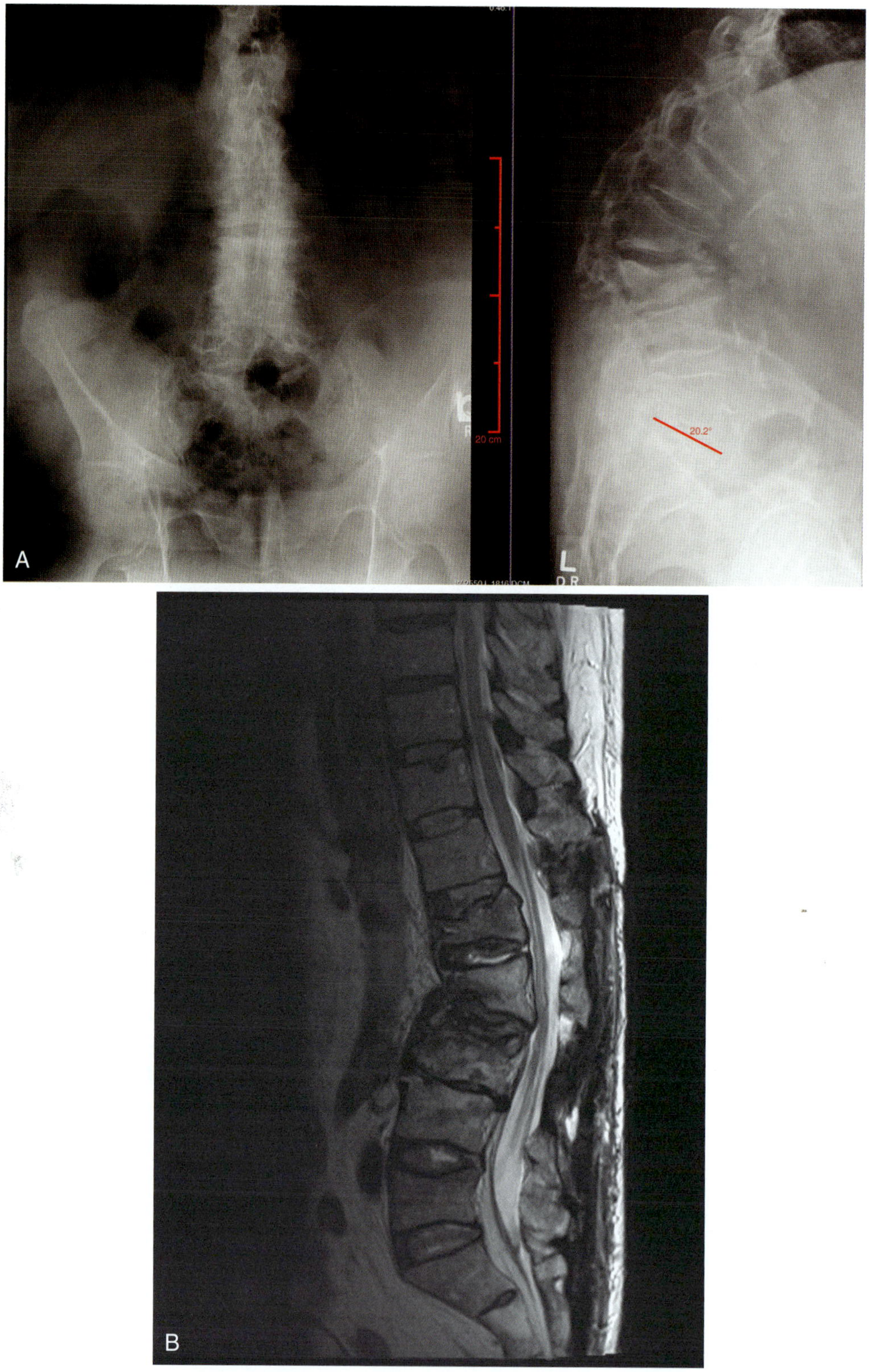

• **Fig. 22.5** **A**. A 65-year-old male patient status post (s/p) with multiple lumbar laminectomies, attempted fusions, and removal of symptomatic implants, who now exhibited symptoms of profound sagittal imbalance requiring a walker to hold himself upright. Standing plain radiographs demonstrate profound sagittal imbalance and degenerative processes: posteroanterior (PA) *(left)* and lateral *(right)*. The patient suffered multiple compression fractures from undue stresses secondary to the postlaminectomy syndrome and multiple attempted fusions. Prior to our intervention, the patient's lumbar kyphosis measured 20 degrees. Sagittal imbalance was greater than 30 cm. **B**. Sagittal T2-weighted magnetic resonance image sequence demonstrating profound postlaminectomy and postinsufficiency changes.

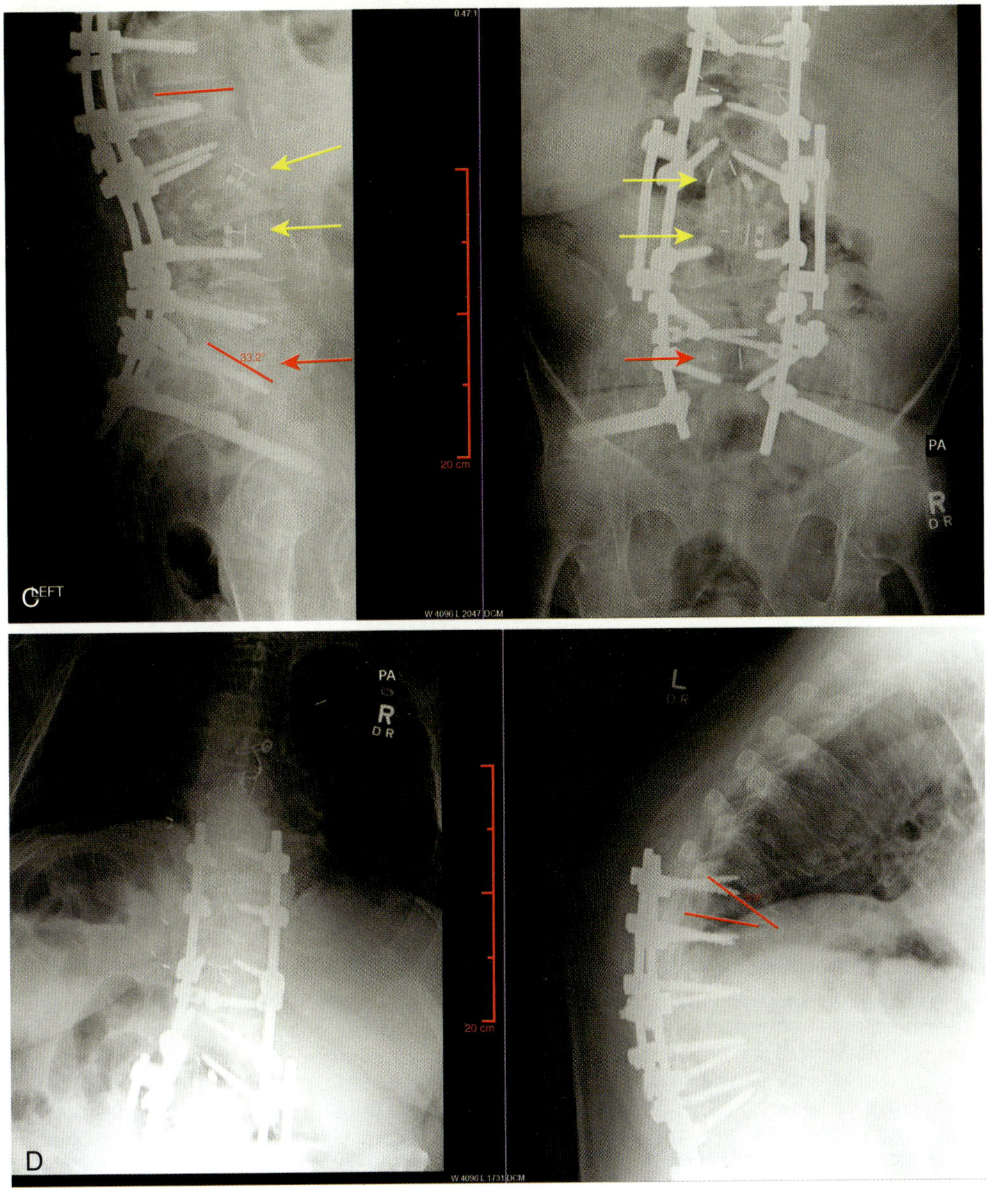

Fig. 22.5, cont'd C. PA *(left)* and lateral *(right)* standing radiographs at 3-months s/p L3 pedicle subtraction osteotomy, with T10-S2 segmental instrumented fusion. Note that interbody polyetheretherketone (PEEK) devices were employed at points of maximal stress, including the lumbosacral junction *(red arrow)* and at levels above and below the pedicle subtraction osteotomy *(yellow arrows)*. A turn-and-rotate cage (Capstone Control; Medtronic, Minneapolis, MN) was used at the lumbosacral junction for its relatively large lordotic contour (12 degrees). **D**. At approximately 4 months postoperative, patient had a fall and sustained compression fracture and screw pullout at proximal junction (T10). PA *(left)* and lateral *(right)* standing radiographs demonstrate screw pullout and 25 degree kyphotic wedging of T10 vertebrae.

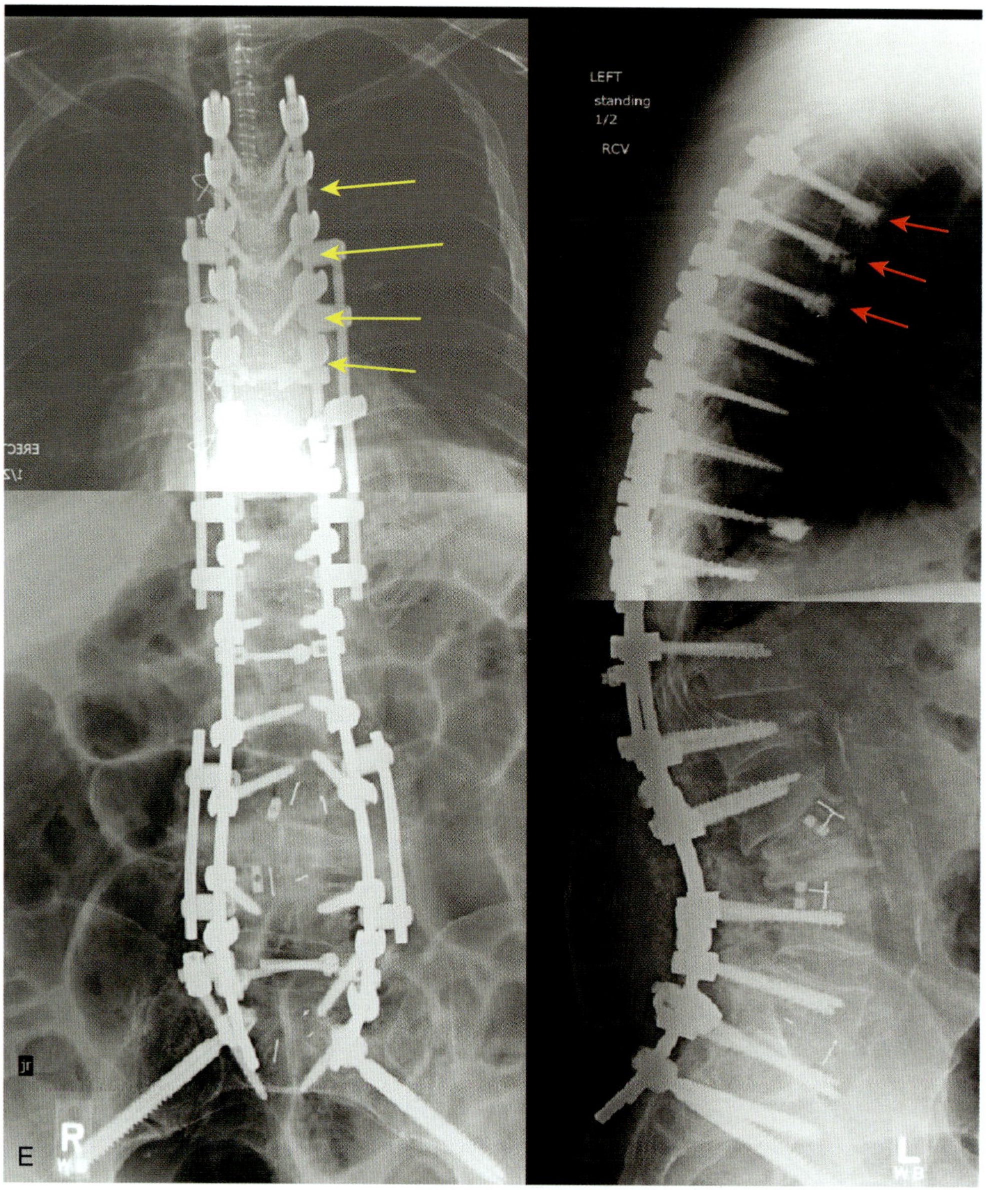

Fig. 22.5, cont'd E. At 6 months following initial pedicle subtraction osteotomy (PSO) procedure, full-length "stitched" radiographs of the thoracolumbosacral spine. Multiple techniques were employed to prevent further failure at new T4 proximal junction, including cemented screw augmentation *(red arrows)*, use of supplemental laminae wiring from T5-9 (*yellow arrows* [not to be confused with superimposed preexisting sternal wires]), use of comparatively elastic titanium rods instead of the cobalt-chromium alloy rods, and slightly exaggerated kyphosis in rods at the top of the construct to avoid sharp transition angles. Fortunately, at nearly 9 months following the osteotomy, the patient has a solid fusion, minimal pain, and walks mostly unassisted with a cane for distance.

Conclusion

The thoracolumbar and lumbosacral junctions are unique anatomic areas of the spine that are susceptible to a variety of "overlap pathology," including trauma, pseudarthrosis, proximal junction kyphosis or failure, and disk herniations. Access to the anterior column or disk at the TL junction is somewhat challenging, and the classic thoracotomy approach is fraught with complications. A direct lateral approach or a transforaminal approach via facetectomies is an alternative way to access the disk space at the TL junction in order to address a variety of pathologies.

References

1. Oda I, Abumi K, Cunningman BW, et al. An in vitro human cadaveric study investigating the biomechanical properties of the thoracic spine. *Spine (Phila Pa 1976)*. 2002;27(3):64–70.
2. Dai LY. Orientation and tropism of lumbar facet joints in degenerative spondylolisthesis. *Int Orthop*. 2001;25(1):40–42.
3. Fujiwara A, Lim T, An H, et al. The effect of disc degeneration and facet joint osteoarthritis on the segmental flexibility of the lumbar spine. *Spine (Phila Pa 1976)*. 2000;25(23):2026–2044.
4. Kuklo TR, Bridwell KH, Lewis SJ, et al. Minimum 2-year analysis of sacropelvic fixation and L5-S1 fusion using S1 and iliac screws. *Spine (Phila Pa 1976)*. 2001;26:1976–1983.

5. Kim YJ, Bridwell KH, Lenke LG, et al. Pseudarthrosis in primary fusions for adult idiopathic scoliosis: incidence, risk factors, and outcome analysis. *Spine (Phila Pa 1976)*. 2005;30(4):468–474.
6. Madan S, Boeree NR. Outcome of posterior lumbar interbody fusion versus posterolateral fusion for spondylolytic spondylolisthesis. *Spine (Phila Pa 1976)*. 2002;27(14):1536–1542.
7. Wang JC, Mummaneni PV, Haid RW. Current treatment strategies for the painful lumbar motion segment: posterolateral fusion versus interbody fusion. *Spine (Phila Pa 1976)*. 2005;30(suppl 16):S33–S43.
8. Wirtz DC, Genius I, Windberger JE, et al. Diagnostic and therapeutic management of lumbar and thoracic spondylodiscitis—an evaluation of 59 cases. *Arch Orthop Trauma Surg*. 2000;120(5):245–251.
9. Klemme WR, Owens BD, Dhawan A, et al. Lumbar sagittal contour after posterior interbody fusion: threaded devices alone versus vertical cages plus posterior instrumentation. *Spine (Phila Pa 1976)*. 2001;26(5):534–537.
10. Baghdadi YM, Larson AN, Dekutoski MB, et al. Sagittal balance and spinopelvic parameters after lateral lumbar interbody fusion for degenerative scoliosis: a case-control study. *Spine (Phila Pa 1976)*. 2014;39(3):166–173.
11. Machino M, Yukawa Y, Ito K, et al. Transforaminal thoracic interbody fusion in the management of lower thoracic spine fracture dislocations: technical note. *J Spinal Disord Tech*. 2013;26(6):E209–E214.
12. Uribe JS, Smith WD, Pimenta L, et al. Minimally invasive lateral approach for symptomatic thoracic disc herniation: initial multicenter clinical expertise. *J Neurosurg Spine*. 2012;16:264–279.
13. Wang J, Zhou Y, Zhang ZF, et al. Disc herniation in the thoracolumbar junction treated by minimally invasive transforaminal interbody fusion surgery. *J Clin Neurosci*. 2014;21(3):431–435.
14. Rao RD, Bagaria V. Anterior approaches to the thoracolumbar spine. *Orthopaedic Knowledge Online Journal*. 2005;3(6). http://www.aaos.org/OKOJ/vol3/issue6/SPI018. Accessed May 2017.
15. Nair SK, Petko M, Hayward MP. Aetiology and management of chylothorax in adults. *Eur J Cardiothorac Surg*. 2007;32(2):362–369.
16. Kibuule LK, Herkowitz HN. Thoracic spine: surgical approaches. In: Herkowitz HN, Garfin SR, Eismont FJ, et al., eds. *Rothman and Simeone: The Spine*. 6th ed. Philadelphia, PA: Elsevier Saunders; 2011:318–338.
17. Stambough JL, Clouse EK. Vascular complications in spinal surgery. In: Herkowitz HN, Garfin SR, Eismont FJ, et al., eds. *Rothman and Simeone: The Spine*. 6th ed. Philadelphia, PA: Elsevier Saunders; 2011:1728–1776.
18. Arnold PM, Anderson KK, McGuire Jr RA. The lateral transpsoas approach to the lumbar and thoracic spine: a review. *Surg Neurol Int*. 2012;3(suppl 3):S198–S215.
19. Kwon B, Kim DH. Lateral lumbar interbody fusion: Indications, outcomes, and complications. *J Am Acad Orthop Surg*. 2016;24(2):96–105.
20. Melissano G, Civilini E, Bertoglio L, et al. Angio-CT imaging of the spinal cord vascularization: a pictorial essay. *Eur J Vasc Endovasc Surg*. 2010;39(4):436–440.
21. von Glinski KS, Krettek C, Blauth M, et al. Hepatic ischemia as a complication after correction of post-traumatic gibbus at the thoracolumbar junction. *Spine (Phila Pa 1976)*. 2000;25(8):1040–1044.
22. Meredith DS, Kepler CK, Huang RC, et al. Extreme lateral interbody fusion (XLIF) in the thoracic and thoracolumbar spine: technical report and early outcomes. *HSS J*. 2013;9(1):25–31.
23. Kim YJ, Bridwell KH, Lenke LG, et al. Pseudarthrosis in long adult spinal deformity instrumentation and fusion to the sacrum: prevalence and risk factor analysis of 144 cases. *Spine (Phila Pa 1976)*. 2006;31(20):2329–2336.
24. Shufflebarger HL, Clark CE. Thoracolumbar osteotomy for postsurgical sagittal imbalance. *Spine (Phila Pa 1976)*. 1992;17(suppl 8):S287–S290.
25. Chang KW, Tu MY, Huang HH, et al. Posterior correction and fixation without anterior fusion for pseudoarthrosis with kyphotic deformity in ankylosing spondylitis. *Spine (Phila Pa 1976)*. 2006;31(13):E408–E413.

23

Evidence-Based Report on Interbody Fusions of the Lumbar Spine

JULIE L. CHAN, ROBERT G. WHITMORE, AND ZOHER GHOGAWALA

Introduction

Lumbar fusion is a commonly performed procedure for various spine conditions, including spondylolisthesis, degenerative disk disease, dynamic instability, or lumbar spondylosis. Despite numerous studies, significant debate remains regarding the most effective surgical technique for lumbar fusion. Specifically, use of an interbody graft in lumbar fusion is an area of controversy. Although an interbody graft potentially provides the benefits of improved fusion rate and restoration of foraminal height, it is also associated with increased complications and costs. In this chapter, key studies are reviewed which compare posterolateral fusion with an interbody graft versus posterolateral fusion alone in regard to effect on fusion, clinical outcomes, and cost-effectiveness. Together, the current evidence generally supports the use of an interbody graft in lumbar fusion as a cost-effective means to achieve solid fusion and improved clinical outcome. However, further studies are required to confirm the use of an interbody graft as superior to methods that rely on posterolateral fusion alone.[1]

Surgical Indications

Rationale for Using Interbody Grafts

The use of an interbody graft was first adopted after evidence suggested that persistent back pain may be related to diskogenic disease, and interbody placement may reduce motion-related pain by adding structural stability.[2–4] Posterolateral fusion has historically been used to reduce segmental motion. However, stabilization of the load-bearing portion of the spine, namely the anterior column, may be more effective in achieving fusion than fusion across the facet joints alone. Interbody graft use in lumbar fusion is supported by a number of class II and III studies which demonstrate increased fusion rate, restoration of foraminal height, preservation of biomechanical properties, reduced reoperation rate, and cost-effectiveness. High quality class I evidence for or against interbody fusion is lacking. Conversely, a number of analyses demonstrate no difference in clinical outcome and emphasize negative effects of interbody grafts, such as increased intraoperative duration, length of stay, and complications.[5,6] In addition, there are multiple variables of interbody grafts, such as graft composition, bone material within the interbody, and different types of interbody grafts including expandable cages, that have yet to be rigorously evaluated (Fig. 23.1).

Increased Rate of Fusion

The main rationale for using an interbody graft in lumbar fusion is the potential to improve fusion rate. Physiologically, interbody

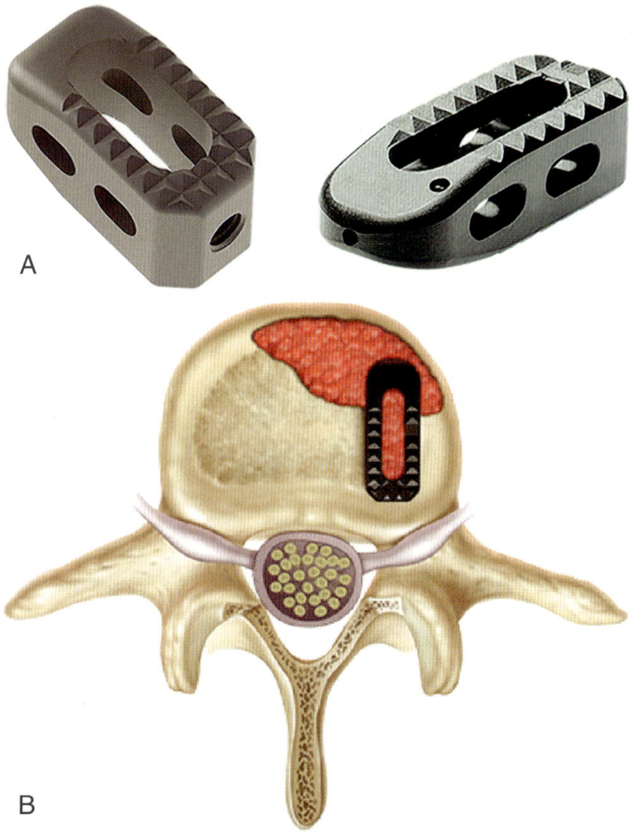

• **Fig. 23.1** Examples of standard cage *(left)* and bulleted titanium cage *(right)* (A). Graphic representation of cage placement during posterior lumbar interbody fusion with additional graft material loaded within and surrounding the cage (B). (Images courtesy of DePuy Synthes, Raynham, MA.)

placement provides increased surface area for fusion as well as ample vascular supply following adequate decortication of the endplates. There are two randomized controlled clinical trials and a meta-analysis that support improved fusion with interbody compared with posterolateral fusion alone (Table 23.1). The two key randomized studies supporting interbody fusion over posterolateral fusion are those by Christensen et al.[7] and Fritzell et al.[8] In 2002, Christensen et al. demonstrated a significant increase in fusion rate in circumferential versus posterolateral fusion alone.[7] This randomized clinical trial evaluated 148 patients with severe chronic low back pain who underwent either posterolateral fusion with Cotrel-Dubousset instrumentation (posterolateral fusion [PLF]) or circumferential fusion with posterolateral fusion plus retroperitoneal insertion of a Brantigan cage (anterior lumbar interbody fusion [ALIF]). Patients were followed over the course of 8 years and 1 year postoperative static radiographs were evaluated. For patients who underwent PLF, continuous intertransverse bony bridges on at least one side were assessed, whereas ALIF was evaluated by continuous bone structure surrounding Brantigan cages and absence of migration of the cage. Overall, patients who underwent additional interbody placement for severe chronic back pain demonstrated significantly increased fusion rate (92%) over those with posterolateral fusion alone (80%) (P <.04). In a similar comparison, Fritzell et al.[8] demonstrated improved fusion with internal fixation when comparing anterior lumbar interbody fusion or posterior lumbar interbody fusion (ALIF/PLIF) versus PLF or PLF with variable screw placement and internal fixation (PLF+PSF). This prospective randomized multicenter study evaluated 294 patients who underwent one of the above treatments (or no surgery) for chronic low back pain. Patients were diverse and collected from 19 different centers. At 2 years after surgery, radiologists evaluated bony fusion on a 3-point scale, ultimately demonstrating that use of interbody graft improved fusion rate (91% and 87%) over posterolateral fusion alone (72%) (P <.004).[8]

In addition to these randomized studies, a recent meta-analysis also supports improved fusion with interbody placement. Luo et al.[9] evaluated nine different studies, focusing on the clinical effectiveness of PLIF versus PLF for isthmic spondylolisthesis. In this study, fusion rate was evaluated in 421 patients and found to be significantly lower for PLF than PLIF with an odds ratio of 0.29 (0.14,0.58; P = .005).

TABLE 23.1 Summary of Evidence for Interbody Fusion

Level of Evidence	Study Type	Reference	Description	Conclusion
I	Prospective randomized trial	Christensen et al., 2002	Prospective randomized clinical study analyzing ALIF vs. instrumented PLF in severe chronic low back pain.	Circumferential fusion demonstrated higher fusion rate with decreased reoperation rate.
II	Prospective comparison	Fritzell et al., 2002	Multicenter randomized study comparing PLF vs. PLF with variable screw placement and internal fixation (PLF+PSF) vs. ALIF/PLIF for severe chronic low back pain.	Internal fixation improved fusion rate compared with posterolateral fusion only.
I	Prospective randomized study	Kim et al., 2006	Prospective randomized study compared PLF vs. PLIF vs. PLF+PLIF.	No difference in fusion rate between the groups. PLIF demonstrated better sagittal balance than PLF alone.
I	Randomized clinical trial	Videbaek et al., 2011	Randomized controlled clinical trial compared ALIF + instrumented PLF vs. instrumented PLF for severe back pain.	No difference in sagittal balance.
I	Randomized clinical trial	Thalgott et al., 2009	Randomized clinical trial which compared ALIF+instrumented PLG vs. instrumented PLF for severe back pain.	Freeze-dried graft was inferior to frozen graft with a higher potential for pseudoarthrosis.
III	Retrospective review	Hsieh et al., 2007	Retrospective overview of medical records and radiographs to evaluate ALIF vs. TLIF.	ALIF is superior to TLIF in restoration of foraminal height, local disk angle, and lumbar lordosis.
II	Prospective nonrandomized clinical study	Oliviera et al., 2010	Prospective study evaluating XLIF for degenerative lumbar conditions with stenosis.	XLIF is an effective method to decompress the spine and increase foraminal height.
I	Randomized controlled trial	Soegaard et al., 2007	Cost-utility evaluation of a randomized trial comparing ALIF vs. PLF with instrumentation.	ALIF is significantly more cost-effective over a long-term analysis.
III	Retrospective review	Macki et al., 2015	Retrospective review of patients who underwent first-time lumbar fusion.	PLF +PLIF/TLIF was associated with greater spondylolisthesis correction as well as reduced reoperation compared to PLF alone.
III	Retrospective review	Bydon et al., 2015	Retrospective cost analysis.	PLIF demonstrated decreased reoperation rate, improved long-term cost savings, and better functional outcomes compared with PLF.

ALIF, anterior lumbar interbody fusion; *PLF*, posterolateral fusion; *PLIF*, posterior lumbar interbody fusion; *PSF*, pedicle screw fixation; *TLIF*, transforaminal lumbar interbody fusion.

Foraminal Height Restoration

Another argument for interbody use is that it restores foraminal height (Fig. 23.2). Hsieh et al.[10] compared the change in foraminal height between two different interbody placement methods. When comparing ALIF versus transforaminal lumbar interbody fusion (TLIF), the authors demonstrated that an anterior approach was superior, restoring foraminal height by 18.5%, whereas TLIF decreased foraminal height by 0.4%.[10] One possible explanation for this suboptimal increase in foraminal height with TLIF may be compression along the pedicle screws with a dorsal approach. Several studies report a significant increase in foraminal height when a direct lateral approach is used. In a small nonrandomized study, patients who underwent eXtreme lateral interbody fusion (XLIF) for central or lateral lumbar stenosis experienced an increase (13.5%) in foraminal height.[11] Similarly, a recent retrospective study by Alimi et al.[12] demonstrated that single-level XLIF was effective for unilateral foraminal stenosis with a significant increase in foraminal height after placement of the graft (18 ± 0.5 vs. 11 ± 0.5 mm, P <.001).

Biomechanical Principles of Interbody Grafts

Spinal biomechanics are important to consider during lumbar fusion. Use of interbody cages and placing the graft under

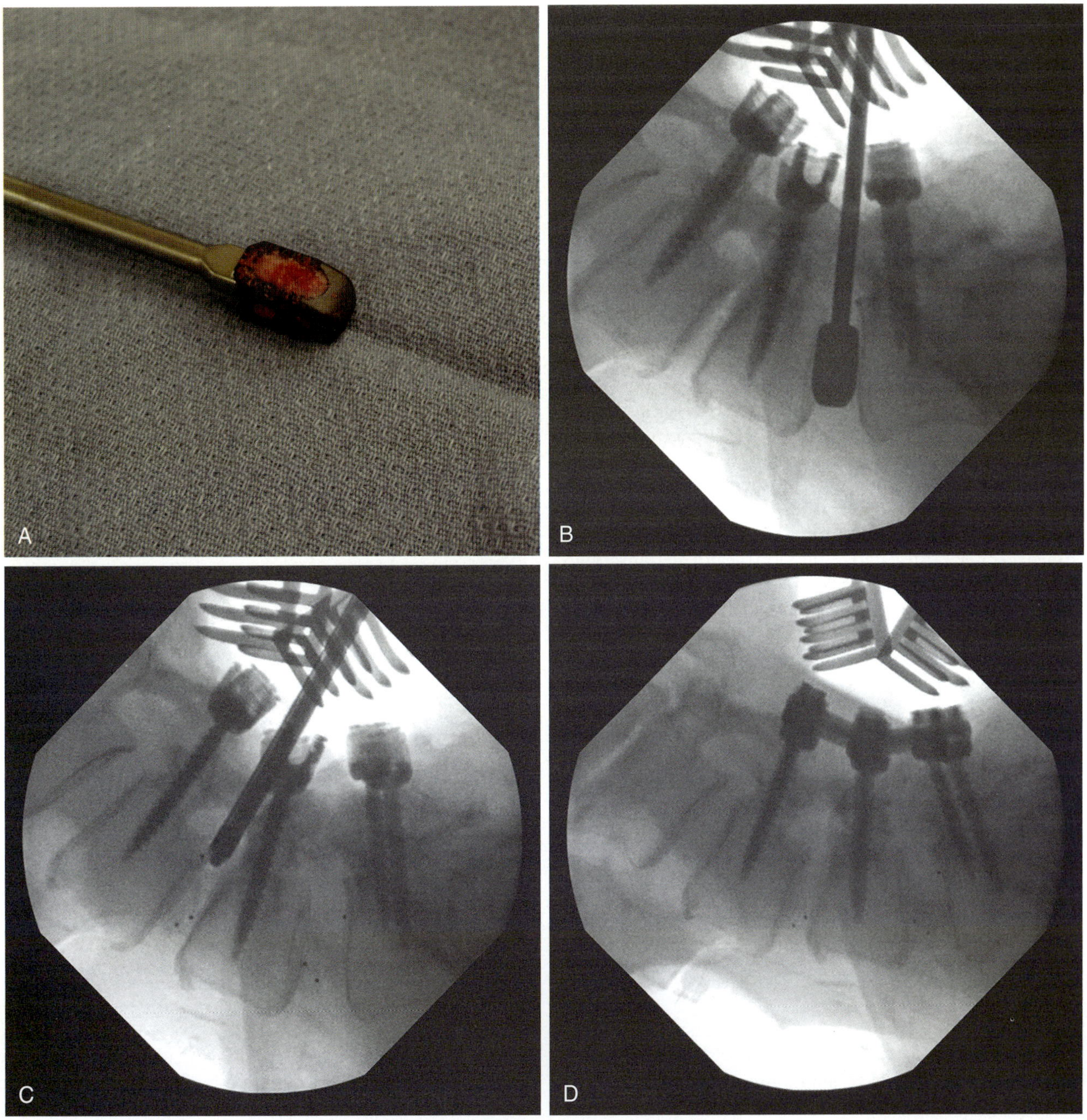

• **Fig. 23.2** **A.** Polyetheretherketone (PEEK) interbody cage loaded with allograft and bone morphogenetic protein. **B.** Distraction of the L5-S1 disk space. **C** and **D.** Radiolucent PEEK interbody cage placement at L4-5 and L5-S1.

compression may ultimately improve fusion and healing rate based on Wolff's law.[13] In addition, regional and global sagittal balance must be either preserved or restored to achieve good outcome following lumbar fusion and reduce the likelihood of adverse complications.[14] Macki et al.[15] demonstrated lumbar fusion with interbody graft (PLIF or TLIF) was more effective in reducing spondylolisthesis (13.06%) compared with traditional posterolateral fusion alone (5.67%) (P <.001). Kim et al.[16] compared the use of 1- or 2-level PLIF, PLF, and PLIF+PLF in the management of degenerative lumbar disease. After 3 years of follow-up, patients who underwent PLIF or PLIF+PLF demonstrated postoperative improvement in lumbar lordosis and segmental angle (P <.05, P <.05); however, those who underwent PLF alone did not demonstrate any significant improvement.[16] Similarly, a meta-analysis by Zhou et al.[17] also demonstrated better restoration of spinal alignment with interbody use. Despite these results, there are conflicting studies which evaluated spinopelvic parameters of pelvic tilt and lumbar lordosis, and demonstrated no difference in sagittal balance between PLF and ALIF.[18]

Limitations

Clinical Improvement

A number of studies have attempted to quantify the level of clinical improvement interbody fusion provides over traditional posterolateral lumbar fusion. In 2007, Soegaard et al.[19] analyzed data from the 2002 Christensen study, demonstrating that interbody fusion was clinically superior to posterolateral fusion alone. In this analysis, the authors included the Dallas pain questionnaire (DPQ), the Oswestry Disability Index (ODI) and overall general health measured by Short Form-36 (SF-36). Those who underwent interbody fusion had a postoperative mean ODI score of 28 compared with 40 for those who underwent posterolateral fusion, suggesting significantly less disability after interbody fusion (P <.004). SF-36 scores confirmed greater postoperative physical health in those who underwent ALIF compared with PLF (39 vs. 33, P = .005). In addition, at the 5- to 9-year follow-up, those who underwent interbody fusion had significantly less back pain measured by VAS pain scale (3 vs. 6, P <.05). Most recently, a study by Glassman et al.[20] utilized the National Neurosurgical Quality and Outcomes Database (N^2QOD) to evaluate interbody use (TLIF) versus PLF for isthmic or degenerative spondylolisthesis. Cases within each group were propensity-matched and change in ODI evaluated, demonstrating those who underwent interbody fusion had significant reduction in disability at 3 (19.4 vs. 26.0, P = .009) and 12 months (20.8 vs. 29.3, P = .001) postoperatively.[20] In a conflicting study, Hoy et al.[21] conducted a randomized clinical trial of 100 patients comparing TLIF and PLF for low back pain with radiculopathy. At 2 years after surgery, no statistically significant difference was seen in daily activity, work ability, mental health, or back pain/radiculopathy when using ODI, DPQ, and SF-36.[21]

Cost-Effectiveness

Use of an interbody graft adds significantly to the implant costs of lumbar fusion, and several studies have evaluated whether this additional cost is associated with improved outcomes. These studies also account for the costs of reoperation. In 2007, Soegaard et al.[19] evaluated the data generated in the 2002 Christensen et al. study from a long-term economic perspective, and concluded that interbody fusion is less expensive from a societal perspective. Specifically, the reoperation rate was significantly reduced with interbody use (P <.009), with a 7% reoperation rate in circumferential fusion versus 22% in instrumented posterolateral fusion. The lower reoperation rate for circumferential fusion also significantly contributed to its lower cost compared with posterolateral fusion alone (P <.001).[19] In addition, loss of productivity costs were also greater in patients who underwent posterolateral fusion only, with a reduced rate of return to work (11.1% vs. 44.4%) and reduced workforce productivity ($175,640 vs. $145,883). Additional cost variables favored interbody use, including outpatient visits (P <.023), comorbidity-related surgeries (P <.025), and transportation (P <.008). Similarly, a retrospective review of 103 patients by Bydon et al.[22] demonstrated that interbody use was associated with reduced repeat surgery. This study evaluated patients at 2 years postoperative and compared instrumented PLF versus PLIF/TLIF for spondylolisthesis. The authors demonstrated that PLF was associated with increased (26.51%) reoperation rate compared with lumbar fusion with interbody graft (9.26%) for 137 patients undergoing first-time surgery for lumbar spondylolisthesis (P = .13).[22]

SURGICAL TECHNIQUE

Step 1: Position patient prone, preferably on a Jackson table in lordotic position.
Step 2: Confirm the correct operative level with lateral x-ray.
Step 3: Dissect the paraspinal musculature starting with a midline incision.
Step 4: Perform appropriate laminectomies, and foraminotomies, if indicated. Set aside bone and morselize for future placement into interbody and disk space.
Step 5: Perform thorough diskectomies. Retract the crossing nerve root medially with a nerve root retractor. Incise the annulus of the disk with an 11 blade, mobilize the disk space with a spreader or paddle, then remove the disk fragments with a pituitary.
Step 6: Prepare the disk space to interbody placement with shavers or rasps to further mobilize and remove the disk and decorticate the endplate. Place a spacer into the disk space, and confirm appropriate placement and size of implant with a lateral x-ray.
Step 7: Prepare interbody cage, fill with autograft from above (see Figs. 23.1 and 23.2). Alternative sources of bone graft material may be iliac crest, allograft, or bone substitutes.
Step 8: Place interbody into disk space and pack interbody with surrounding bone autograft.
Step 9: Repeat for adjacent levels as necessary.
Step 10: Place pedicle screws and rods for instrumented fusion.
Step 11: Decorticate lateral to instrumentation and onlay remaining autograft and/or cadaver bone.
Step 12: Closure

Interbody Graft Composition

Multiple different types of interbody grafts are commercially available. These vary in composition, shape, size, and function, and include newer technologies such as expandable cages. The composition of the interbody graft is of particular interest in regard to fusion effectiveness. The composition of interbody grafts includes allograft, PEEK, and titanium, each of which has its advantages. Allograft provides the greater surface area for bone contact, but may fracture on insertion or subside significantly. Titanium was originally chosen for cages for its structural and porous similarity to bone.[23,24] PEEK was introduced as an alternative as it has a similar density to bone and is radiolucent, allowing for accurate assessment of fusion.[25,26] Despite PEEK's advantages in decreased incidence of allergic reaction and MRI artifact, it may be associated with a higher rate of nonunion compared to titanium. This may, in part, be owing to its poor ability to integrate with osseous formation as titanium is more effective in promoting osteoblasts and bone morphogenetic protein (BMP) formation.[27] The superiority and use of titanium versus PEEK remains controversial. Nemoto et al.[28] retrospectively analyzed 48 patients who underwent a single-level TLIF, noting that fusion rate was superior with titanium (100%) compared to PEEK (76%) cages. Titanium grafts allow for maintenance of disk height and early growth of bone into the graft, but are difficult to assess for fusion postoperatively. Unlike the study by Nemoto et al.[28], Tanida et al.[29] found similar fusion rates (82.8% and 80.4%) for titanium and PEEK 2 years after TLIF.

The bone material within the interbody graft likely influences fusion rate to a great extent. Thalgott et al.[30] demonstrated that freeze-dried femoral ring allograft (FRA) was inferior to frozen FRA for ALIF. Fusion was determined by blinded radiologists who assessed bridging bone on computed tomography, mobility on flexion/extension films, and the degree of FRA incorporation. In this study of 50 patients, those who received frozen allograft had a significantly better fusion rate. Many additional bone formulations have been used within an interbody graft, including iliac crest, local autogenous bone from harvested spinous process and lamina, demineralized bone matrix, and newer stem cell-based technologies. There is insufficient evidence in support of one of these bone formulations over another at the present time.

Closure

Secured wound closure is paramount to preventing hardware infection. The wound should be closed in layers, starting with reopposition of the lumbosacral fascia with snug 0 Vicryl. If desired, Vancomycin powder may be distributed over the hardware and above the deep fascial layer to reduce the potential for hardware infection. The subdermis should be closed with 2-0 or 3-0 Vicryl. Skin closure may be approached in a number of ways. For small incisions such as in minimally invasive surgery (MIS) techniques, subcuticular Monocryl or Dermabond may be utilized. Larger incisions may require staples, and if a cerebrospinal fluid leak was encountered, use of nylon suture is preferable.

Postoperative Care

Follow-up and Incision Care

Postoperatively, patients should keep the wound clean and dry with daily cleansing. Ideally, patients should follow up at 2 weeks for incision healing as well as at 1, 3, 6, and 12 months postoperatively with plain x-rays to evaluate fusion progression.

Activity and Brace Use

Patients should refrain from heavy lifting for 10 weeks postoperatively, and may return to exercise as tolerated. Although patients may wear a brace for comfort, postoperative bracing is not recommended because bracing after instrumented lumbar fusion does not improve clinical outcome or fusion rate.[31,32]

Complications/Side-Effects

Unforeseen circumstances may occur and are of particular concern regarding interbody use during posterior instrumented fusion. Although standard operative risk concerns, such as durotomy, infection, and hemorrhage apply, some studies suggest these risks are increased during interbody fusion compared with posterolateral fusion alone.[33] Li et al.[34] compared intraoperative blood loss in 40 patients undergoing instrumented PLF versus TLIF for degenerative scoliosis, demonstrating a significant increase with interbody placement (1,166.7±554.1 vs. 1,673±922.4 mL, P = .048) Other studies, such as that by Luo et al. demonstrated no difference in weighed mean difference (WMD) in blood loss between instrumented PLF and PLIF for lumbar isthmic spondylolisthesis (WMD: 121.17 (-152.68,395.01), P = .39).[9] Unique to interbody fusion where meticulous disk space dissection must take place, prudent complications include adjacent segment disease (ASD) and neurologic injury owing to over-distraction. Vascular injury is also another potential complication of lumbar interbody fusion. The example here is a 31-year-old male patient with grade 2 L5-S1 spondylolisthesis and bilateral L5 radiculopathy. During diskectomy of the L4-5 disk space, the anterior longitudinal ligaments were violated with subsequent injury to the left iliac artery (Fig. 23.3). The patient was taken to the vascular surgery operating room where a stent was deployed and the remainder of the case completed with resolution of bilateral radiculopathy.

Outcomes

Future Studies and Alternative Fusion Methods

Although a body of evidence supports the use of interbody fusion over posterolateral fusion alone in the lumbar spine, number of class III studies did not arrive at similar conclusions. Pradhan et al.[35] and Kim et al.[16] demonstrated no significant difference in fusion rate, whereas Videbaek et al.[18] demonstrated no difference in sagittal balance between the various techniques. Pradhan et al.[35] reviewed 122 patients who underwent anterior interbody or posterior intertransverse lumbar fusion for degenerative disk disease (DDD) or spondylolisthesis and found no difference in fusion rate between interbody use (95%) and posterolateral approach (91%). Further evidence also indicated that interbody use may cause an increased rate of ASD[36] as well as increased operative time and complications.[9] Lee et al. analyzed 490 patients who underwent 3 or fewer levels in lumbar fusion. Although they found the average annual incidence of ASD to be consistently low (1.2%), PLIF was associated with a higher incidence of ASD (11.7% at 10 years) compared with 6.7% following PLF (P = .048).[36] The authors propose that this increased incidence of ASD may be related to improved arthrodesis, permitting increased rigidity which is subsequently transmitted as increased stress on the adjacent levels.[37–39] These data are in line with other studies demonstrating that fusion rate may not translate to improved patient outcomes.[40.41]

Alternative Approaches

Traditional PLIF and TLIF are likely the most commonly used methods for implementing an interbody device in lumbar fusion. However, some studies advocate the technique of full 360 degree circumferential fusion over posterior-only methods. The anterior approach (ALIF) may augment traditional posterolateral fusion, but it does have additional risks such as retrograde ejaculation

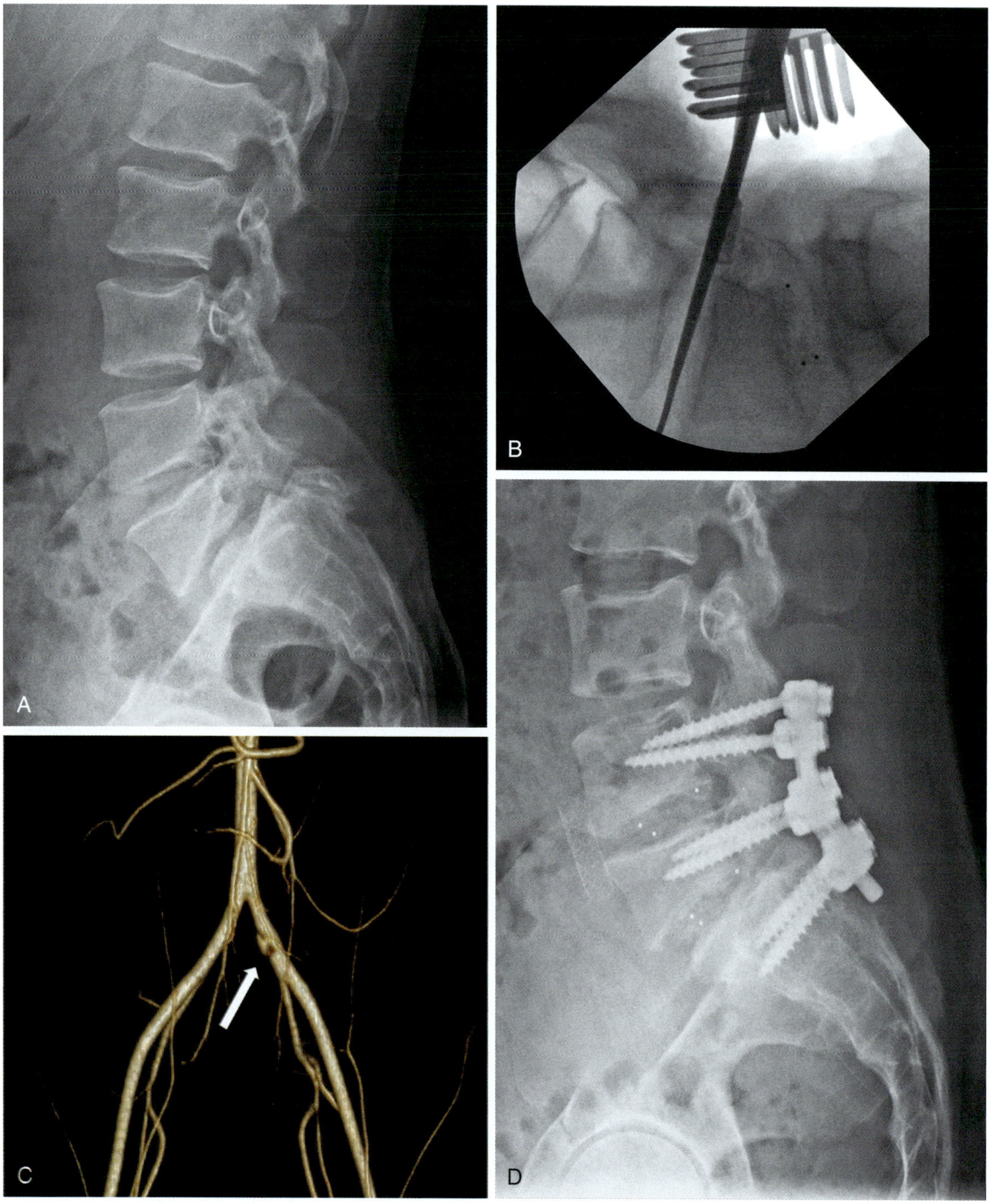

• **Fig. 23.3** Preoperative imaging demonstrating grade 2 L5-S1 isthmic spondylolisthesis with bilateral L5 radiculopathy (A). Intraoperative radiograph with Penfield 4 demonstrating violation of the anterior longitudinal ligaments beyond the L4-5 disk space (B) and angiogram demonstrating subsequent left iliac artery injury (*arrow*, C). Postoperative radiograph demonstrating correction of spondylolisthesis (D).

for men, as well as vascular and abdominal injuries. Christensen et al.[7] utilized ALIF in addition to PLF to compare the effect of interbody use with good results as described above. Future comparative studies are required to determine if there is further benefit to ALIF over PLIF or TLIF when considering interbody fusion. A recent systematic review by Schroeder et al.[42] evaluating arthrodesis at L5-S1 suggests TLIF fusion rate is superior to ALIF or axial interbody methods ($P = .005$). Further analysis showed that when correcting for bilateral instrumentation, there is no difference between the methods ($P > .05$), and they all provide significant fusion rate overall (99.2, 97.2, 90.5%).[42]

In addition to anterior and axial methods, there is also the lateral interbody fusion (LLIF) approach, also known as direct lateral, far lateral, extreme lateral, and extraforaminal approaches (DLIF, FLIF, XLIF, ELIF), which can also be used to correct coronal deformity. This method is suggested to provide a minimally invasive route to the disk space that avoids major vessels with larger graft placement, high fusion rates, and overall better recovery time.[43–45] Currently, no level 1 evidence suggests superiority of the direct lateral approach over other conventional approaches[46]; however, a number of studies demonstrate level 2 evidence that the lateral approach is a safe and effective technique for minimally invasive interbody fusion. Sembrano et al.[47] compared 2-level contiguous lumbar interbody fusion utilizing the MIS-TLIF and XLIF approaches. In this prospective trial, 55 patients were randomized to either of the approaches, demonstrating similar operative times and length of stay. Those patients who underwent direct lateral approach experienced decreased blood loss ($P < .001$); however, they also experienced increased postoperative complications including hip flexion weakness (31% vs. 0%).[47] Additional analysis on the same cohorts showed that those patients who underwent XLIF demonstrated less subsidence at 24 months postoperatively ($P = .002$) and increased postoperative disk space magnitude compared with MIS-TLIF ($P < .05$).[43] Given the MIS nature of this lateral approach, it may be an option for those who present a higher preoperative risk as Rodgers and Rodgers[48] found octogenarians who underwent XLIF experienced less complications, blood loss, and hospital length of stay compared with traditional open PLIF ($P < .0001$) as well increased home discharge rate versus skilled nursing facility (SNF) (92.5% vs. 0%).

Although a number of studies support the benefits of this approach, it is not without complications, such as increased nerve injury, as suggested in the extensive review by Ahmadian et al.[49] In an effort to further optimize the lateral approach, an oblique lateral interbody fusion (OLIF) has been proposed which utilizes a lateral position with dissection anterior to the psoas.[50] As evidenced by the numerous techniques available to access the lumbar interbody space, it is clear that the approach is an evolving process. At present time, studies have not demonstrated superiority of the lateral approach over traditional interbody fusion methods, and additional studies are needed to determine the overall safety profile and efficacy of these newer approaches in the acute and long-term postoperative periods.

Conclusion

Although many studies support interbody use in lumbar fusions to improve fusion rate, sagittal balance, and reduce overall costs, significant debate remains. Future studies are needed to further strengthen the evidence supporting interbody use in patients undergoing fusion for lumbar pathology.

References

1. Mummaneni PV, Dhall SS, Eck JC, et al. Guideline update for the performance of fusion procedures for degenerative disease of the lumbar spine. Part 11: interbody techniques for lumbar fusion. *J Neurosurg Spine*. 2014;21(1):67–74.
2. Freemont AJ, Peacock TE, Goupille P, et al. Nerve ingrowth into diseased intervertebral disc in chronic back pain. *Lancet*. 1997;350(9072):178–181.
3. Rolander SD. Motion of the lumbar spine with special reference to the stabilizing effect of posterior fusion. An experimental study on autopsy specimens. *Acta Orthop Scand*. 1966;(suppl 90):1–144.
4. Zdeblick TA, Smith GR, Warden KE, et al. Two-point fixation of the lumbar spine. Differential stability in rotation. *Spine (Phila Pa 1976)*. 1991;16(suppl 6):S298–S301.
5. Wang JC, Mummaneni PV, Haid RW. Current treatment strategies for the painful lumbar motion segment: posterolateral fusion versus interbody fusion. *Spine (Phila Pa 1976)*. 2005;30(suppl 16):S33–S43.
6. McAnany SJ, Baird EO, Qureshi SA, et al. Posterolateral fusion versus interbody fusion for degenerative spondylolisthesis: a systematic review and meta-analysis. *Spine (Phila Pa 1976)*. 2016;41(23): E1408–E1414.
7. Christensen FB, Hansen ES, Eiskjaer SP, et al. Circumferential lumbar spinal fusion with Brantigan cage versus posterolateral fusion with titanium Cotrel-Dubousset instrumentation: a prospective, randomized clinical study of 146 patients. *Spine (Phila Pa 1976)*. 2002;27(23):1683–2674.
8. Fritzell P, Hagg O, Wessberg P, et al. Chronic low back pain and fusion: a comparison of three surgical techniques—a prospective multicenter randomized study from the Swedish Lumbar Spine Study Group. *Spine (Phila Pa 1976)*. 2002;27(11):1131–1141.
9. Luo J, Cao K, Yu T, et al. Comparison of posterior lumbar interbody fusion versus posterolateral fusion for the treatment of isthmic spondylolisthesis. *J Spinal Disord Tech*. 2015;24(8):1621–1630.
10. Hsieh PC, Koski TR, O'Shaughnessy BA, et al. Anterior lumbar interbody fusion in comparison with transforaminal lumbar interbody fusion: implications for the restoration of foraminal height, local disc angle, lumbar lordosis, and sagittal balance. *J Neurosurg Spine*. 2007;7(4):379–386.
11. Oliveira L, Marchi L, Coutinho E, et al. A radiographic assessment of the ability of the extreme lateral interbody fusion procedure to indirectly decompress the neural elements. *Spine (Phila Pa 1976)*. 2010;35(suppl 26):S331–S337.
12. Alimi M, Hofstetter CP, Tsiouris AJ, et al. Extreme lateral interbody fusion for unilateral symptomatic vertical foraminal stenosis. *Eur Spine J*. 2015;24(suppl 3):346–352.
13. Mummaneni PV, Haid RW, Rodts GE. Lumbar interbody fusion: state-of-the-art technical advances. Invited submission from the Joint Section Meeting on Disorders of the Spine and Peripheral Nerves, March 2004. *J Neurosurg Spine*. 2004;1(1):24–30.
14. Glassman SD, Bridwell K, Dimar JR, et al. The impact of positive sagittal balance in adult spinal deformity. *Spine (Phila Pa 1976)*. 2005;30(18):2024–2049.
15. Macki M, Bydon M, Weingart R, et al. Posterolateral fusion with interbody for lumbar spondylolisthesis is associated with less repeat surgery than posterolateral fusion alone. *Clin Neurol Neurosurg*. 2015;138:117–123.
16. Kim K-T, Lee S-H, Lee Y-H, et al. Clinical outcomes of 3 fusion methods through the posterior approach in the lumbar spine. *Spine (Phila Pa 1976)*. 2006;31(12):1351–1357.
17. Zhou ZJ, Zhao FD, Fang XQ, et al. Meta-analysis of instrumented posterior interbody fusion versus instrumented posterolateral fusion in the lumbar spine. *J Neurosurg Spine*. 2011;15(3):295–310.
18. Videbaek TS, Bunger CE, Henriksen M, et al. Sagittal spinal balance after lumbar spinal fusion: the impact of anterior column support results from a randomized clinical trial with an eight- to thirteen-year radiographic follow-up. *Spine (Phila Pa 1976)*. 2011;36(3): 183–191.
19. Soegaard R, Bünger CE, Christiansen T, et al. Circumferential fusion is dominant over posterolateral fusion in a long-term perspective: cost-utility evaluation of a randomized controlled trial in severe, chronic low back pain. *Spine (Phila Pa 1976)*. 2007;32(22): 2405–2414.
20. Glassman SD, Carreon LY, Ghogawala Z, et al. Benefit of transforaminal lumbar interbody fusion vs posterolateral spinal fusion in lumbar spine disorders: a propensity-matched analysis from the National Neurosurgical Quality and Outcomes Database Registry. *Neurosurgery*. 2016;79(3):397–405.
21. Høy K, Bünger C, Niederman B, Helmig P, Hansen ES, Li H, et al. Transforaminal lumbar interbody fusion (TLIF) versus posterolateral instrumented fusion (PLF) in degenerative lumbar disorders: a randomized clinical trial with 2-year follow-up. *Eur Spine J*. 2013;22(9):2022–2029.
22. Bydon M, MacKi M, Abt NB, et al. The cost-effectiveness of interbody fusions versus posterolateral fusions in 137 patients with lumbar spondylolisthesis. *Spine J*. 2015;15(3):492–498.

23. Rapuano BE, Lee JJ, MacDonald DE. Titanium alloy surface oxide modulates the conformation of adsorbed fibronectin to enhance its binding to alpha(5) beta(1) integrins in osteoblasts. *Eur J Oral Sci.* 2012;120(3):185–194.
24. Cheng A, Humayun A, Cohen DJ, et al. Additively manufactured 3D porous Ti-6Al-4V constructs mimic trabecular bone structure and regulate osteoblast proliferation, differentiation and local factor production in a porosity and surface roughness dependent manner. *Biofabrication.* 2014;6(4):045007.
25. Toth JM, Wang M, Estes BT, et al. Polyetheretherketone as a biomaterial for spinal applications. *Biomaterials.* 2006;27(3):324–334.
26. Vadapalli S, Sairyo K, Goel VK, et al. Biomechanical rationale for using polyetheretherketone (PEEK) spacers for lumbar interbody fusion—a finite element study. *Spine (Phila Pa 1976).* 2006;31(26): E992–E998.
27. Olivares-Navarrete R, Gittens RA, Schneider JM, et al. Osteoblasts exhibit a more differentiated phenotype and increased bone morphogenetic protein production on titanium alloy substrates than on poly-ether-ether-ketone. *Spine J.* 2012;12(3):265–272.
28. Nemoto O, Asazuma T, Yato Y, et al. Comparison of fusion rates following transforaminal lumbar interbody fusion using polyetheretherketone cages or titanium cages with transpedicular instrumentation. *Eur Spine J.* 2014;23(10):2150–2155.
29. Tanida S, Fujibayashi S, Otsuki B, et al. Vertebral endplate cyst as a predictor of nonunion after lumbar interbody fusion: comparison of titanium and polyetheretherketone cages. *Spine (Phila Pa 1976).* 2016;41(120):E1216–E1222.
30. Thalgott JS, Fogarty ME, Giuffre JM, et al. A prospective, randomized, blinded, single-site study to evaluate the clinical and radiographic differences between frozen and freeze-dried allograft when used as part of a circumferential anterior lumbar interbody fusion procedure. *Spine (Phila Pa 1976).* 2009;34(12):1251–1256.
31. Yee AJ, Yoo JU, Marsolais EB, et al. Use of a postoperative lumbar corset after lumbar spinal arthrodesis for degenerative conditions of the spine. A prospective randomized trial. *J Bone Joint SurgAm.* 008;90(10):2062–2068.
32. Dailey AT, Ghogawala Z, Choudhri TF, et al. Guideline update for the performance of fusion procedures for degenerative disease of the lumbar spine. Part 14: brace therapy as an adjunct to or substitute for lumbar fusion. *J Neurosurg Spine.* 2014;21(1):91–101.
33. Kasis AG, Marshman LA, Krishna M, et al. Significantly improved outcomes with a less invasive posterior lumbar interbody fusion incorporating total facetectomy. *Spine (Phila Pa 1976).* 2009;34(6): 572–577.
34. Li FC, Chen QX, Chen WS, et al. Posterolateral lumbar fusion versus transforaminal lumbar interbody fusion for the treatment of degenerative lumbar scoliosis. *J Clin Neurosci.* 2013;20(9):1241–1245.
35. Pradhan BB, Nassar JA, Delamarter RB, et al. Single-level lumbar spine fusion: a comparison of anterior and posterior approaches. *J Spinal Disord Tech.* 2002;15(5):355–361.
36. Lee JC, Kim Y, Soh J-W, et al. Risk factors of adjacent segment disease requiring surgery after lumbar spinal fusion: comparison of posterior lumbar interbody fusion and posterolateral fusion. *Spine (Phila Pa 1976).* 2014;39(5):E339–E345.
37. Weinhoffer SL, Guyer RD, Herbert M, et al. Intradiscal pressure measurements above an instrumented fusion. A cadaveric study. *Spine (Phila Pa 1976).* 1995;20(5):526–531.
38. Lee CK, Langrana NA. Lumbosacral spinal fusion. A biomechanical study. *Spine (Phila Pa 1976).* 1984;9(6):574–581.
39. Sudo H, Oda I, Abumi K, et al. Biomechanical study on the effect of five different lumbar reconstruction techniques on adjacent-level intradiscal pressure and lamina strain. *J Neurosurg Spine.* 2006;5(2):150–155.
40. Moller H, Hedlund R. Instrumented and noninstrumented posterolateral fusion in adult spondylolisthesis—a prospective randomized study: part 2. *Spine (Phila Pa 1976).* 2000;25(13):1716–1721.
41. Park Y, Ha JW, Lee YT, et al. The effect of a radiographic solid fusion on clinical outcomes after minimally invasive transforaminal lumbar interbody fusion. *Spine J.* 2011;11(3):205–212.
42. Schroeder GD, Kepler CK, Millhouse PW, et al. L5/S1 fusion rates in degenerative spine surgery: a systematic review comparing ALIF, TLIF, and axial interbody arthrodesis. *Clin Spine Surg.* 2016;29(4):150–155.
43. Isaacs RE, Sembrano JN, Tohmeh AG, et al. Two-year comparative outcomes of MIS lateral and MIS transforaminal interbody fusion in the treatment of degenerative spondylolisthesis: part II: radiographic findings. *Spine (Phila Pa 1976).* 2016;41(suppl 8):S133–S144.
44. Youssef JA, Mcafee PC, Patty CA, et al. Minimally invasive surgery: lateral approach interbody fusion results and review. *Spine (Phila Pa 1976).* 2010;35(suppl 26):S302–S311.
45. Ozgur BM, Aryan HE, Pimenta L, et al. Extreme Lateral Interbody Fusion (XLIF): a novel surgical technique for anterior lumbar interbody fusion. *Spine J.* 2006;6(4):435–443.
46. Barbagallo GMV, Albanese V, Raich AL, et al. Lumbar Lateral Interbody Fusion (LLIF): comparative effectiveness and safety versus PLIF/TLIF and predictive factors affecting LLIF outcome. *Evid Based Spine Care J.* 2014;5(1):28–37.
47. Sembrano JN, Tohmeh A, Isaacs R. Two-year comparative outcomes of MIS lateral and mis transforaminal interbody fusion in the treatment of degenerative spondylolisthesis: part I: clinical findings. *Spine (Phila Pa 1976).* 2016;41(suppl 8):S123–S132.
48. Rodgers WB, Gerber EJ, Rodgers JA. Lumbar fusion in octogenarians the promise of minimally invasive surgery. *Spine (Phila Pa 1976).* 2010;35(suppl 26):355–360.
49. Ahmadian A, Deukmedjian AR, Abel N, et al. Analysis of lumbar plexopathies and nerve injury after lateral retroperitoneal transpsoas approach: diagnostic standardization. *J Neurosurg Spine.* 2013;18(3):289–297.
50. Woods KRM, Billys JB, Hynes RA. Technical description of oblique lateral interbody fusion at L1 to L5 (OLIF25) and at L5-S1 (OLIF51) and evaluation of complication and fusion rates. *Spine J.* 2017;17(4):545–553.

Index

Note: Page numbers followed by "f" indicate figures, "t" indicate tables and "b" indicate boxes.

M